Skeletal Developmental Anatomy for Students of Chiropractic

Skeletal and Developmental Anatomy for Students of Chiropractic

Robert A. Walker, PhD
Department of Anatomy
New York Chiropractic College
Seneca Falls, New York

C. Owen Lovejoy, PhD
Department of Anthropology and
School of Biomedical Sciences
Kent State University
Kent, Ohio

M. Elizabeth Bedford, PhD
Department of Anatomy
New York Chiropractic College
Seneca Falls, New York

William Yee, DC, LAc
New York Chiropractic College
Seneca Falls, New York

Illustrations by William Yee

F. A. Davis Company • Philadelphia

F. A. Davis Company
1915 Arch Street
Philadelphia, PA 19103
www.fadavis.com

Printed in the United States of America

Last digit indicates print number: 10 9 8 7 6 5 4 3 2 1

Acquisitions Editor: Margaret Biblis
Developmental Editor: Susan Rhyner
Production Editor: Jessica Howie Martin
Cover Design: Louis J. Forgione
Cover Illustration: William Yee

As new scientific information becomes available through basic and clinical research, recommended treatments and drug therapies undergo changes. The authors and publisher have done everything possible to make this book accurate, up to date, and in accord with accepted standards at the time of publication. The authors, editors, and publisher are not responsible for errors or omissions or for consequences from application of the book, and make no warranty, expressed or implied, in regard to the contents of the book. Any practice described in this book should be applied by the reader in accordance with professional standards of care used in regard to the unique circumstances that may apply in each situation. The reader is advised always to check product information (package inserts) for changes and new information regarding dose and contraindications before administering any drug. Caution is especially urged when using new or infrequently ordered drugs.

Library of Congress Cataloging-in-Publication Data

Skeletal and developmental anatomy for students of chiropractic / Robert A. Walker . . .
[et al.]; illustrations by William Yee.
    p. ; cm.
Includes bibliographical references and index.
ISBN 0-8036-0766-0 (pbk. : alk. paper)
    1. Chiropractic. 2. Human skeleton—Growth. 3. Human anatomy. 4. Bones—Growth. 5. Musculoskeletal system.   I. Walker, Robert A. 1958–
    [DNLM: 1. Bone Development. 2. Bone and Bones—anatomy & histology. 3. Chiropractic. 4. Muscle, Skeletal—anatomy & histology. WE 200 S62675 2002]
RZ242 .S575 202
612.7—dc21

                                                                        2001058163

Preface

This book contains a detailed description of the osseous and ligamentous anatomy of the human skeleton, with special emphasis on the spine. Although a number of textbooks describe human osteology in general terms, none treats osseous anatomy in the detail needed for clinical practitioners, basic sciences instructors in health care curricula, and serious students of human skeletal anatomy. Most books of this type generally ignore the ligaments of the axial skeleton and give, at best, cursory treatment to important ligaments of the appendicular skeleton. Most do not address the anatomy of the vertebral column in the detail provided in this text. We have prepared this book with the chiropractic student specifically in mind, although we anticipate that it will be of use to other health care professional students and advanced undergraduate and graduate students in programs in which knowledge of human skeletal anatomy is essential.

We have collectively taught human osteology, either as a stand-alone course or as part of a general human gross anatomy course, more than 50 times. This includes courses taught to undergraduate and graduate students in biological anthropology and biomedical sciences as well as to chiropractic, dental, medical, and physical therapy students. This text is based on our experiences in teaching human osteology in all these contexts. As a result, we take what we believe to be both a unique and useful approach to human osteology and trust that students will find it useful.

Robert A. Walker, C. Owen Lovejoy, M. Elizabeth Bedford, William Yee

Acknowledgments

We thank members of the faculty of the New York Chiropractic College (NYCC) Department of Anatomy for their editorial comments and factual and typographic corrections: J. Donald Dishman, D.C.; Thomas M. Greiner, Ph.D.; Mike Lentini, D.C.; Raj Philomin, M.D., Ph.D.; Maria Thomadaki, D.C.; Brigitte Tremblay, D.C.; Narayan Vijayashankar, M.D.;Roger O. Walter, Ph.D.; and Michael Zumpano, Ph.D. Fiona Jarrett-Thelwell, D.C., of the Radiology group of the NYCC Diagnosis Department contributed a great deal of useful information and checked the manuscript for consistency with the NYCC Radiology instructional program.

We also thank our colleagues in the Biological Anthropology Program at Kent State University, the Anatomy Department at the Northeast Ohio Universities College of Medicine, Bruce Latimer and the Physical Anthropology Department of the Cleveland Museum of Natural History, and Jerome C. Rose of the Department of Anthropology at the University of Arkansas at Fayetteville. We thank Barry Yee for his assistance in the preparation of the illustrations, Debbie Kelly for her assistance in the preparation of the text, and Carl Jagos for his constant support.

The following members of the NYCC faculty reviewed all or parts of the manuscript: Deborah Barr, DSc; Lisa Bloom, DC; Dale J. Buchberger, DC, DACBSP; Brian Cunningham, DC; John L. Decicco, DC.; Greg DeMaille, DC; J. Donald Dishman, DC; Maggie Finn, DC; Lillian M. Ford, DC; Thomas M. Greiner, PhD; Sandy Hartwell-Ford, DC; Jim Inzerillo, DC; Fiona Jarrett-Thelwell, DC; Mike Lentini, DC; Raj Philomin, PhD, MD; Julie Plezbert, DC; Bob Ruddy, DC; Veronica Sciotti, PhD; Bill Sherwood, DC; Judy Silvestrone, DC; Bob Story, DC; Maria Thomadaki, DC; Brigitte Tremblay, DC; Lee Van Dusen, DC; Narayan Vijayashankar, MD; Roger O. Walter, PhD; and Michael Zumpano, PhD.

The authors also thank the reviewers who read the manuscript for F. A. Davis: Barclay W. Bakkum, DC, PhD; Paul Barlett, PhD; Craig L. Mekow, MS; Michael D. Reife, DC; Patricia A. Rogers, DC; and Carlos F. Soniera, MD, MSc. Their many comments have improved the manuscript greatly. We thank the following individuals who reviewed the manuscript at various stages during its development: Tal Simmons, PhD, Department of Anthropology, Western Michigan University; Sue Firkins, MS, and Melanie McCollum, PhD, Department of Anatomy, Case Western Reserve University Medical School.

Special thanks are due to Sue Firkins, MS, formerly of the Department of Anatomy of NYCC. Sue has carefully proofread every version of this work since its origins as a manual at NYCC in the early 1990s. Her many careful readings and suggestions for clarifications and corrections have added invaluable insights and made significant improvements. Thomas Greiner, PhD, and Michael Zumpano, PhD, both of the NYCC Anatomy Department, provided invaluable commentary on the embryology and development of the craniofacial region. Narayan Vijayashankar, MD, and Raj Philomin, MD, also of the NYCC Anatomy Department, provided many insights throughout the preparation of the manual. J. Donald Dishman, DC; Maria Thomadaki, DC; and Brigitte Tremblay, DC, of the NYCC Anatomy Department have through the years and multiple early versions of the manual kept it focused on the needs of future clinicians.

The authors acknowledge and thank New York Chiropractic College, particularly the Division of Academic Affairs, for use of facilities, computer equipment, audiovisual assistance, secretarial support, and encouragement. We specifically thank Glenn Fried, MDiv, Associate Provost for Academic Affairs, and John DeCicco, DC, former Dean of Academic Affairs. The authors also wish to thank Kenneth W. Padgett, DC, President of NYCC; G. Lansing Blackshaw, PhD, Executive Vice President and Provost, NYCC; and Mr. John Pecchia, Vice President for Business Affairs, NYCC.

Support for William Yee in preparing the illustrations was provided by the Department of Anatomy and the Division of Academic Affairs at NYCC.

We thank Sandy Reinhardt, former Senior Medical Editor, and Margaret Biblis, Acquisitions Editor, at F. A. Davis. Without them, this project would not have become a reality. We especially thank Roberta Massey, our original Developmental Editor. Through her efforts, the text has been greatly improved. We appreciate all her hard work.

Finally, we thank the many students who have used previous versions of this work. Their comments and suggestions have greatly aided in making improvements. The manual began as a laboratory handout in the gross anatomy program at NYCC in Seneca Falls, New York. Early versions were used in courses at both NYCC and Kent State University. Dr. Walker and Dr. Bedford had been Dr. Lovejoy's graduate students at Kent State University. Much of the inspiration for this book came from course work and research that Dr. Walker and Dr. Bedford had participated in with Dr. Lovejoy. Dr. Bedford and Dr. Walker have worked together for many years teaching human gross anatomy at NYCC and elsewhere. Dr. Yee is a former student of Dr. Bedford and Dr. Walker and a 1999 graduate of NYCC.

Contents

Chapter 1

Introduction: Anatomical Terminology

This text is a general overview of the gross anatomy of the human skeletal system. In particular, it concentrates on the axial skeleton and treats its principal ligaments in great detail.

The vertebral skeleton is becoming progressively more important in clinical practice. It and its associated structures serve as the organizing axis of this book. After a brief introduction to the vertebral column as a whole, we begin a detailed description at the top of the cervical spine and proceed down the column to the thoracic, lumbar, sacral, and coccygeal regions.

After examining the vertebral column, we view and discuss its closely associated structures: the ribs, costal cartilages, and sternum. From there we proceed to the clavicles and scapulae, which attach the upper limbs to the axial skeleton. After examining the osseous and ligamentous pectoral girdle, we continue with an examination of the skeleton of the upper limbs. We then consider the pelvis and its ligaments, followed by the skeleton of the lower limbs. After an examination of the postcranium, we examine the osteology of the cranium.

We suggest that you refer frequently to the many detailed line drawings that accompany the text. The purpose of these drawings is to elucidate the structures described in the text. Often a line drawing gives a clearer idea of the location and nature of structures, such as crests or protuberances, than does a photograph. Where greater detail is needed to illustrate the structures, photographs are provided.

To understand the osteology of the human skeleton, some basic understanding of anatomical terminology is necessary.

All human anatomical terminology is relative to the *anatomical position* (Figure 1–1). In the anatomical position, the subject is assumed to be standing. The legs are

Figure 1-1   Person standing in the anatomical position.

together and the feet are flat on the surface, with the toes facing forward. The subject's face and eyes are directed forward as well. The arms are allowed to hang at the subject's sides, with the palms facing forward and the hands held open with the fingers pointing downward and thumbs pointing away from the body. Parts of the body are always indicated as if the subject were standing in the position just described.

The cardinal anatomical directions are based on this anatomical position. With the subject in the anatomical position, the upward direction (toward the head) is described as *superior*. The direction toward the feet is defined as *inferior*. These directions are not absolute but are relative to other parts of the body. In the anatomical position, the knees are superior to the feet but inferior to the chest. In human anatomy, a common synonym for superior is *cranial* (Latin: "toward the head") and a common synonym for inferior is *caudal* (Latin: "toward the tail"). The terms *cranial* and *caudal* are more frequently encountered in embryology and comparative anatomy.

Whereas *superior* and *inferior* describe one very important axis of the human body, *anterior* and *posterior* define another very important axis. *Anterior*, in human anatomy, means toward the front side, or face side, of the body. *Posterior* refers to the back side of the body. Using Figure 1–2A through C, note the locations of the *scapulae* (shoulder blades) and *sternum* (breast bone). The scapulae are located posteriorly, whereas the body of the sternum is located anteriorly. The sternum is anterior to the thoracic vertebrae, whereas the thoracic vertebrae are posterior to the sternum. In human anatomy, a common synonym for anterior is *ventral* (the "belly" side), and a common synonym for posterior is *dorsal* (the "back" side). The terms *ventral* and *dorsal*, like *cranial* and *caudal*, are more frequently encountered in embryology and comparative anatomy.

This is a good point at which to introduce a basic difference between human anatomy and the anatomy of other terrestrial and amphibious vertebrates (tetrapods, or vertebrates with four limbs). Humans are peculiar in a few respects, one of the most important being our obligatory bipedal style of locomotion (habitually moving by means of only the two "hind" limbs). As one consequence of this type of locomotion, humans carry their trunks erect over the pelvis. As a result, the vertebral column is held perpendicular to the ground, whereas other tetrapods, supported by forelimbs and hindlimbs, carry the vertebral column, running along the long axis of the trunk, parallel to the ground (Figure 1–3). As a result, in a tetrapod, the cranial end of the body is anterior, rather than superior, and the caudal end is posterior, rather than inferior. Also, in tetrapods, inferior is ventral, whereas superior is dorsal (as in the dorsal fin of a fish or whale).

Two more important relative terms of direction are *medial* and *lateral*. When we describe a structure as being medial, we mean that it is closer to the midline or in the direction of the midline of the body. When we describe a structure as lateral, we mean that it lies farther from the midline of the body. Again, these are relative terms. Refer back to Figure 1–1, representing the anatomical position. Note the thumbs and the fingers of the hands. The thumbs are lateral to the fingers; conversely, the other digits are medial to the thumbs. Likewise, the ears are lateral to the cheeks, whereas the cheeks are lateral to the nose; conversely, the cheeks are medial to the ears but lateral to the nose. The term *median* refers to structures that lie in the midline of the body. *Median* is an absolute term. The nose is a median structure, as is the vertebral column.

Another pair of terms of relationship are *proximal* and *distal*, and they are used extensively in the descriptions of the limbs. *Proximal* means closer to the point of

(*Text continues on page 7*)

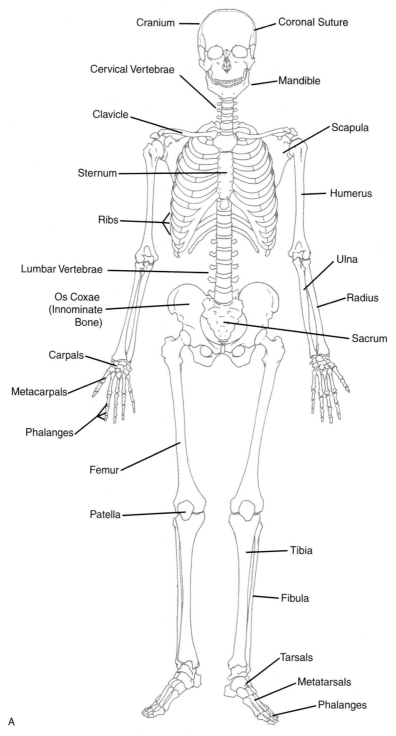

Figure 1-2 The human skeleton: (*A*) anterior.

Figure 1-2 *(Continued)* *(B)* posterior.

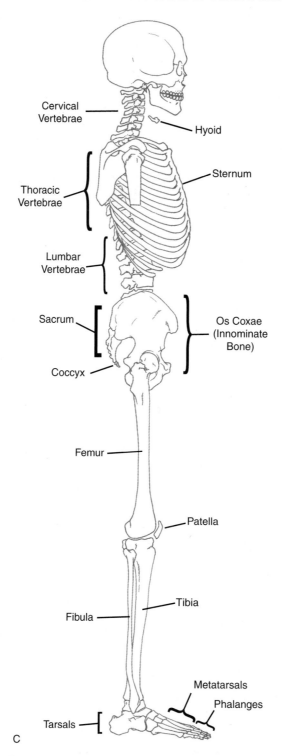

Figure 1-2 (*Continued*) (*C*) lateral.

Dorsal

Caudal

Cranial

Ventral

Figure 1-3 The horse, illustrating the anatomical position of a tetrapod, or four-legged vertebrate.

origin or midline of the body, whereas *distal* refers to being farther from the point of origin or midline of the body. Like most of the other terms we have examined, *proximal* and *distal* are relative terms; for example, the elbow joint is more proximal than the wrist joint, but it is distal to the shoulder joint.

In addition to these anatomical terms of relationship, some basic planes of anatomy should be understood (Figure 1–4). The three basic anatomical planes are *sagittal*, *coronal*, and *transverse* (or *horizontal*). If we return to the anatomical position, a sagittal plane divides the body into left and right portions. A sagittal plane is a plane that passes parallel to the plane of the sagittal suture of the cranium (see Fig. 1–2B). The sagittal plane that passes directly through the midline of the body and divides the body into equal left and right halves is called the midsagittal plane or median plane. Other sagittal planes that lie to one side or the other of the midline of the body and divide the body into unequal left and right portions are referred to as *parasagittal planes*. A coronal plane is a plane that lies parallel to the plane of the coronal suture (see Fig. 1–2A), which runs from side to side across the top of the skull. Coronal planes divide the body into anterior and posterior portions. A horizontal, or transverse, plane divides the body into superior and inferior portions. The three

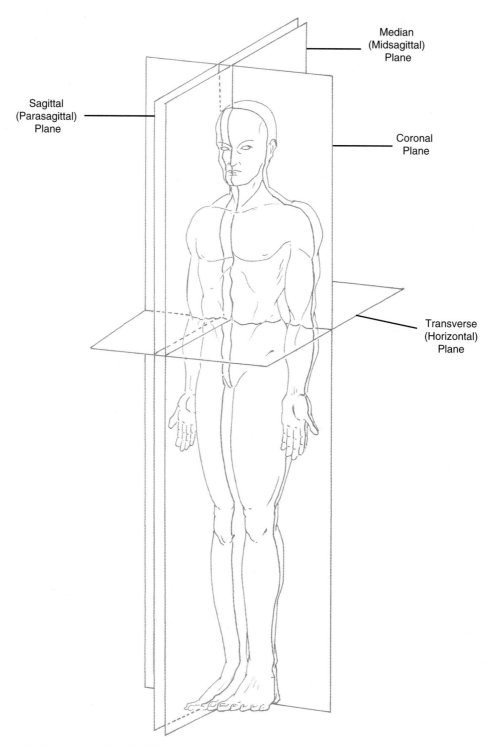

Median
(Midsagittal)
Plane

Sagittal
(Parasagittal)
Plane

Coronal
Plane

Transverse
(Horizontal)
Plane

Figure 1-4   Basic anatomical planes.

anatomical planes are *orthogonal* to one another (they meet one another at 90-degree angles). *Sections* through the body or a body part are generally defined according to one of these planes. An *oblique section* is a section that meets one or more of the anatomical planes at less than a 90-degree angle.

These are the principal anatomical terms needed to understand basic anatomical descriptions. Note that these terms may be combined—as in *superoinferior, superolateral, anteroposterior*, and so forth—to describe directions through the body or a portion of the anatomy.

Chapter 2

Bone: The Anatomy and Growth of the Skeletal System

The skeletal system is closely related functionally to the *muscular system* and the *articulations* (joints). The skeletal and muscular systems are often together referred to as the *musculoskeletal system*. The appendix of this book lists origins and insertions of the principal muscles of the trunk, limbs, and masticatory apparatus.

FUNCTIONS OF THE SKELETAL SYSTEM

The skeletal system functions closely with other body systems in a variety of ways. It supports the soft tissues of the body and protects delicate structures such as the brain and the heart. It also acts as a system of levers for muscular action. Without relatively rigid levers for attachments, muscular contraction could not create movement or perform work.

The skeleton acts as a storage area for minerals, particularly calcium and phosphorus. Bone is highly vascular, allowing rapid exchange of minerals between bone and blood.

The skeletal system also provides a site for blood cell production (hematocytopoiesis). In children, red marrow, where hematocytopoiesis occurs, is found in all bones of the skeleton. By adulthood, it is restricted to the vertebrae, ribs, sternum, scapulae, clavicles, pelvis, cranial bones, and proximal ends of the humeri and femora. It is replaced by yellow marrow (composed principally of fat) in other bones of the adult.

STRUCTURE OF THE SKELETAL SYSTEM

There are many forms of connective tissue. They are found throughout the body and perform numerous functions. They are often broken down into two types: loose and dense. *Loose connective tissue* has a higher proportion of cells and a lower amount of extracellular material. It is found extensively throughout the body and does not have a characteristic form; its fibers are randomly arranged and loosely packed. *Dense connective tissue* contributes to specific structures and generally has a very high proportion of extracellular material relative to the number of cells.

The skeletal system is generally composed of three specialized types of connective tissue: *fibrous tissue,* which is the primary element of tendons and ligaments; *cartilage*; and *bone,* or *osseous, tissue.* All of these tissues involve cells with the primary role of producing and maintaining extracellular matrix, the basic substance in which the cells of the individual tissue type become embedded. The cells are usually housed in small spaces called *lacunae.*

There are three principal differences between bone and cartilage. The first is that hydroxyapatite crystals are deposited preferentially in bone but, under most circumstances, not in cartilage. The second is that the collagen fibers in bone matrix are arranged in a highly organized, specific arrangement (except within primitive or woven bone, as described later), whereas collagen fibers in cartilage are more often randomly arranged (except in some forms of fibrocartilage). The third is that bone is a highly vascular tissue with a rich blood supply, whereas cartilage is avascular. This is clinically important because it allows bone to heal more readily than does cartilage. The rich vascular network within and around bone is a result of the ossification process—that is, the formation of bone tissue—and a function of the highly organized lamellar ("layered") design of mature bone.

Characteristics of Cartilage

Different types of cartilage are distinguished by the kinds of fibers embedded in their extracellular matrices. As mentioned, cartilage is avascular. It therefore receives nourishment primarily through osmosis and diffusion. The human body contains three types of cartilage: hyaline cartilage, fibrocartilage, and elastic cartilage (Figure 2–1).

Hyaline cartilage (*hyaline* means "glassy") has no fibers that are visible to the naked eye or with a light microscope, and the cartilage appears clear and smooth. Hyaline cartilage does, however, contain very fine collagen fibers. As we will see, the developmental models, or *anlagen* (singular *anlage*), for most bones of the skeleton are composed of hyaline cartilage. Furthermore, the *epiphyseal growth plates* of growing bones and the *articular cartilages* of synovial joints—a type of joint covered by a protective membrane and containing a lubricating fluid called *synovial fluid*—are composed of hyaline cartilage.

Fibrocartilage contains large amounts of collagen fibers and is an important structural cartilage. It does not form part of the bones but is found in joints. The annulus fibrosus of the intervertebral disc is composed of fibrocartilage, and fibrocartilage is characteristic of the general class of joints called *symphyses.*

Elastic cartilage contains large amounts of a structural protein called *elastin.* As the name implies, elastin is a highly elastic protein and is thus capable of

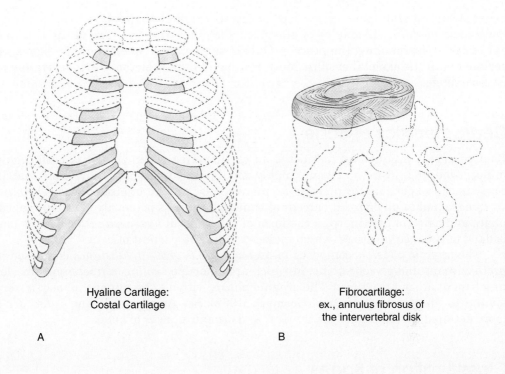

Hyaline Cartilage:
Costal Cartilage

A

Fibrocartilage:
ex., annulus fibrosus of
the intervertebral disk

B

Elastic Cartilage:
ex., cartilage of the nose

C

Figure 2-1   Three types of cartilage: (*A*) hyaline cartilage (costal cartilage), (*B*) fibrocartilage (annulus fibrosus of the intervertebral disc), and (*C*) elastic cartilage (cartilage of the nose).

being stretched and distorted without losing its original shape. It is said to have a low *elastic modulus*. Examples of elastic cartilage are the cartilage of the external ear and that surrounding the nostrils. Only a small amount of elastic cartilage is associated with the skeletal system. Most cartilage in the skeleton is either hyaline or fibrocartilage.

Characteristics of Bone

Bone matrix is unique and distinct from cartilage matrix in that it is both highly mineralized and, in mature bone, highly regular in its arrangement. Bone matrix consists of two portions, or phases: a mineral phase and an organic phase. The *mineral phase* makes up 65 to 70 percent of bone and consists primarily of calcium phosphate and calcium carbonate in the form of the mineral *hydroxyapatite*. This is embedded in the *organic phase,* which makes up 30 to 35 percent of bone.

The organic phase is composed of an *amorphous ground substance* composed of proteoglycans and glycoproteins, in which are embedded *collagen fibers* and smaller numbers of other fiber types. The organic phase, without the mineral phase, is very similar to fibrocartilage matrix (Cormack, 1992). See Avioli and Krane (1998) for a more detailed description of the mineral and organic phases of bone.

Classification of Bones

Bones can be classified by shape. There are various schemes, but probably the one most commonly used classifies bones as long, short, flat, irregular, or sesamoid (Figure 2–2).

LONG BONES: The morphology of long bones is what most people envision when they think of a bone. A long bone consists of a tubular shaft, called the *diaphysis*, with expanded ends, called the *epiphyses*. The major bones of the upper and lower limbs, for example, are long bones, as are the bones of the fingers and toes *(phalanges)*, the bones of the palm *(metacarpals)*, and the bones of the sole of the foot *(metatarsals)*.

SHORT BONES: Short bones are essentially "cubes" of bone, restricted to the wrist *(carpus)* and ankle *(tarsus)*.

FLAT BONES: Flat bones are platelike bones consisting of a "sandwich" of two outer, dense bone tables with spongelike bone between them. The bones of the cranial vault that protect the brain are the best examples.

IRREGULAR BONES: Irregular bones are bones of irregular shape that do not fit the other categories. Vertebrae are good examples.

SESAMOID BONES: Sesamoid bones (i.e., resembling a sesame seed) are a special class of bone that develops in the tendons of muscles. The primary function of large, regularly occurring sesamoids is to move a tendon away from the center of a joint, thus increasing the moment arm of the muscle that acts across the joint. The moment arm is the distance from the center of rotation, or fulcrum, to the point of application of the muscular force. The greater the moment arm, the greater the mechanical efficiency of the muscle.

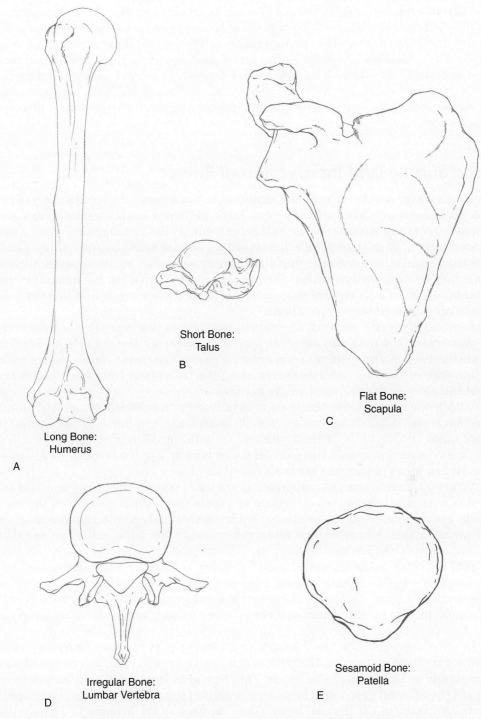

Figure 2-2   Classification of bones by shape: (*A*) long (humerus), (*B*) short (talus), (*C*) flat (scapula), (*D*) irregular (lumbar vertebra), and (*E*) sesamoid (patella).

Current evidence suggests that most sesamoids are genetically determined, although it is possible that the development of some sesamoids may be in response to stresses applied to a tendon as it crosses a bone. The *patella* (kneecap) in the tendon of the quadriceps femoris muscle is the largest and best example of a sesamoid bone. Other sesamoid bones known as *fabellae* are frequently found in the gastrocnemius muscle of the calf, at the ball of the foot in the flexor hallucis brevis muscle, and elsewhere. Refer to the appendix for muscle origins, insertions, and principal actions.

Blood Supply and Innervation of Bone

Bone is a highly vascular tissue, meaning that it has a very rich blood supply. Every bone has at least one *nutrient artery,* the principal blood supply to the bone. As we shall see, the vascularization of the anlage, or model of the forming bone, is an essential step in bone formation. The nutrient artery—or arteries, because there can be more than one—passes into the *medullary (marrow) cavity* of the bone through an opening in the *compact bone* called the *nutrient foramen.* Within the medullary cavity, branches of the nutrient artery spread throughout the marrow and line the *inner (endosteal) surface* of the compact bone.

Additionally, a rich network of *subperiosteal vessels* lies beneath the *periosteum,* the membrane that lines the outer surface of the compact bone. These derive from the nutrient artery, from *metaphyseal arteries,* from *epiphyseal arteries*—all of which are branches of systemic arteries surrounding the bone—and from the muscles that invest the outer, or fibrous, layer of the periosteum.

Within the substance of the bone matrix itself is a network of small channels, called *haversian canals,* that contain small arterioles or capillaries. They are the ultimate blood supply to the bone tissue and its cells, or *osteocytes.* In a typical long bone, these haversian canals run parallel to the long axis of the bone. They are interconnected in turn via transverse canals called *Volkmann's canals.*

Volkmann's canals carry small arterial branches inward from the periosteal vessels and outward from endosteal vessels to *anastomose,* or network, with the small vessels in haversian canals. Additional Volkmann's canals connect adjacent haversian canals with one another and allow the vessels within the haversian canals to anastomose with one another.

Still other vascular channels, called *primary osteons* or *nonhaversian canals,* transmit blood vessels. These vessels were originally subperiosteal vessels that became encased in bone matrix by subperiosteal deposition of bone during bone growth. Ultimately, in human bone, most of these primary osteons are replaced by haversian bone, that is, a secondary form of bone that repairs or replaces existing bone.

In some instances, the blood supply to a bone or part of a bone may be lost because of trauma. Fractures to the neck of the femur, for instance, can cause a loss of blood supply to the head of the femur. This loss of blood supply can lead to tissue death in the affected portion of the bone, a condition referred to as *aseptic necrosis;* it is frequently seen in the femoral head. Veins accompany the arteries in all instances to provide drainage from the bone tissue.

Bones and joints receive innervation as well. Joints in general are innervated by the same nerves that innervate the muscles crossing these joints. There is a wide network of sensory nerves in the periosteum of bone. Myelinated and nonmyelinated nerve fibers run with the nutrient artery and branch into the marrow and into the haversian canals. Innervation of bones is particularly rich near the articular surfaces of long bones.

Morphology of Bone

The anatomy of a typical long bone is described in this section. Similar parts are present in all bones, although the relative shapes and sizes of the parts vary from bone to bone (Figure 2–3).

The tubular shaft of long bones is the diaphysis. The broadened ends of the diaphysis adjacent to the metaphyses and epiphyses are referred to as the *diaphyseal funnel*. The *epiphyses* (singular: *epiphysis*) are the expanded proximal and distal ends of a long bone that have played a primary role in its development from the original anlage. Often multiple growth centers are found at one or both ends of long bones.

Sometimes a distinction is made between the growth centers that take part in joint formation (epiphyses) and those that serve primarily as sites of muscle insertion (*apophyses,* or "traction epiphyses"). The *metaphyses* compose the transitional zone between the tubular shaft of the diaphysis and the expanded epiphyses and apophyses. In many long bones, an epiphysis is of considerably greater diameter than its diaphysis, and the metaphysis can be identified as the flared zone of the bone that joins the epiphysis with the diaphysis.

The surfaces of the bones that take part in a synovial articulation are covered by *hyaline articular cartilage*. Joints between long bones or between a long bone and another bone, such as the scapula, typically involve the epiphyses of these bones. The hyaline cartilage creates a very smooth surface, which is lubricated by the synovial fluid. This allows the joint to move smoothly and freely.

Except for the joint surfaces, the entire external surface of a bone is covered by a fibrous membrane, the *periosteum* (literally, "surrounding the bone"). The periosteum consists of two layers: an inner osteogenic layer and an outer fibrous layer. Each has unique properties and functions.

The *osteogenic layer* is in contact with the external bone surface. It is referred to as the osteogenic layer because it contains osteoprogenitor cells that may differentiate into *osteoblasts,* the cell type that forms bone matrix. The production of bone matrix deep to the osteogenic layer of the periosteum is referred to as *subperiosteal apposition*. It is through this subperiosteal apposition that bones grow in diameter. Any time the periosteum is pulled away from the surface of a bone, subperiosteal apposition occurs. It is in part this tearing away of the periosteum from a bone shaft during a fracture that triggers bone deposition and healing.

Similarly, if an infection occurs under the periosteum *(periostitis)*, the periosteum can be lifted away from the bone and bone will be deposited as healing occurs. This is referred to as a *periosteal scab*. This is frequently seen, particularly in archeological bone, on the tibia and other areas in which the skin lies just above the bone.

Advanced infection of bones, which includes infection in the marrow cavity as well as beneath the periosteum, is known as *osteomyelitis*. Severe cases of osteomyelitis involve formation of massive amounts of bone callus beneath both the periosteum and the endosteum. The tibia is a frequent site of osteomyelitis partly because it lies so close to the skin and is frequently injured. Severe cases of osteomyelitis have become very rare because of effective antibiotic treatment.

The outer layer of the periosteum is the *fibrous layer*. It consists of dense, irregular connective tissue. Tendons of muscles insert into the fibrous layer of the

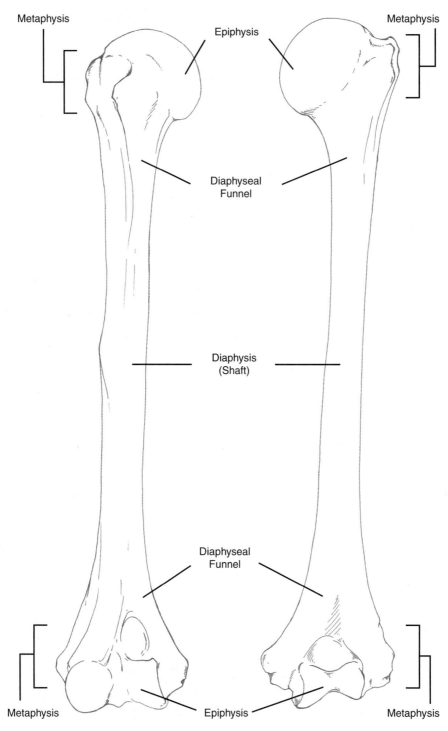

Figure 2-3   The morphology of a typical long bone.

periosteum. These fibers, which also extend into the underlying bone matrix, are known as *Sharpey's fibers*.

Within the diaphysis of a long bone, and extending into the epiphyses of mature bones, is the medullary cavity, or marrow cavity. Many organs are described as having an outer cortex and an inner medulla. In the case of bones, the outer compact bone is the *cortex*, often described as *cortical bone,* whereas the *medulla* of the bone is composed of the marrow. As a result, the cavity inside the diaphysis is referred to as the *medullary cavity* because it contains the bone's medulla.

The *endosteum* of a bone is a membrane very similar in composition to the osteogenic layer of the periosteum. The endosteum, however, lines the internal surface of the cortical bone, separating it from the bone marrow within the medullary cavity. Osteogenic cells of the endosteum help supply *osteoblasts* (bone-forming cells) for the repair of fractures. The endosteum also provides osteoblasts for the formation of new *haversian systems* (or *secondary osteons*) in the bone remodeling process (discussed later). Unlike the periosteum, the endosteum normally has no fibrous layer or a poorly developed one.

All bones have one or more nutrient arteries, the principal blood supply to the bone. The principal nutrient artery invades the anlage of the bone early in the ossification process and becomes surrounded by the forming bone. The passage left for the artery in the newly formed bone is termed the *nutrient foramen*. There is usually one nutrient foramen in the diaphysis of a long bone for the *primary center of ossification* and one or more in each epiphysis for the *secondary centers of ossification* located there. Veins accompany the nutrient arteries.

Microscopic Structure of Bone

Woven Bone

Woven bone consists of bone in which the collagen fibers of the bone matrix are arranged in a haphazard manner without a preferred orientation. It is found only in specific circumstances, such as in the bone callus formed during fracture repair or in the centers of ossification in forming bones. Woven bone is also known as *primitive* or *immature* bone.

Unlike trabecular and compact bone, woven bone is not lamellar. Although in lamellar bone the collagen fibers of the bone matrix are highly organized parallel to one another, in woven bone the collagen fibers have no specific fiber orientation. Woven bone is considered immature because it is the first type of bone laid down in the cartilage or mesenchymal bone model (anlagen) when the process of *ossification,* or bone formation, begins. Woven bone is also the type of bone laid down in the *bone callus* that forms around a healing fracture.

Ultimately, nearly all woven bone is remodeled away and replaced by lamellar bone. Small amounts of woven bone may remain, however, near cranial sutures, tooth sockets, and tendon and ligament attachments, as well as in the bony labyrinth of the ear. Usually, however, in these locations the woven bone is present in patches surrounded by lamellar bone.

A second type of immature bone is termed *coarsely bundled bone* (Cormack, 1987) or *parallel-fibered bone* (Enlow, 1969), in which thick collagen bundles are arranged parallel to one another and *osteocytes* ("resting" bone cells) occur between the collagen bundles.

Lamellar Bone

Lamellar ("layered") *bone* is mature bone and takes the form of either compact bone or trabecular bone. *Compact bone* is the dense bone that makes up the cortex of the shaft of the diaphysis *(cortical bone)* and the thin layer of bone beneath articular cartilage *(subchondral bone)*. *Trabecular bone* is generally found at the ends of long bones supporting the subchondral articular surface, in the bodies of the vertebrae, or between the bony plates forming the exterior of flat bones.

TRABECULAR BONE

Trabecular, or *cancellous,* bone is also known as spongy bone because it appears to be made up of a series of intersecting small pillars or beams (Latin: *trabeculae* means little beams) with a great deal of space between them, similar in appearance to a sponge. In contrast to compact bone, in which osseous tissue predominates over empty space per volume of bone, the situation is reversed in spongy bone.

Trabecular and compact bone are histologically very similar. Trabecular bone is very common under the thin shell of compact bone that underlies articular cartilage (subchondral bone). Although the shaft of a long bone is often subjected to bending and torsion, its articular ends are subjected almost exclusively to compression, allowing the subchondral bone to be supported by trabecular bone without a significantly increased probability of failure.

At the same time, the elastic modulus of cancellous bone is significantly lower than that of compact bone. This means that the cancellous bone is more easily deformed or has more "give." Hyaline cartilage cannot be repaired; once it is damaged, it loses some of its capacity to ensure friction-free motion within the joint. Therefore it is very important that it be protected from damage during the imposition of very high forces. The greater elasticity of cancellous bone therefore serves the very important function of preventing its overlying cartilage from being excessively compacted during the application of high compressive loads.

Trabeculae are generally so arranged that they maximize their capacity to resist the loads typically imposed upon the joint. This feature is largely the result of the sensitivity of the growth plate by which trabeculae are formed to the forces to which the growth plate is subjected during development. As noted, the articular surfaces at the ends of long bones are supported almost entirely by trabecular networks. Another example is the bodies of vertebrae, which are essentially thin-walled "drums" of bone filled with trabeculae.

CIRCUMFERENTIAL LAMELLAR BONE

Circumferential lamellar bone is a form of mature, compact bone that contains primary osteons (Figure 2–4). Both this type of bone and haversian bone have matrices that are composed of lamellae in which collagen fibers have a specific orientation. The principal differences between circumferential lamellar bone and haversian bone are the organization of their lamellae and their developmental origins. Circumferential lamellar bone is a form of mature bone in which the lamellae extend around the circumference of the shaft of a bone and lie in layers deep to its periosteum. In each individual lamella, most of the collagen fibers are organized parallel to one another. *Lacunae* (singular: *lacuna*), the small spaces in the bone matrix occupied by osteocytes, or "resting" bone cells, lie in the plane between adjacent lamellae.

Haversian Systems (secondary osteons)

Primary Osteons   Circumferential Lamellar Bone

Figure 2–4   Photomicrograph of circumferential lamellar bone.

Circumferential lamellar bone forms by the process of *subperiosteal apposition (deposition)*. Throughout the period of growth, the bone grows in diameter by the addition of lamellae around the shaft. Each lamella is in some ways analogous to the growth ring of a tree, although this analogy should not be carried too far: you cannot determine skeletal age simply by counting circumferential lamellae.

Osteoprogenitor cells in the osteogenic layer of the periosteum differentiate into osteoblasts, which then begin laying down bone matrix beneath the periosteum. Osteoblasts that become covered over by bone matrix formed by faster-moving osteoblasts become encased in lacunae and become osteocytes. Again, these osteocytic lacunae come to lie in the plane between adjacent lamellae.

Beneath the periosteum is a rich network of small arteries. As new lamellae are laid down, some of these arteries become covered over by the advancing bone and hence come to lie in small, osseous tunnels. A few concentric lamellae may be laid down around the blood vessel within these tunnels. The bony tunnels encasing these blood vessels are termed *primary osteons*, *primitive osteons*, or "nonhaversian canals." They are termed *primary osteons* because they form as the bone itself is forming, as distinguished from *secondary osteons*, or *haversian systems,* that form in already existing bone. The arteries within these primary osteons help supply blood to the osteocytes within their lacunae.

Because bone is a highly rigid material impermeable to osmosis and diffusion, the osteocytes must be able to receive oxygen and nutrients and dispose of waste products. Each osteocyte has a great number of hairlike cellular processes that come into contact with other osteocytes. These cellular processes pass through minute channels in the bone matrix called *canaliculi* (Latin: "little channels"). The canaliculi and cellular processes of the osteocytes nearest a blood vessel communicate with it, and other osteocytes in turn communicate with that osteocyte and other osteocytes. As a result, all osteocytes are connected with either another osteocyte or a blood vessel; therefore, nutrients can reach the cells and waste products can be eliminated.

The orientation of collagen fibers in the lamellae of mature bone has important consequences for the mechanical properties of the bone. The mineral deposited in the bone matrix and around the collagen fibers gives bone its *compressive strength,* the ability to bear weight or resist compression. The collagen fibers provide bone matrix with its *tensile strength,* its ability to resist tension or being pulled upon.

Collagen is a tough structural protein found throughout the skeleton and throughout connective tissue in general. There are many different subtypes, depending on the tissue in which the collagen is located and its stage of development, but all have in common a high tensile strength. Many collagen fibers within a typical long bone lie parallel with the long axis of the bone shaft and thus provide the bone with great tensile strength. Under a muscle, tendon, or ligamentous attachment, the collagen fibers in the bone are usually oriented along the directions in which those structures apply tension to the bone. (As noted before, the specialized collagen fibers that connect these structures to bone are called Sharpey's fibers.) Although the overall arrangement of fibers gives overall tensile strength to the bone, the arrangement of fibers in the individual lamellae of circumferential lamellar bone, in combination with the hydroxyapatite crystals, also provides the bone with torsional strength.

Lamellar bone thus has design features to resist all the principal forces to which it is normally subjected: compression, tension, and torsion. When the design parameters of the bone are exceeded, the result is a fracture. Because of its random arrangement of collagen fibers, woven bone has less resistance to tension and torsion than does lamellar bone. (We forego a lengthy discussion of the mechanical properties of bone here. See Currey, 1984, and references cited therein for a detailed discussion of the mechanical properties of bone.)

HAVERSIAN BONE

The basic unit of haversian bone is the *secondary osteon* or *haversian system* (Figures 2–5 and 2–6). Haversian bone is secondary lamellar bone. Recall that circumferential lamellar bone forms as a bone grows in diameter. As one ages, however, microfractures and other types of damage occur within that circumferential lamellar bone. If these microfractures and other insults to the integrity of lamellar bone are allowed to go unchecked, the bone ultimately fails; therefore, such insults to lamellar bone must be repaired. The body responds by the formation of secondary osteons. They are referred to as *secondary osteons* because they form within bone that already exists, as opposed to *primary osteons*, which are formed at the same time as the lamellar bone within which they exist (see Fig. 2–4).

A secondary osteon forms within a *resorption space* (Figure 2–7) carved out within the compact bone by *osteoclasts*, cells specialized for the destruction of bone matrix. Osteoclasts resorb the bone around the insult. In long bones, this forms a long, narrow channel that generally follows the long axis of the diaphysis of the bone.

Resorption spaces in cross-section demonstrate scalloped edges. The scallops are known as *Howship's lacunae* (Figure 2–8) and represent the spaces occupied by the osteoclasts as they resorb away the bone.

Obviously, if this process were allowed to continue unchecked, the remaining bone matrix would start to resemble Swiss cheese and the bone would become very much weakened. This, in fact, is precisely what happens in *osteoporosis,* in which the

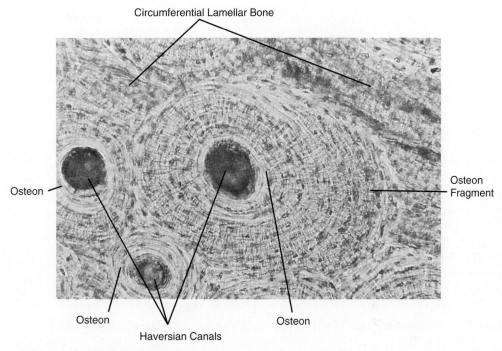

Figure 2–5   Photomicrograph of haversian bone.

Figure 2–6   Photomicrograph of haversian bone, osteon fragments.

Figure 2-7   Photomicrograph of resorption space, osteons, and interstitial lamellae.

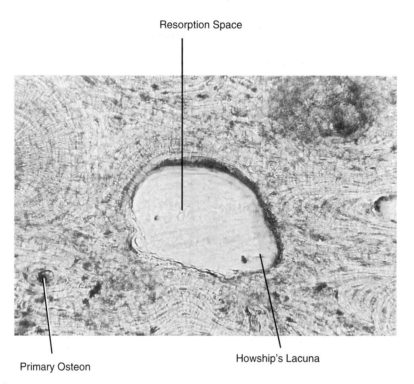

Figure 2-8   Photomicrograph of resorption space demonstrating Howship's lacunae.

bone mass is substantially reduced and bones become easily subject to fracture. To prevent the bone matrix from becoming extremely weak, the resorption space formed at the site of a microfracture or other insult is eventually filled in with new lamellar bone formed by osteoblasts.

We have already noted that lamellar bone contains a rich blood supply, initially in the form of the arteries within primary osteons and the subperiosteal vessels, as well as branches of the nutrient arteries. After the formation of the resorption space, blood vessels grow into the space and bring with them osteoblasts. These osteoblasts then begin the process of forming lamellar bone inside the resorption space, filling it from the *outside inward*. The lamellar bone that forms inside the resorption space eventually forms a secondary osteon or haversian system (Figure 2–9). The space that remains in the center contains an arteriole and a venule, or sometimes only a single capillary. This channel in the center of the secondary osteon is known as the *haversian canal*. Haversian systems contain no lymph vessels; only periosteal tissue is supplied with lymphatics.

On average, human haversian systems are approximately 300 microns (0.3 mm) in diameter, although their size can vary a great deal with age and location within the skeleton (Walker, 1989, 1993, 1997, 1998, Walker & Lovejoy, 1999; Walker et al., 1994).

With increased skeletal remodeling with age, almost all circumferential lamellar bone is converted to haversian bone. Although this slightly weakens the bone, it greatly increases its vascularity. In haversian bone, there is, on average, an arteriole

Large Haversian Canal of a Young Haversian System

Small Haversian Canal of an Older Haversian System

Lamellae of Secondary Osteon

Volkmann's Canal

Figure 2-9   Photomicrograph of secondary osteon or haversian system.

and venule every 0.3 mm in each haversian canal. This increased vascularity of haversian bone allows for a very rapid and efficient exchange of minerals, particularly calcium and phosphorus, between blood and bone. Individual haversian systems also probably prevent the spread of cracks within the bone (Currey, 1984).

As circumferential lamellar bone is remodeled away and replaced by haversian bone, some patches or islands of circumferential lamellar bone may remain between haversian systems. Such isolated patches of circumferential lamellae are referred to as *interstitial lamellae* (see Fig. 2–6). With increasing age and increasing amounts of remodeling, eventually older haversian systems begin to be remodeled away and are replaced by newer haversian systems. Remnants of older haversian systems are also a form of interstitial lamellae (see Figs. 2–6 and 2–7). When it is apparent that these patches are remnants of partially eroded older haversian systems, they are known as *fragmentary osteons* or *osteon fragments* (see Fig. 2–6). The numbers of complete and fragmentary haversian systems have a weak correlation with age at death but appear to be more highly correlated with mechanical factors (Walker et al., 1994, and references therein).

Bone *cortex,* or *compact bone,* is formed by the dense bone of the shaft of the diaphysis. Compact bone is not limited to just the cortex of long bones, but it is most abundant at the diaphysis. The greatest mass of bone in the adult skeleton is compact bone. It can be in the form of either haversian bone or circumferential lamellar bone. Specific structures found within haversian systems include those described in the following paragraphs.

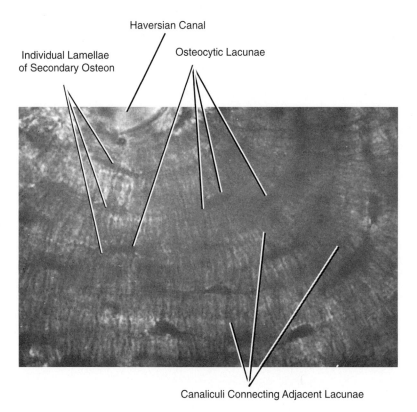

Figure 2–10   Photomicrograph of lamellae, lacunae, and canaliculi within a haversian system.

LAMELLAE: As with circumferential lamellar bone, the bone formed inside the haversian system is lamellar (Figure 2–10; see also Fig. 2–9) and is very similar in its organization to circumferential lamellar bone. However, they exist at different levels of magnitude. Although circumferential lamellae may surround the entire shaft of the femur, for example, the lamellae within a haversian system generally have a total circumference of far less than a millimeter. As with circumferential lamellae, the collagen fibers in any given lamella are usually parallel to one another.

LACUNAE: As in circumferential lamellar bone, osteocytes reside in osteocytic lacunae (Figure 2–11; see also Fig. 2–10) within secondary osteons. The lacunae are located at the interface between individual lamellae that make up the secondary osteon. Again, these represent osteoblasts that have become entrapped within bone matrix by more rapidly advancing osteoblasts.

CANALICULI: Canaliculi (see Figs. 2–10 and 2–11) join adjacent osteocytes with one another and connect the innermost osteocytes with the blood vessels in the haversian canal. As with canaliculi in circumferential lamellar bone, these canaliculi contain osteocytic cellular processes that pass oxygen and nutrients to, and drain metabolic wastes away from, osteocytes. In cross-section, a secondary osteon somewhat resembles a spider web, with the haversian canal at the center, surrounded by concentric rings formed by the planes between lamellae, with canaliculi radiating out from the central haversian canal toward the outside perimeter of the osteon. Osteocytic lacunae are located along the planes of intersection between adjacent lamellae and resemble flies caught in the spider's web.

Figure 2-11 Photomicrograph of lamellae, lacunae, and canaliculi within a haversian system.

HAVERSIAN CANALS: As has been noted, the haversian canals (see Figs. 2–9 through 2–11) occupy the central space of the haversian system and usually contain an arteriole and a venule.

VOLKMANN'S CANALS: Volkmann's canals (see Fig. 2–9) are similar to haversian canals but are oriented perpendicular to them. Volkmann's canals transmit blood vessels and nerve fibers between adjacent haversian canals, connect the vessels within the outermost haversian canals to the subperiosteal blood vessels, and connect the innermost haversian canals with endosteal blood vessels and branches of the nutrient arteries. Unlike haversian canals, Volkmann's canals are not lined by concentric lamellae, and they are oriented perpendicular to the long axis of the diaphysis rather than parallel to it, as are haversian canals.

SKELETAL REMODELING

Skeletal modeling and remodeling are the processes by which bone undergoes changes in shape and size with growth and development during normal aging and in the course of disease processes. The formation of bone from the development of the anlage through ossification of the model is known as *modeling. Remodeling* is change that occurs secondary to that. The development of primary osteons and circumferential lamellar bone, for example, is a result of the modeling process. The development of haversian bone, by contrast, is the result of the remodeling process.

Both modeling and remodeling occur through the action of bone cells. As has already been alluded to, there are three types of bone cells. These are the osteoblasts, the osteoclasts, and the osteocytes. Each has a specific role in the metabolism of bone. Because we are more concerned with bone morphology than bone cell biology in this text, we present here only a cursory description of bone cell types. See any recent histology text or *Gray's Anatomy* for more detail regarding the histology and cell biology of the osteoblast, osteoclast, and osteocyte.

OSTEOBLASTS (CREATE BONE): Osteoblasts are mononuclear cells that are found as a monolayer of cells on the surfaces of growing or remodeling bone. Osteoblasts arise from *osteoprogenitor cells* that are in turn derived from pluripotential stromal stem cells (undifferentiated cells with the potential to differentiate into a wide range of cell types) found throughout the bone marrow and in other connective tissues. As has already been noted, these osteoprogenitor cells are also found beneath the periosteum and endosteum. Osteoblasts synthesize, deposit, and mineralize bone matrix (Rodan and Rodan, 1984; Simmons and Grynpas, 1990).

OSTEOCYTES ("RESTING" BONE CELLS IN LACUNAE): Osteocytes are the principal type of cell in mature bone matrix. They derive from osteoblasts that have ceased or reduced their production of bone matrix and have become enclosed in bone matrix formed by other osteoblasts. They retain connections with each other and with blood vessels under the periosteum and endosteum through the network of canaliculi described earlier. The exact functions of osteocytes are not entirely clear, but it is assumed that they have an important role in the maintenance of bone. The deaths of the osteocytes within an area of bone matrix lead to the resorption of that matrix by osteoclasts.

Osteocytes probably are involved in the repair of fractured trabeculae by splinting them with microscopic amounts of bone callus. They may also act as sensors of the local mechanical and chemical state of bone and initiate the resorption or deposition of bone matrix in the locality (Lanyon, 1993a, 1993b). Additionally, they probably play a role in mineral exchange with the bone at the level of the canaliculi and lacunae. Their activities are dependent on a large number of factors, many of which are currently unknown but which certainly include circulating levels of hormones such as calcitonin and parathyroid hormone.

OSTEOCLASTS (REMOVE BONE MATRIX): Osteoclasts are large, polymorphous, polynucleated cells often containing 15 to 20 or more nuclei. They are found on surfaces of bone undergoing active resorption and reside in pits on the bone surface called *Howship's lacunae* or *resorption bays*. Osteoclasts are responsible for the removal of bone matrix, but the exact mechanism by which they do so is not known; it is likely through a combination of demineralization of the bone matrix and phagocytosis of the remaining matrix.

Unlike osteoblasts and osteocytes, osteoclasts do not arise from osteoprogenitor cells but from the fusion of mononuclear cells that originate in the bone marrow or other hematopoietic tissue. They show some similarity and relationship to the macrophages of the blood, which also arise in hematopoietic tissue. Osteoclasts respond to changes in parathyroid hormone and vitamin D levels, as well as to factors released by osteoblasts and other cell types. It has been speculated that when osteoclasts have completed their bone-resorbing activities, they may dissociate back into mononuclear precursor cells.

BONE LINING CELLS: Bone lining cells contain flattened, epithelium-like cells that are particularly abundant in adults. They are found lining surfaces of bone that are undergoing neither deposition nor resorption (Miller and Jee, 1987, 1992). They form a continuous layer overlying the resting bone surface and are in contact with adjacent osteocytes. They line the internal surface of the marrow cavity and line the walls of haversian canals. These cells may be either once-active osteoblasts that can potentially be reactivated or a form of osteoprogenitor cells.

Bones grow and change their shape by two processes that are mediated by the cell types just discussed. These two processes are deposition and resorption. The result of the combined action of these two processes is skeletal modeling and remodeling.

DEPOSITION (APPOSITIONAL GROWTH): Deposition is the process whereby osteoblasts lay down new bone matrix on some pre-existing surface. In mature bone, this is bone laid down on existing bone surfaces. In growing bone, osteoblasts may deposit bone on calcified hyaline cartilage (during *endochondral ossification*) or in mesenchyme (during *intramembranous ossification*). This is referred to as appositional growth, in contrast to interstitial growth, in which growth occurs from within the tissue.

In nonmineralized connective tissues, such as cartilage, the cells may produce new extracellular matrix that causes the matrix around the lacuna containing the cell to stretch and grow in volume. Because the extracellular matrix of cartilage and other connective tissues is usually unmineralized, this process can occur, and the matrix grows in volume essentially from the inside out. This is *interstitial growth*. Bone, on the other hand, has a highly mineralized matrix, preventing interstitial growth. Bone can therefore grow in mass only by the deposition of bone on pre-existing surfaces *(appositional growth)*.

RESORPTION (ABSORPTION OF OLD BONE MATRIX): Resorption is coupled with the process of bone deposition. As noted previously, bone resorption is carried out by specialized cells called *osteoclasts*. If, during growth and development, deposition were unaccompanied by resorption, a long bone would be as solid as a tree trunk, with no medullary cavity present. However, as a bone shaft expands in diameter by subperiosteal deposition, bone is at the same time removed from the endosteal surface of the compact bone, and the medullary cavity grows in conjunction with the growth in the diaphyseal diameter of the bone. In general, throughout most of life, deposition and resorption of bone remain coupled. When they become uncoupled—that is, when deposition outstrips resorption (osteopetrosis) or when resorption outstrips deposition (osteoporosis)—metabolic bone diseases are indicated.

The coupling of bone deposition and resorption throughout life results in bone remodeling. While a young bone is undergoing growth in length and diameter, subtle changes in shape are occurring as well. As the diaphysis grows in length, the epiphyses are pushed away from the center of the shaft. Consequently, the diaphysis, particularly in the metaphyseal region, undergoes changes in shape while the bone grows in length.

LAWS OF BONE GROWTH AND DEPOSITION

Bone growth can be described as following some fairly regular patterns. These patterns have been described as laws or principles. These laws are in reality more descriptions than prescriptions, but they are nonetheless so prevalent in discussions of bone tissue that the student must be familiar with their general definitions and meanings. Two of the most important are Wolff's law and the Heuter-Volkmann principle.

Wolff's Law

Wolff's law (Wolff, 1869, 1892), also referred to more grandiosely as the law of bone transformation, is an old tenet of the study of bone growth that essentially states that *bone is laid down where needed to resist compressive and tensile forces and is removed where not needed in order to achieve the greatest economy of tissue.*

Although this is still more or less a commonly held view by some researchers, more recent evidence suggests that a great deal of bone formation is genetically determined and is not the result of local environmental factors and mechanical loading (Bertram and Swartz, 1991; Swartz et al., 1998). Bone is certainly known to be responsive to mechanical stimuli and, in the absence of loading, bone tissue is rapidly removed by altered bone metabolism. However, it is now clear that the "signal" that causes osteoblasts to synthesize new matrix or osteoclasts to remove matrix is highly complex and is not simply proportional to the loads to which the bone is subjected.

Strain studies of bone, in which gauges are placed upon the bone surface and the deformation of the bone is measured at different points along its surface, show that bone metabolic activity and loading do not bear a simple relationship. In fact, it is not yet known whether the bone signal is mechanical (such as shear forces acting over cell surfaces or deformation of their bodies) hydrodynamic, electrical, or some complex combination of these factors.

Heuter-Volkmann Principle

The *Heuter-Volkmann principle* states that *there is a direct relationship between static compressive forces parallel to the longitudinal axis of a long bone and the rate of growth of the epiphyseal cartilage.*

It has long been known from a variety of experiments in which bone shapes are intentionally altered, such as the removal of a triangular segment of its shaft, that differential growth within the growth plates of epiphyses and apophyses can cause a change in the bone's eventual shape. The angle in the human knee joint, usually referred to as *valgus*, that causes the femoral shaft to angle superolaterally from the joint as it approaches the pelvis is probably the specialized result of habitual loading during bipedal walking, because this angle increases with age and does not develop normally in children with severe developmental insults, such as the various forms of myodysplasia.

Simon and colleagues (Simon, 1983; Simon et al., 1984) demonstrated that increased, intermittent, compressive forces enhance limb bone growth in rats, initially using experimental bipedalism and later using chronic centrifugation to simulate increased weight and compression. Using experimental bipedalism, growth plates that normally would have ceased or almost ceased growth were instead unossified and growing and contained active columns of *chondrocytes,* or cartilage cells. Low levels of chronic centrifugation significantly increased limb bone length. This research suggests that compressive forces may be important factors in regulating the growth of epiphyseal cartilage and even long bone lengths, although a great deal of work remains to be done before we reach a more complete understanding of the ways in which mechanical signals are perceived and responded to by the cells of the growth plate.

BONE FORMATION AND GROWTH

Formation of bone is termed *ossification.* Ossification differs profoundly from simple *calcification,* which is simply the deposition of calcium salts in a tissue. This occurs as one part of ossification, a term that implies actual bone formation, and includes the orderly arrangement of collagen fibers in the organic bone matrix in lamellae, as has been discussed. Some tissues undergo calcification without ossification; for example, calcium salts are simply deposited in the hyaline cartilage matrix of the thyroid cartilage without the presence of lamellar structures and other features common to true bone tissue.

BASIC EMBRYOLOGY OF THE SKELETAL AND ARTICULAR SYSTEMS

The skeleton and the articulations derive from *mesoderm*, or embryonic connective tissue. With the formation of the notochord and the neural tube, the mesoderm lateral to these two median embryonic structures thickens into two columns of *paraxial mesoderm*. (For further details of embryology, see Larson, 1993; Moore and Persaud, 1992; Sadler, 1995; or a similar general embryology text.) At approximately 20 days in utero, this paraxial mesoderm begins to organize itself into 42 to 44 segments.

Initially, the segmented paraxial mesoderm is in the form of loose, whirl-like groups of cells termed *somitomeres*. With the exception of the first seven somitomeres that form in the cranial region, the somitomeres further organize themselves into compact aggregates of cells termed *somites*. Externally, somites appear as a series of pairs of beadlike elevations along the dorsal surface of the embryo. Each somite becomes divided into a ventromedial part called the *sclerotome* and a dorsolateral part called the *dermomyotome*, from which derive *myotomes* and *dermatomes* that in turn give rise to most of the voluntary musculature and skin.

The *sclerotomal cells* soon surround the neural tube and form the primordia, or anlagen, of the vertebrae and ribs. The cells probably do not actually migrate but, because of differential growth of other structures, are shifted in position relative to the neural tube. The developing vertebral column replaces the *notochord*, the stiffening dorsal rod of the embryo characteristic of the animal phylum Chordata, to which vertebrates belong, and takes on its support function while it also protects the spinal cord.

The sclerotomal cells give rise to the vertebral column and its associated ligaments (see Chap. 3). Each sclerotome divides, so that the superior half of one sclerotome unites with the inferior half of the adjacent sclerotome; for example, the inferior half of the T1 sclerotome unites with the superior half of the T2 sclerotome to form the T1 vertebra. This results in the vertebra's being a half step off from the *meristic* (segmental) pattern of the body and thereby provides a pathway for the spinal nerve and blood vessels, so that they do not become encased within the bone.

Unlike somites, the cranial somitomeres are not perfectly segmental and do not cleanly divide into sclerotome, myotome, and dermatome. The somitomeres are responsible, along with the top four "occipital" somites, for the formation of the neurocranium. This is done in a fashion very similar to the formation of the vertebrae, although they must protect a portion of the central nervous system with a much larger diameter than the spinal cord: the brain.

Although the bones of the ribs and vertebral column develop from paraxial or somitic mesoderm, those of the limbs, pelvic girdle, and most of the pectoral girdle develop from *lateral plate mesoderm*. This tissue lines the lateral margins of the embryo and gives rise to paired limb buds. These buds emerge in response to a complex cascade of signaling molecules and are guided by a number of cell-signaling regions that develop within each bud. All the bones of the limbs and girdles develop in response to this complex cascade. Shortly after initiation of the limb bud, primitive muscle cells, or *promyoblasts*, migrate from the somites into the forming bud and become organized into dorsal and ventral muscle blocks. Shortly thereafter, each muscle block begins to split into smaller and smaller segments, which of course are at the same time rapidly expanding by growth. These eventually give rise to all the muscles of each limb. Shortly after this process begins, neurites from the developing spinal cord spread into the limb to innervate each of its muscles.

Mesenchyme is a diffuse network of cells forming embryonic mesoderm from which all connective tissues, including bone, develop. The anlagen of bones initially form as *mesenchymal condensations,* which may undergo direct, or *intramembranous*, ossification or may be transformed into cartilage, which then undergoes *endochondral* ossification. These mesenchymal cells have the ability to differentiate into other cell types, including *fibroblasts* that produce collagen and other fibers, *chondroblasts* that produce cartilage matrix, and *osteoblasts* that produce bone matrix. Some of the mesenchyme of the head region is derived from *neuroectoderm*, or *neural crest cells*, that gives rise to cranial bones of *branchial arch* origin. The ossification of the cranium is discussed in detail in Chapter 8.

Shortly after the anlagen of the bones of the limbs begin to form, they become progressively separated from one another at points where additional special signaling molecules are expressed. These are the presumptive *joints (articulations,* or *arthroses)* of the skeleton. *Synovial joints* differentiate from the *interzonal mesenchyme* between the anlagen of developing bones. Peripherally, the mesenchymal cells become transformed into the fibrous joint capsule and the ligaments of the joint, whereas within, the cells disappear to form the joint cavity, a process called *cavitation.* Some mesenchymal cells give rise to the synovial membranes that line the internal aspects of the joint capsules of synovial joints. In *cartilaginous joints,* the interzonal mesenchyme differentiates into hyaline cartilage or fibrocartilage, but no joint cavity develops. In either case, the ends of the bones participating in the joint remain covered by hyaline cartilage. In the case of *fibrous joints,* the interzonal mesenchyme differentiates into a dense fibrous connective tissue, forming ligaments that bind the bones together.

TWO TYPES OF OSSIFICATION

Ossification is the process whereby bone tissue is formed. This includes the formation of bone matrix and, in the case of lamellar bone, the highly organized network of collagen fibers in the bone matrix. Ossification also includes the deposition of calcium salts (calcification) in the form of hydroxyapatite in the matrix. Unlike calcification, ossification occurs only within the skeleton in normal circumstances. There are two types of ossification, differentiated by the type of tissue in which the bone is formed: endochondral (or intracartilaginous) ossification, in which bone forms in a hyaline cartilage anlage, and intramembranous (or mesenchymal or dermal) ossification, in which bone forms in a mesenchymal membrane.

Endochondral ossification occurs throughout the postcranial skeleton and is therefore the more common or more typical type of ossification. We discuss endochondral ossification in detail first and then examine intramembranous ossification. Intramembranous ossification occurs only in the sides and top of the skull and in the clavicles.

Endochondral Ossification

We first discuss the pattern of endochondral ossification as exemplified in a typical long bone with an epiphysis at either extremity of the diaphysis (Figure 2–12). The pattern of endochondral ossification is similar in other, more irregularly shaped bones, such as vertebrae or hip bones. Once the pattern is understood in a typical long bone, such as the tibia, it is much more readily understood in irregular bones.

Cartilage Model or Anlage

Endochondral ossification begins with the presence of a hyaline cartilage anlage (model). Such models begin as vague condensations of mesenchyme. Soon thereafter

Figure 2-12 Steps in endochondral ossification.

cells around the periphery of the presumptive anlagen begin to express cell adhesion molecules and begin to form into a membrane that eventually becomes the perichondrium. Cells in the interior of the presumptive anlagen continue to mitose and to synthesize collagen and other matrix molecules. Soon a hyaline cartilage anlage, or model, of the bone is formed.

Bone Collar Development

Soon after the perichondrium surrounding the anlage appears, it differentiates into a periosteum; the cells of its deep layer metamorphose into osteoprogenitor cells that begin to synthesize osteoid (unmineralized bone matrix) rather than cartilaginous matrix. The activity of these new osteoblasts causes bone to be laid down around the periphery of the cartilage model. This first bone laid down around the outside of the cartilage model is very similar to the intramembranous ossification that takes place elsewhere in the skeleton. Growing bone around the outside of the cartilage model in a long bone quickly takes the form of a *bone collar*. Osteogenic cells of the periosteum differentiate into osteoblasts that begin producing bone around the outside of the shaft of the anlage.

As the bone collar develops, mitosis within the center of the anlage continues and the cells lying most deeply begin to suffer a loss of ready transport of materials because the anlage is avascular. This signals a change in these cells, which undergo apoptosis (disintegration) and eventual calcification. At about this point in development, a branch of the arterial supply of the new periosteum migrates into the "nodule" of calcifying cartilage, carrying with it osteoprogenitor cells from the periosteum. This constitutes the nutrient artery of the bone diaphysis and its primary center of ossification.

Vascularization

As just noted, when the bone collar begins to develop, the future nutrient artery invades the center of the anlage. Via this arterial route, osteoprogenitor cells are carried into the center of the anlage, where they differentiate into osteoblasts and begin forming bone. As the cartilage model continues to grow in diameter and length by means of interstitial and appositional growth, chondrocytes (cartilage cells) in the center of the anlage continue to apoptose. As they do so, they leave behind a matrix of hyaline cartilage. During the process of *apoptosis*, the chondrocytes in the center of the anlage hypertrophy and their lacunae coalesce, compressing the remaining cartilage matrix into a series of flattened plates known as *spicules*, which are in reality the remaining walls of the chondrocytic lacunae. This remaining cartilage undergoes calcification through the deposition of calcium salts. It does not undergo ossification.

Formation of the Primary Center of Ossification

The ossification process is highly dependent upon vascularization (Cormack, 1987, and references therein). The vasculature carries osteoprogenitor cells and osteoclasts to the developing center of ossification. Osteoclasts may be involved in carving a path through the bone collar, and chondroclasts may cut through calcified cartilage matrix to create spaces through which the nutrient artery can pass. Once inside the diaphysis, branches of the nutrient artery ramify, forming *osteogenic buds*. These osteogenic buds consist of blind-ended capillaries surrounded by osteoprogenitor cells and osteoclasts.

The osteoprogenitor cells then differentiate into osteoblasts, which begin the task of laying down woven bone on the *calcified cartilage spicules* left behind after the death of the hypertrophied chondrocytes. Once this process has begun in the center of the diaphysis, the *primary center of ossification* has been formed. This occurs at about the same time as the initial formation of the bone collar and the invasion of the anlage by the nutrient artery.

Branches of the nutrient artery continue to ramify through the center of the shaft of the anlage as the anlage continues to grow. Subperiosteal deposition continues around the outside of the developing bone shaft, causing the bone to continue to grow in diameter. By the processes just described, the primary ossification center begins to spread throughout the center of the presumptive bone. The woven bone and the calcified cartilage matrix upon which it rests can be considered a temporary scaffolding that will be remodeled away as the diaphysis and the contained forming medullary cavity continue to grow.

Medullary Cavity Formation

The formation of the medullary (marrow) cavity is a consequence of the formation of the primary center of ossification. The primitive medullary cavity first forms when the lacunae of hypertrophied chondrocytes in the center of the anlage begin to coalesce. After the nutrient vasculature has invaded the anlage and the primary center of ossification begins to form, the medullary cavity begins to grow. As we have seen, the first bone deposited within the primary center is woven bone laid down over calcified cartilage matrix. However, remodeling of this material begins almost immediately. As this bone is formed around the perimeters of the primitive marrow cavity and more bone is laid down *on* the bone collar around the outside of the diaphysis, chondrocytes surrounding the periphery of the forming ossification center now begin to hypertrophy and apoptose, leaving behind more calcified cartilage matrix.

Osteoclasts and chondroclasts remove the older matrix and woven bone surrounding the early medullary cavity, and the process begins to repeat itself farther up and down the shaft of the bone. This process continues until at some point the only remaining cartilage that has not undergone this process is the epiphyseal plate. At the same time, lamellar bone is being laid down around the margins of the forming medullary cavity as well as beneath the periosteum. Later, when the epiphyseal plate has synostosed with the diaphysis, the medullary cavity will extend from the diaphysis into the epiphyses.

Thickening and Lengthening of the Bone Collar

While the primary center of ossification is enlarging and the medullary cavity is expanding, the subperiosteal bone collar continues to grow in length and diameter. Of course, while the outside diameter of the shaft is increasing, osteoclastic activity continues to enlarge the medullary cavity so that it keeps pace in relative size with the enlarging bone collar. Generally, the epiphyses of a long bone are wider than the midshaft of the diaphysis. As the diaphysis approaches the epiphysis (or as the bone collar approaches the epiphysis), the diaphysis widens to match the transverse diameter of the epiphysis. This broadened portion of the diaphysis is referred to as the *diaphyseal funnel*.

The *metaphysis* is at the broadest aspect of the diaphyseal funnel subjacent to the epiphysis. As the bone collar lengthens and thickens, bone is constantly removed from its inner surface by osteoclastic action and redeposited on its periosteal surface to keep the bone collar growing in both diameter and length. It is of some interest that this scenario must be reversed in the region of the diaphyseal funnel. There the overall diameter of the shaft just below the metaphysis must actually be reduced as the bone lengthens in order to maintain a smooth transition between the diaphysis and metaphysis; that is, the diaphyseal funnel must be moved farther from the center of the bone as it lengthens.

Work in recent years on bone development has confirmed that much of the genetic information involved in bone formation is maintained and expressed within its growth plates, and this fact accounts for the remarkable ability of a bone to make these kinds of adjustments as it grows in length.

Formation of Secondary Centers of Ossification in the Epiphyses

At some point well after the formation of the primary center of ossification, secondary centers of ossification begin to appear in the epiphyses. The process that occurs here is similar in all respects to the formation of the primary center: Each secondary center undergoes hypertrophy and apoptosis of its chondrocytes, a nutrient artery invades it, calcification of the cartilage matrix begins, and the formation of true bone follows. A secondary center differs from a primary center only in the time of its occurrence, not in terms of its structure. In a typical long bone, one or more secondary centers are at both the proximal and the distal ends of the bone, or epiphyses. Eventually, all of the hyaline cartilage in the epiphysis is replaced by bone by the mechanisms already described, with two exceptions. First, until growth in length of the bone ceases, the *epiphyseal plate* remains cartilaginous. Second, a thin layer of hyaline cartilage remains covering the surfaces of the epiphyses that participate in synovial joints. In a sense, the hyaline articular cartilage is the sole remnant of the cartilage anlage that survives into adulthood.

Development of the Epiphyseal Plate

The epiphyseal plate comes into existence after primary and secondary ossification centers have appeared. The epiphyseal plate develops from the plate of hyaline cartilage that remains between the primary and secondary ossification centers and forms the *epiphyseal growth plate*. This growth plate has a distinct, layered structure. From the epiphyseal side to the diaphyseal side of the epiphyseal plate, four cartilaginous zones may be distinguished (Figure 2–13).

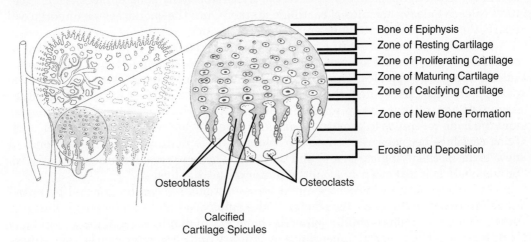

Bone of Epiphysis
Zone of Resting Cartilage
Zone of Proliferating Cartilage
Zone of Maturing Cartilage
Zone of Calcifying Cartilage

Zone of New Bone Formation

Erosion and Deposition

Osteoblasts   Osteoclasts

Calcified
Cartilage Spicules

Figure 2-13   The four cartilaginous zones of the epiphyseal plate.

Zone of resting cartilage: Also referred to as the zone of reserve cartilage, the zone of resting cartilage is the layer of the epiphyseal plate closest to the epiphysis. The chondrocytes, or cartilage cells, in this layer are relatively quiescent, essentially being held in reserve for later growth of the epiphyseal plate. However, as the bottom of this layer, nearer the diaphysis, is approached, some cells are beginning to undergo active mitosis. At this point, the first zone merges into the second zone.

Zone of proliferating cartilage: The second zone is a zone of actively mitosing chondrocytes and is hence referred to as the zone of proliferating cartilage. These cells continue to produce extracellular matrix, and through the interstitial growth of the cartilage in this zone, the bone continues to grow in length. So long as the epiphyseal plate remains active and unossified, the bone is capable of continued growth in length. As the proliferative zone grows in thickness, the epiphysis is pushed farther from the center of the diaphysis.

A few cells in the layer nearest the epiphysis remain constant as the zone of resting cartilage, whereas the remainder continue to mitose and transform. The mitosing cells form columnar arrangements throughout the epiphyseal plate, with resting cells nearest the epiphysis, whereas cells become increasingly active toward the diaphyseal side of the zone. Columns of extracellular matrix mark the spaces between columns of cells. Toward the bottom of this zone (nearer the diaphysis) is a transition to the third zone of the epiphyseal plate.

Zone of maturing cartilage: The third zone is referred to as the zone of maturing cartilage or the zone of hypertrophying cartilage. Within this zone, the same sorts of changes take place as those in the center of the primary and secondary centers of ossification. Chondrocytes within the maturing zone grow in size and undergo cell death. The lacunae of adjacent chondrocytes within the column begin to merge as the cells hypertrophy, and the columns of extracellular matrix between the lacunae become compressed. At the extreme diaphyseal side of the third zone, the remaining cartilage spicules begin to undergo calcification, just as is seen in the primary and secondary centers of ossification. This marks the transition to the fourth zone.

Zone of calcifying cartilage: The layer of the epiphyseal plate nearest the diaphysis is known as the zone of calcifying cartilage. Again, just as in the primary and secondary centers of ossification, once the hypertrophying cells enlarge, their lacunae coalesce to leave spicules of cartilage matrix. Once the chondrocytes undergo cell death, these remaining cartilage spicules become calcified.

At this point, we can say there is a fifth zone, a *zone of bone formation* or *zone of ossification,* wherein osteoblasts start laying down woven bone around the exposed calcified cartilage spicules. The epiphyseal plate does not remain static. As one side of the plate becomes ossified, the other side, the epiphyseal side, continues to produce new cartilage, so that the epiphysis is continually pushed away from the diaphysis and the bone continues to grow in length as a result. What was once the zone of calcifying cartilage becomes ossified, the previous layer of maturing cartilage becomes a new layer of calcifying cartilage, and so forth. The epiphyseal plate constantly rebuilds itself as it moves away from the center of the diaphysis.

At some genetically predetermined time—although it can be affected by nutritional status, disease, and other factors—the epiphyseal plate undergoes *synostosis,* during which it becomes solidly joined by bone to the diaphysis, and growth in bone length ceases. The times of appearance of primary and secondary centers of ossification and the times of epiphyseal union differ from bone to bone and between boys and girls. (For a summary of these times, see Krogman and Iscan, 1986.) Such patterns of appearance of ossification centers and union of epiphyses can, in fact, be used to estimate biological age in radiographs of children or from unidentified skeletal remains.

Synostosis of Primary and Secondary Ossification Centers

As has been noted, the epiphyseal plate continues to exist until growth at the plate ceases and the epiphysis synostoses with the diaphysis. It should be remembered that the process of endochondral ossification is a continuous process throughout life and that one phase blends into the next without sharp demarcation.

Nearly all epiphyseal plates synostose by 21 years of age. The last to fuse is usually the epiphyseal plate at the sternal end of the clavicle, which may remain open until 25 years of age or more, although active bone growth within the pubic symphysis may continue into the fourth decade of life; a small, irregular epiphysis called the *ventral rampart* usually appears on the medial aspect of each pubic bone in the latter phases of the third decade of life and fuses in the early part of the fourth. Once all epiphyseal plates have fused, no further growth in stature or bone length can occur. If the epiphyseal plate undergoes early synostosis because, for example, of a fracture through the plate, the bone will not grow to its normal length.

Not all bones formed by endochondral ossification follow so closely the presented model. We have described the process in a typical long bone with a primary center of ossification in the diaphysis and secondary centers of ossification in the epiphyses. However, not all endochondral bones take this form. A typical vertebra, for example, has *three* primary centers of ossification and *five* secondary centers. The *body* of a typical vertebra represents one of the primary centers, the *centrum,* whereas the *neural,* or *vertebral, arch* is formed by two primary centers that fuse in the midline to form the *spinous process* and fuse anteriorly with the body (Figure 2–14). In

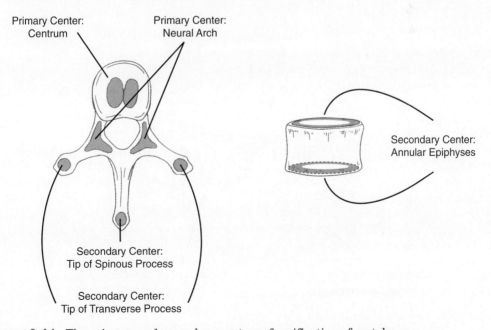

Figure 2–14   The primary and secondary centers of ossification of vertebrae.

addition, a typical vertebra has secondary centers at the tips of each transverse process, one at the tip of the spinous process and two ring-shaped annular epiphyses that cap the top and bottom of the cylinder of the body of the vertebra, for a total of *five* secondary centers. Each secondary center is separated from its primary center by an epiphyseal growth plate. The same processes occur there as occur in a typical long bone, but the forms of the elements involved are substantially different. *Spina bifida* occurs when the two halves of the neural arch fail to fuse with each other. As a result, the secondary center at the tip of the spinous process does not develop, the two halves of the neural arch do not meet, and the spinal cord is either exposed or covered only by soft tissue.

Another good example of endochondral ossification in a less typical bone is the ossification of the *os coxae* (hip bone or innominate bone; Figure 2–15). The innominate is usually described as developing from three separate bones: the *ilium*, the *ischium*, and the *pubis*. In reality, these are three primary centers of ossification for the os coxae. They are separated from one another in the *acetabulum*, the socket for the head of the femur, by a Y-shaped epiphyseal plate. Again, this has the elements of an epiphyseal plate but is greatly modified in shape. In addition, the innominate has

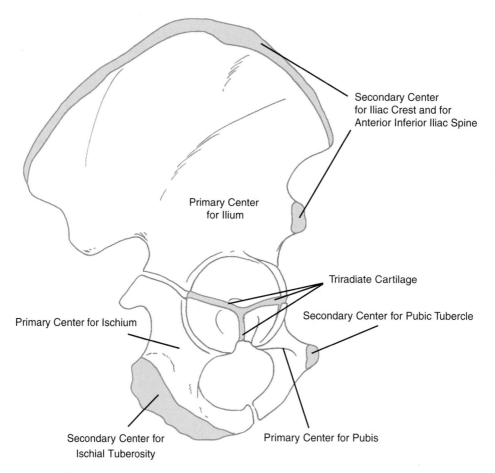

Figure 2-15   Centers of ossification of the os coxae.

a number of secondary centers, all separated from the rest of the bone by epiphyseal growth plates. These include, but are not limited to, the *iliac crest*, the *ischial tuberosity*, and the ventral rampart of the *pubic symphyseal surface*, as just discussed. Additionally, the *anterior inferior iliac spine* develops as a secondary center of ossification under the superior attachment of the rectus femoris muscle. Such a secondary center under a muscle attachment is known as a *traction epiphysis* or *apophysis*.

Intramembranous Ossification

Intramembranous ossification (mesenchymal or *dermal ossification)* is a somewhat less complicated form of ossification than endochondral ossification. It is restricted to most of the clavicle and the flat bones of the cranial vault. Intramembranous ossification is the direct ossification of highly vascular connective tissue, and it spreads outward from a primary center of ossification.

Osteoprogenitor cells differentiate to osteoblasts in the highly vascular center of a mesenchymal membrane anlage. The mesenchymal membrane is free to continue to grow in size at its margins. Ossification, however, continues outward from

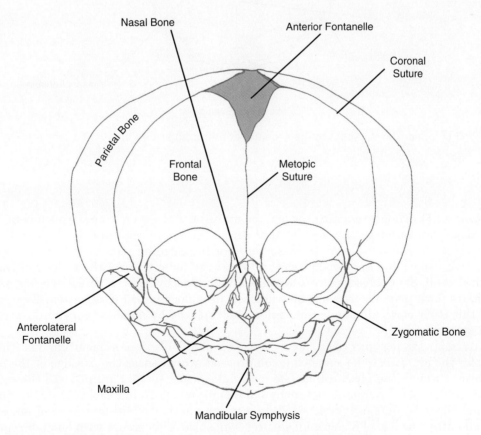

Figure 2-16   Bone development in the neonatal cranium, anterior view.

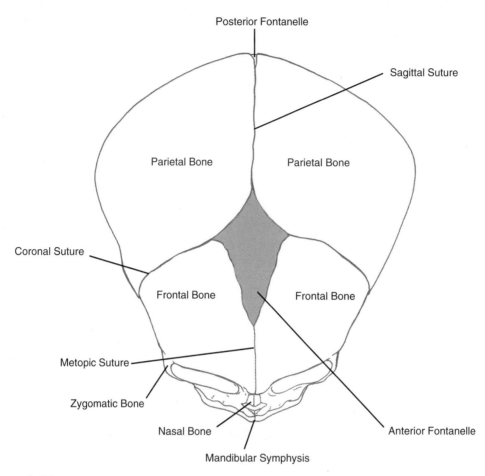

Figure 2-17   Bone development in the neonatal cranium, superior view.

the center of the bone, reaching toward the margins of the membrane. Woven bone is laid down surrounding the vessels that enter the membrane and form primitive trabeculae. At the outer and inner surfaces of the forming membrane bone, these primitive trabeculae are joined together by woven bone to form the early compact cortical shell. Some blood vessels become surrounded by bone in this newly formed cortex to form primary osteons, as was seen in endochondral ossification. Eventually, this early cortical bone is remodeled and replaced by lamellar bone and haversian systems.

At birth, the margins of the bones of the cranial vault remain membranous. This enables the cranium to be somewhat compressed, which eases the passage of the fetal head through the birth canal. The fontanelles (soft spots; Figures 2–16 through 2–18) are formed of remnant mesenchymal membrane. With increasing maturity, the cranial bones become fully ossified and meet one another at sutures. Very often, especially after the age of 35, cranial sutures synostose. This occurs with enough regularity that estimates of age at death can be obtained from the pattern of cranial suture closure (Meindl and Lovejoy, 1985).

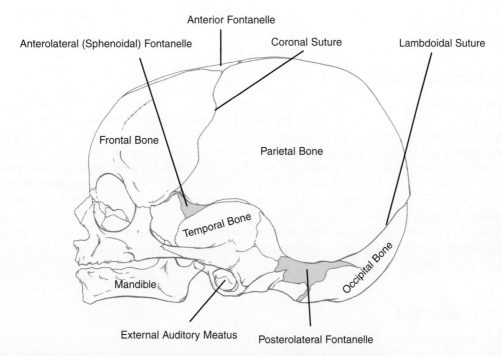

Figure 2-18   Bone development in the neonatal cranium, lateral view.

TYPICAL DISORDERS OF BONE GROWTH AND REMODELING

So far, we have outlined the normal progress of ossification and bone growth and development. Bone metabolism is subject to the effects of many factors, including nutrition, hormones, vitamins, mechanical loading, and genetic disturbances. (For a good summary of bone metabolism, endocrinology, and metabolic bone disease, see Avioli and Krane, 1998.) Some clinically important problems related to bone growth, development, and remodeling are briefly discussed here.

Rickets

Rickets is a disease of childhood in which the bone matrix that forms is not calcified or is incompletely calcified. Uncalcified bone matrix is called *osteoid*. Osteoid is normally calcified rapidly after its production. In rickets, the osteoid does not calcify or at best is only poorly calcified. The resulting bone is very weak in compression. A telltale characteristic of rickets in a young child is bowing of the femurs.

There are different varieties of rickets. The most common is *vitamin D-deficiency rickets*. Vitamin D (1,25 dihydroxycholecalciferol) is necessary for calcification of bone. Adequate amounts of vitamin D are normally acquired through the diet or synthesized by the body. Ordinarily, vitamin D-deficiency rickets responds to vitamin D supplementation.

Vitamin D-resistant rickets are forms of rickets in which the bone does not respond to vitamin D supplementation. These forms of rickets are a result of problems with other steps in the metabolic pathways of calcification rather than to vitamin D deficiency.

Osteomalacia

Osteomalacia is sometimes referred to as the adult form of rickets. Its etiology is similar. It may result from vitamin D deficiency or other causes. The net result is that the osteoid that is formed is not adequately mineralized. Of course, adults do not possess epiphyseal growth plates, so the manifestation of the disease is not the same as in rickets. Most new bone formation in adults occurs during remodeling and thus within haversian systems. In osteomalacia, new haversian systems form but remain unmineralized or poorly mineralized. The result is that the newly formed bone is weaker than the surrounding healthy bone. This can be caused by inadequate calcium in the diet, vitamin or hormonal problems, or pregnancy and lactation, when calcium is diverted to the fetus during growth of the fetal skeleton or to the infant through lactation.

Osteoporosis

Osteoporosis (Figures 2–19 through 2–21) is not a single disease but a number of conditions that all result in a similar presentation. Osteoporosis can be most directly defined as *a condition in which the amount of actual bone matrix per unit volume is reduced*. As the name implies, osteoporotic bone has greatly increased porosity. Spaces develop within the bone, and compact bone of the diaphyses of long bones becomes thinner, a condition referred to as *cortical involution*. Not only does cortical bone become thinner, but the remaining cortex becomes increasingly porous and weak (Walker, 1989, and references therein). In fact, in advanced cases of osteoporosis, the bone may become so thin and weak that it undergoes fracture under body weight alone. There are a number of subtypes of osteoporosis with different underlying causes.

A   B

Figure 2-19   Osteoporosis. Cross-section of two femora at their midshafts, anterior at top. (*A*) A normal, healthy adult femur. (*B*) A femur with advanced osteoporosis. Note the thin cortex and increased porosity, particularly anteroposteriorly.

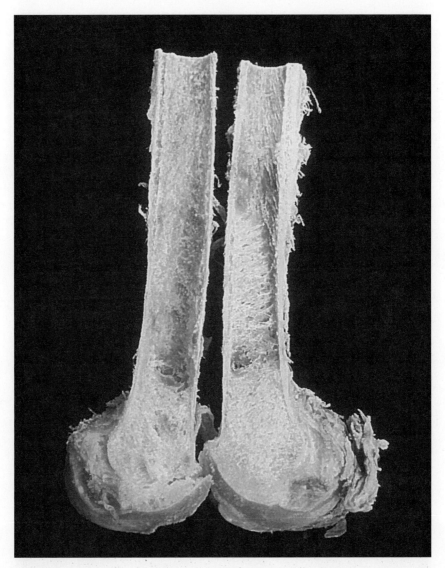

Figure 2-20   Disuse osteoporosis. These two femora are from the same individual. The femur on the left is from a leg that was amputated at the knee, whereas the femur on the right is from the patient's intact leg.

Postmenopausal Osteoporosis

The most common and generally the best-known type of osteoporosis is *postmenopausal osteoporosis.* Estrogens and androgens (i.e., testosterone) are both *anabolic,* meaning that they promote tissue formation for bone. At menopause, there is a dramatic decrease in the production and circulating levels of estrogen. In women who originally have low bone mass, low calcium intake, and/or may have been less physically active before menopause, this can result in a dramatic decrease in bone mass (Gardsell et al., 1991).

Figure 2-21   Osteoporosis in the clavicle. This figure represents through radiographs progressive bone loss in the clavicle with age. The youngest individual is represented at the top.
(Source: Walker, RA, and Lovejoy, CO [1985]. Radiographic changes in the clavicle and proximal femur and their use in the determination of skeletal age at death. *American Journal of Physical Anthropology, 68,* 73. Copyright © 1985, Wiley-Liss, Inc. Reproduced by permission of Wiley-Liss, Inc.,
a subsidiary of John Wiley & Sons, Inc.)

Postmenopausal osteoporosis appears to occur with higher frequencies among populations of European origin, although it can, and does, occur in people of all ancestries (Armelagos, 1969; Chalmers and Ho, 1970; Mangaroo et al., 1985; Martin et al., 1987; Ross et al., 1990; Slemenda and Johnston, 1990; Walker, 1991). It can be prevented, or at least the level of severity can be decreased, by adequate calcium intake and adequate exercise both before and after menopause.

Senile Osteoporosis

Senile osteoporosis is the osteoporosis of old age. Senile osteoporosis affects both men and women. The effects in older women are worse than in older men, primarily because they suffer the combined effects of *both* postmenopausal and senile osteoporosis.

Disuse Osteoporosis

As the name implies, *disuse osteoporosis* (see Fig. 2–20) is a form of osteoporosis that results from a lack of, or decrease in, applied external mechanical loads. Generally, bone requires a minimum mechanical signal ("minimum functional strain") to be maintained at normal levels. Prolonged bed rest can result in significant reductions in bone mass, as can immobilization of a limb in a cast. Even the removal of the forces of gravity results in a loss of bone mass. Space flight, even for relatively short periods, can result in a significant decrease in bone mass. Luckily, disuse osteoporosis is entirely reversible as long as it is not associated with paralysis or other conditions that prevent a body part from being loaded.

Idiopathic Osteoporosis

Idiopathic osteoporosis is osteoporosis that does not have a readily observed cause. Idiopathic osteoporosis may strike anyone at any age. Loss of bone mass may result from a decrease in osteoblastic activity, from an increase in osteoclastic activity, or from a combination of both osteoblastic and osteoclastic activity.

Different bones show different levels of susceptibility to osteoporosis. The vertebral column, especially in the thoracic region, shows an especially high susceptibility to osteoporosis. Vertebrae in older people, especially older women, may become so highly osteoporotic that they undergo compression fractures of the vertebral body. This results in a severe *kyphosis,* an anteriorly concave vertebral curvature of the thoracic vertebral column, sometimes referred to colloquially as a "dowager's hump" (Figure 2–22). If the kyphosis is severe enough, it can compromise the ability of the heart and lungs to function properly.

Osteopetrosis

Osteopetrosis (marble bone disease) is almost the opposite of osteoporosis. In osteopetrosis, abnormally large amounts of bone matrix are produced and abnormally high mineralization of bone matrix takes place. As a result, osteopetrotic bone appears almost entirely chalky white in radiographs. Because the amount of bone mineral is abnormally high relative to the amount of collagen fibers in the bone matrix, the bone is very brittle and easily fractured.

Figure 2-22   Kyphosis of the thoracic vertebral region. Anterior is to the left.

Osteopetrotic bones demonstrate very thick cortical bone, dense networks of cancellous bone, and large amounts of calcified cartilage. Experimentally, hypervitaminosis D in rats can present a similar condition. This condition is rare in humans but is sometimes seen in infants with fatal anemia and as an inherited autosomal recessive trait.

Paget's Disease

Paget's disease (osteitis deformans) has a presentation similar to osteopetrosis but is a more localized phenomenon. Bone affected by Paget's disease shows thickened cortical bone and coarse, thickened trabeculae. It may be restricted to a single bone or may have multiple foci within a single individual. It is not, however, systemic, as is osteopetrosis.

Osteogenesis Imperfecta

The name *osteogenesis imperfecta* literally means "imperfectly formed bone." In this disorder, the collagen of the bone matrix is affected. As a result, the bone is soft and brittle. Osteogenesis imperfecta is inherited as an autosomal dominant trait.

Ankylosing Spondylosis

Bony *ankylosis* is an abnormal condition in which joints become immobilized by the production of bone across the joint, thus uniting the bones solidly to one another. The condition may be genetic or may be induced by trauma, disease, or surgery (e.g., vertebral fusion). *Ankylosing spondylosis* is specifically the pathological ankylosis of the vertebral column.

Bone tissue responds to many hormonal influences (calcitonin, parathyroid hormone, and growth hormone, for example), and disorders of hormonal equilibrium can cause changes in the skeletal system, including many of the aforementioned conditions. Other conditions may result as well. Decreased amounts of growth hormone result in dwarfism. Increased amounts of growth hormone during childhood before the closure of epiphyseal growth plates result in gigantism. Generally, this condition is the result of disorders of the pituitary gland and is referred to as *pituitary gigantism*.

Increased amounts of growth hormone after the closure of the epiphyseal plates cannot cause any further growth in bone length, but it can cause increased amounts of subperiosteal bone deposition, resulting in the coarsening of facial features and increased bone diameters. This disorder is known as *acromegaly*.

References

Armelagos, G (1969). Disease in ancient Nubia. *Science, 163,* 255–259.

Avioli, LV, and Krane, SM (Eds) (1998). *Metabolic Bone Disease and Clinically Related Disorders* (3rd ed). Academic Press, New York.

Bertram, JE, and Swartz, SM (1991). The "law of bone transformation": A case of crying Wolff? *Biological Reviews of the Cambridge Philosophical Society, 66,* 245–273.

Chalmers, J, and Ho, KC (1970). Geographical variations in senile osteoporosis. *Journal of Bone and Joint Surgery, 52B,* 667–675.

Cormack, DH (1992). *Essential Histology.* Lippincott-Raven, Philadelphia.

Cormack, DH (Ed) (1987). *Hamm's Histology* (9th ed). JB Lippincott, Philadelphia.

Currey, J (1984). *The Mechanical Adaptations of Bone.* Princeton University Press, Princeton, NJ.

Enlow, DH (1969). The bone of reptiles. In C Gans (Ed), *Biology of the Reptilia* (Vol 1, pp 45–80). Academic Press, New York.

Gardsell, P, Johnell, O, Nilsson, BE, and Sernbo, I (1991). Bone mass in an urban and a rural population: A comparative, population-based study in southern Sweden. *Journal of Bone and Mineral Research, 6,* 67–75.

Krogman, WM, and Iscan, MY (1986). *Human Skeleton in Forensic Medicine* (2nd ed). Charles C Thomas, Springfield, IL.

Lanyon, LE (1993a). Osteocytes, strain detection, bone modelling and remodelling. *Calcified Tissue International, 53* (2, Suppl 1), S102-S107.

Lanyon, LE (1993b). Skeletal responses to physical loading. In GR Mundy and TJ Martin (Eds), *Physiology and Pharmacology of Bone* (pp 485–505). Springer-Verlag, Berlin.

Larson, WJ (1993). *Human Embryology* (3rd ed). Churchill Livingstone, New York.

Mangaroo, J, Glasser, JH, Roht, LH, and Kapadia, AS (1985). Prevalence of bone demineralization in the United States. *Bone, 6,* 135–139.

Martin, DL, Magennis, AL, and Rose, JC (1987). Cortical bone maintenance in an historic Afro-American cemetery sample from Cedar Grove, Arkansas. *American Journal of Physical Anthropology, 74,* 255–264.

Meindl, RS, and Lovejoy, CO (1985). Ectocranial suture closure: A revised method for the determination of skeletal age at death based on the lateral-anterior sutures. *American Journal of Physical Anthropology, 68* (1), 57–66.

Miller, SC, and Jee, WSS (1987). The bone lining cell: A distinct phenotype? *Calcified Tissue International, 41,* 1–5.

Miller, SC, and Jee, WSS (1992). Bone lining cells. In BK Hall (Ed). *Bone: Vol 4. Bone Metabolism and Mineralization* (pp 1–19). CRC Press, Boca Raton, FL.

Moore, KL, and Persaud, TVN (1992). *The Developing Human: Clinically Oriented Embryology* (6th ed). Williams and Wilkins, Baltimore.

Rodan, GA, and Rodan, SB (1984). Expression of the osteoblastic phenotype. In WA Peck (Ed), *Bone and Mineral Research Annual 2* (pp 244–285). Elsevier, Amsterdam.

Ross, PD, Wasnich, RD, and Davis, JW (1990). Fracture prediction models for osteoporosis prevention. *Bone, 11,* 327–331.

Sadler, TW (1995). *Langman's Medical Embryology* (7th ed). Lippincott-Williams and Wilkins, Baltimore.

Slemenda, CW, and Johnston, CC, Jr (1990). Osteoporotic fractures. In DJ Simmons (Ed), *Nutrition and Bone Development* (pp. 131–147). Oxford University Press, New York and Oxford.

Simmons, DJ, and Grynpas, MD (1990). Mechanisms of bone formation *in vivo*. In BK Hall (Ed), *Bone: Vol 1. The Osteoblast and the Osteocyte* (pp 193–302). Telford Press, Caldwell, NJ.

Simon, MR (1983). The effect of dynamic loading on the growth of the epiphysial growth plate of the rat. *Acta Anatomica, 101,* 176–183.

Simon, MR, Holmes, KR, and Olsen, AM (1984). The effects of quantified amounts of increased intermittent compressive forces for 30 and 60 days on the growth of limb bones in the rat. *Acta Anatomica, 120,* 173–179.

Swartz, SM, Parker, A, and Huo, C (1998). Theoretical and empirical scaling patterns and topological homology in bone trabeculae. *Journal of Experimental Biology, 201,* 573–590.

Walker, RA (1989). *Assessment of Cortical Bone Dynamics and Skeletal Age at Death from Femoral Cortical Histomorphology.* Unpublished doctoral dissertation, School of Biomedical Sciences, Kent State University, Kent, OH.

Walker, RA (1991). *Variation in Femoral Cortical Thickness in Three Human Populations.* Paper presented at the 60th annual meeting of the American Association of Physical Anthropologists, Milwaukee, Wisconsin. (Abstract published in *American Journal of Physical Anthropology,* Suppl 12, p 179, 1991)

Walker, RA (1993). *Relationship of Cross-Sectional Biomechanical Properties of Cortical Bone to Histomorphology in White Americans over 50.* Paper presented at the 62nd annual meeting of the American Association of Physical Anthropologists, Toronto, Ontario. (Abstract published in the *American Journal of Physical Anthropology,* Suppl 16, p 202, 1993.)

Walker, RA (1997). *Intraindividual Variation in Cortical Thickness and Histomorphology of the Midshaft Femur.* Paper presented at the 66th annual meeting of the American Association of Physical Anthropologists, St Louis, Missouri. (Abstract published in *American Journal of Physical Anthropology,* Suppl 24, p 234, 1997.)

Walker, RA (1998). *A Survey of Remodeling in the Mammalian Skeleton: A Pilot Study.* Paper presented at the 67th Annual Meeting of the American Association of Physical Anthropologists, Salt Lake City, Utah, April 2, 1998. (Abstract published in the *American Journal of Physical Anthropology,* Suppl 26, pp 224–225, 1998.)

Walker, RA, and Lovejoy, CO (1999). *A Survey of Remodeling in the Vertebrate Skeleton,* Part II. Paper presented at the 68th Annual Meeting of the American Association of Physical Anthropologists, Columbus, Ohio, April 29, 1999. (Abstract published in the *American Journal of Physical Anthropology*, Suppl 28, p 272, 1999.)

Walker, RA, Lovejoy, CO, and Meindl, RS (1994). The histomorphological and geometric properties of human femoral cortex in individuals over 50: Implications for histomorphological determintion of age-at-death. *American Journal of Human Biology, 6,* 659–667.

Wolff, J (1869). Über die Bedeutung der Arichitektur der spongiosen Substanz. *Zentralblatt fur die medizinishe Wissenschaft, VI,* 223–234.

Wolff, J (1892). *Das Gesetz der Transformation der Knochen.* A Hirschwald, Berlin.

Chapter 3

Development of the Vertebral Column

B. Rosenman,* C.O. Lovejoy,* and M. McCollum†

Clinicians concerned with the functioning of the human body often deal solely with adult anatomical complexes. This is especially true of the spinal column because many of its pathologies occur only in adulthood. To fully understand the etiology of many ailments and therefore better diagnose them, however, a basic awareness is required of the processes by which the vertebral column is assembled. This chapter reviews early vertebral column development, with an emphasis on the pattern and processes involved in its creation.

EMBRYOLOGICAL DEVELOPMENT FROM FERTILIZATION TO NEURULATION

How does a single cell develop into a complex, multicellular organism? This process involves a multitude of steps, all of which are precisely determined and coordinated. In this section, we will trace development from the fertilized egg to the creation of the germ layers that give rise to the tissues and structures of the body, including the vertebral column.

---

*School of Biomedical Sciences and Department of Anthropology, Kent State University
†Department of Anatomy, Case Western Reserve University School of Medicine.

Before fertilization, the egg is surrounded by an acellular layer called the *zona pellucida*. This layer serves as one of the barriers to multiple fertilizations by normally allowing the entrance of no more than one sperm. Approximately 1 day after fertilization, the fertilized egg (zygote) initiates a series of cell divisions called *cleavage*. Because they are bounded by the zona pellucida, the resultant daughter cells, or *blastomeres,* become smaller with each subsequent *mitosis,* or cell division. By the 32-cell stage (the fourth day postconception), these blastomeres take on the appearance of a mulberry, hence their designation as the *morula* (Latin: *morum* means "mulberry"). The morula gives rise to the embryo, the *extraembryonic membranes,* and the placenta.

Up to this stage, *embryogenesis* (the process of embryo formation) is roughly similar in all vertebrates. However, from this point on, the process in mammals begins to differ significantly from that in other animals, especially the chick, whose development has been most intensively studied. Until recently, many of the detailed events of mammalian development were poorly understood. Many medical texts continue to use bird development as a general outline in discussing early embryology; this is no longer necessary, however, because current research has greatly expanded our knowledge of mammalian embryogenesis. Here we touch on only some of the principal events in mammalian development.

About two thirds of the cells of the morula lie on its external surface. These are called the *trophectoderm,* also known as the *trophoblast.* The remaining one third of the cells are internal and are called the *inner cell mass.* Collectively, both structures are called the *blastocyst.* Cells of the trophectoderm begin pumping fluid into the interior of the blastocyst, causing formation of a fluid-filled vesicle called the *blastocoele.* The fluid pushes the inner cell mass against one end of the trophectoderm termed the *embryonic pole.*

At the same time, the inner cell mass differentiates into two distinct regions. The outer region, which is in contact with the trophectoderm, is called the *epiblast,* whereas the inner region, called the *primitive endoderm,* borders the blastocoele (Figure 3–1). These events begin at day 3½ and are completed by day 4½ when the zona pellucida ruptures, freeing the blastocyst to interact directly with the uterine wall.

At implantation, day 5½, some of the trophectoderm gives rise to giant cells that invade the uterus. The remainder of the trophectoderm contributes to the *placenta,* which supplies nutrition to the embryo. At the same time, the primitive endoderm spreads over the internal surface of the trophectoderm that is not in contact with the epiblast and forms the *parietal endoderm.* The portion of the primitive endoderm that remains in contact with the epiblast is now called the *visceral endoderm.*

By day 6 the epiblast has assumed a cuplike shape with an internal cavity (U-shaped in cross-section). It is now composed of about 1000 cells, and its external surface is visceral endoderm. At day 6½ the process of *gastrulation* begins. This is the process during which the three primary germ layers *(ectoderm, mesoderm,* and *endoderm)* are formed.

At a point on the circumference of the cup-shaped epiblast, at the future posterior end of the embryo, a localized thickening of cells appears. This is called the *primitive streak.* Cells of the epiblast proliferate and migrate through those of the primitive streak. As they do so, they spread anteriorly and laterally between the epiblast (which soon becomes the embryonic ectoderm) and the visceral endoderm. These cells are the *embryonic mesoderm.* Some epiblast cells penetrate the visceral endoderm layer and isolate it from the remainder of the epiblast. These new epiblast-derived

Figure 3-1   Early embryogenesis. The fertilized egg enters a series of stages: (A) two cell, (B) four cell, (C) morula, (D) blastocyst, and (E) egg cylinder.

cells form the *embryonic endoderm* (Figure 3–2). While these events are occurring, the primitive streak elongates toward the future anterior end of the embryo.

By this point, the simple "cup" of the epiblast has been transformed into one cup with three distinct layers. The internal surface of this cup (the ectoderm) is the dorsal surface of the embryo, and its external surface is the endoderm. Once gastrulation is complete, the formation of the basic body plan is well on its way. The body's primary tissues have been defined, as have its primary axes (craniocaudal, mediolateral [midline to right and left], and dorsoventral). Each germ layer forms different organ systems and tissues: the ectoderm forms epidermis, glands, hair, nails, tooth enamel, neural tissue, and much of the skull. The mesoderm forms the postcranial skeleton; connective tissue; striated muscle; and the urinary, reproductive, and circulatory systems. The endoderm forms the digestive tract, lungs, and several internal organs.

In the final stages of gastrulation, a series of complex foldings takes place that internalizes the embryonic endoderm and externalizes the embryonic ectoderm. In essence, the cup turns inside out. Many of the internal movements are complex, however; for example, the presumptive heart and liver first form anterior to the future head, but the tissues that form the head also fold. As they do so, they move the presumptive heart and liver to their more central location in the developing embryo.

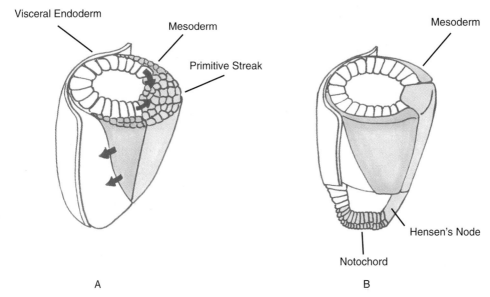

Visceral Endoderm

Mesoderm

Primitive Streak

Mesoderm

Hensen's Node

Notochord

A

B

Figure 3-2   Gastrulation: (A) The primitive streak forms at the future posterior midline of the developing embryo. Epiblast cells pass through the primitive streak and migrate anteriorly and laterally between the epiblast and visceral endoderm to form the mesoderm. Some epiblast cells penetrate and displace the visceral endoderm to become the embryonic endoderm. (B) Hensen's node is formed at the anterior end of the primitive streak. Cells passing through Hensen's node form the notochord, which plays a central role in later development of the neuraxis and vertebral column.

Recall that the primitive streak first forms at the posterior end of the embryo and elongates anteriorly. At its anterior termination is found a condensation of cells traditionally called Hensen's node. Epiblast cells that pass through this node and migrate anteriorly become organized into a solid rod called the *notochord*. The first cells to do so form its anteriormost, or most cranial, portion. The notochord passively elongates posteriorly, or caudally, as these new cells are added.

Once established, the notochord induces (causes to occur by interaction with) overlying ectodermal cells to form a layer called the *neural plate* (Figure 3–3). As with the notochord, formation of the neural plate occurs in a cranial to caudal sequence. Cranially, the neural plate is comparatively broad and gives rise to the three primary components of the developing brain: the prosencephalon (forebrain), mesencephalon (midbrain), and rhombencephalon (hindbrain). Caudal to the rhombencephalon the neural plate forms the spinal cord.

Beginning in the region of the future midbrain and spreading both cranially and caudally, the neural plate begins to fold along its midline. Its two sides, the *neural folds,* both move dorsally. The process is called *neurulation,* and the point of flexure is called the *neural groove.* The two sides then meet and fuse to form the *neural tube.* Upon fusion, the neural groove becomes the *neural canal.* Eventually the neural tube becomes isolated from surface ectoderm and is completely encased in mesoderm.

During neurulation, cells lying along the crests of the neural folds separate and migrate ventrally in the developing embryo. These *neural crest cells* eventually give rise to many diverse structures, including the ciliary and pupillary muscles of the

Figure 3-3   The process of neurulation: (*A*) neural plate, (*B*) neural groove, (*C*) appearance of neural crest, (*D*) completion of neural tube, and (*E*) formation of neural crest.

eye, facial skeleton, parts of the developing teeth, melanocytes of the skin, connective and muscular tissue of the vessels around the heart, adrenal medulla, and various ganglia of the nervous system and their supportive cells. With respect to the vertebral column, neural crest cells form the sensory cell bodies of the dorsal root ganglia.

FORMATION OF THE VERTEBRAL COLUMN

As the notochord is forming during gastrulation (and elongating caudally), the mesoderm flanking the developing neural tube begins to differentiate (Christ and Ordahl, 1995). The mesoderm lying adjacent to either side of the developing *neuraxis,* the presumptive central nervous system and vertebral column, becomes the *paraxial mesoderm* (Figure 3–4). This gives rise to a series of tissue blocks called *somites* (Tam and Trainor, 1994). Lateral to the paraxial mesoderm lies a second sheet of mesodermal cells called the *lateral plate mesoderm.* It gives rise to much of the body wall as well as to the skeleton and connective tissues of the limbs, although not to the limb musculature, which arises from somitic mesoderm and migrates into the limbs (Chevallier, 1978; Chevallier et al., 1977). Finally, lying between the paraxial mesoderm and the lateral plate mesoderm on each side is a band of *intermediate mesoderm.* This gives rise to important structures of the reproductive and urinary systems.

Somite formation proceeds in a strict craniocaudal direction (Christ et al., 2000; Gossler and Hrabe de Angelis, 1998; McGrew and Pourquié, 1998). At any one time, mature somites may be found at the cranial end of the embryo, with newly formed somites budding off from the paraxial mesoderm more caudally. Early in this process electron microscopy can detect swirls of mesenchymal cells in the paraxial mesoderm (Meier, 1979). These "presomites" are called *somitomeres* and are essentially the first stage in somite formation. Somites form when unsegmented paraxial mesenchyme undergoes a process called *epithelialization.* This process is facilitated by the expression of cell adhesion molecules within each somitomere (N-cadherin and fi-

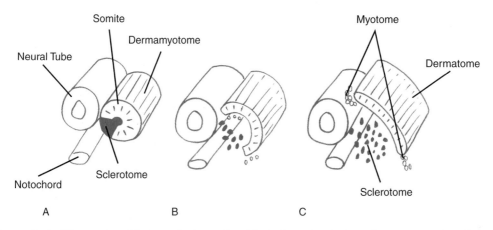

Figure 3–4   The somite: (*A*) A newly formed epithelial somite, before dissociation. (*B*) The sclerotome is beginning to lose its epithelial character, whereas the dermomyotome remains epithelial. (*C*) Sclerotomal cells migrate around the notochord and the dermomyotome has differentiated into its constituent parts, the dermatome and the myotome.

bronectin [Christ and Wilting, 1992; Horikawa et al., 1999; Lash et al., 1984; Linask et al., 1998]).

The early somite is a sphere of epithelial cells surrounded by a thick basement membrane (Solursh et al., 1979). At the center of each somite lies a lumen, termed the *somitocoele,* which contains loose mesenchymal cells that contribute to the formation of several structures, including the intervertebral discs (Huang et al., 1994, 1996). Each somite next undergoes a series of subdivisions (Christ and Wilting, 1992). It is first divided into a cranial and a caudal half by the *intrasegmental fissure* (called *von Ebner's fissure* in older literature). A second division separates each somite into dorsolateral and ventromedial portions. The ventromedial portion becomes a structure called the *sclerotome,* the precursor to the vertebrae, intervertebral discs, and ribs (Christ et al., 1998; Hall, 1977; Huang et al., 2000b). Separated by the intrasegmental fissure, cells in the cranial half of the sclerotome are less dense than those in the caudal half, and the developing axons and neural crest cells therefore migrate through only the cranial half of each sclerotome.

The sclerotome next subdivides into dorsolateral and ventromedial components, each of which further divides to become specific components of vertebral structure. The dorsolateral halves of the sclerotome give rise to the vertebral arch and the ribs. On each side of the future column, dorsolateral sclerotomal cells migrate around the neural tube to reach each other at the dorsal midline, making a complete neural arch around the developing spinal cord. At the same time, the more laterally placed sclerotomal cells expand laterally. In future thoracic vertebrae, these extensions form ribs. In nonthoracic vertebrae, they are smaller and form part of the transverse processes.

As the neural arches take shape, the notochord, which lies ventral to the neural arch, is surrounded only by extracellular matrix. The ventromedial group of sclerotomal cells migrates ventromedially to completely surround the notochord, encasing it in a *perichordal tube,* or *sheath* (Balling et al., 1996). Unlike the cells of the dorsolateral sclerotome, which maintain their segmental identity via the intrasegmental fissures, the perichordal tube loses its segmental borders and becomes one continuous mass of cells. Later, condensations appear in the perichordal tube (Bundy et al., 1998). These then develop into the intervertebral discs, whereas the less dense sections of the tube develop into the vertebral bodies. Whether these condensations are segmental or intersegmental (i.e., whether the vertebra of a specific level corresponds to the original somite level) has been one of the most controversial topics in vertebral column development; therefore, we must examine the theory of *resegmentation* (also known as "Neugliederung"; Figure 3–5).

Remak first proposed resegmentation in the middle of the last century (Verbout, 1976, 1985). He argued that a vertebra is made not from a single somite but from the caudal half of one somite and the cranial half of the somite just caudal to it. Therefore, one vertebra is the union of two adjacent somites. There are some exceptions to this "rule." The first four somites form part of the occipital bone instead of a vertebra (Kant and Goldstein, 1999). In addition, the body of the atlas (C1) has become incorporated into the axis during development, forming the *odontoid process,* or *dens.*

The greatest criticism against resegmentation arises from the fact that no one has directly witnessed the splitting of a somite. However, labeling and quail transplantation studies of somites (Bagnall, 1992a, 1992b; Bagnall et al., 1988a, 1988b, 1989; Ewan and Everett, 1992; Stern and Keynes, 1987) provide evidence that supports resegmentation. The recent work of Huang and colleagues (2000a) definitively shows that the vertebral body, neural arch, pedicles, and transverse processes

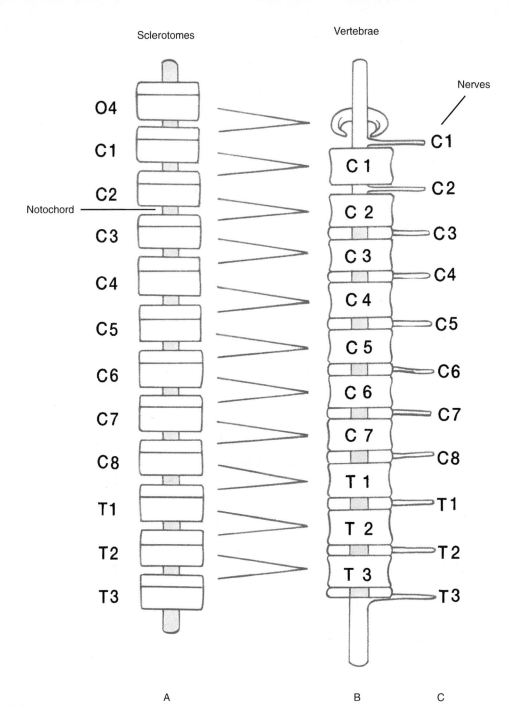

Figure 3-5 Resegmentation: (*A*) Sclerotomes O4 (fourth occipital sclerotome, which contributes to the occipital bone of the skull) through T3 (third thoracic sclerotome) are illustrated. Each sclerotome has surrounded the notochord and has become divided by intrasegmental fissures. (*B*) Vertebrae C1 through T3 after segmentation. Note that each centrum is formed by the union of half of two adjacent sclerotomes, with vertebra C1 being formed by the caudal half of sclerotome C1 and the cranial half of sclerotome C2, and that the notochord persists to eventually become the nucleus pulposus of each vertebral disc. (*C*) The vertebral nerves, each of which supplies a number of structures in the limb and body wall (C5 through T1 contribute to the brachial plexus).

(including the distal ribs) are created by the fusion of two somites. Only the head of the rib is derived from a single somite.

As the perichordal sheath envelops the notochord, the notochordal cells in each of the presumptive vertebra undergo programmed cell death, or *apoptosis.* Those cells in the presumptive intervertebral disc, however, do not die (Walmsley, 1953) but contribute to the formation of the nucleus pulposus, the watery, jellylike deformable center of the intervertebral disc. By birth it appears that cells from the outer annulus fibrosis have replaced most of the notochordal-derived cells of the nucleus pulposus.

The dorsolateral part of the somite remains epithelial. It is termed the *dermamyotome.* It is really two structures: a dorsal *dermatome,* which gives rise to the dermis of the skin of the back, and the underlying *myotome,* which supplies all the muscle cells for the spinal column, body wall, and limbs, but not most of those for the muscles of the head (these cells are derived from the neural crest). Myotome formation is complex and not yet fully understood. Opinions as to the source of myogenic precursor cells differ, and two recent reviews (Kalcheim et al., 1999; Venters et al., 1999) indicate that there may be species-specific differences in the details of myotome formation.

Although it has long been commonly assumed that the epaxial and hypaxial portions of the body's musculature arise from a single muscle cell pool in the myotome, recent studies indicate that this is not the case (Denetclaw and Ordahl, 2000; Ordahl, 1993; Ordahl and Le Douarin, 1992; Williams and Ordahl, 1997). Using chick-quail chimeras and transplantation studies, workers have found that the epaxial muscles originate solely in the medial half of the somite. Furthermore, those myogenic cells that eventually migrate from the somite, such as those that invade the limb bud, are found exclusively in the lateral somite.

DEVELOPMENT: CORE CONCEPTS

Before discussing the molecular controls underlying the processes described previously, we must first address several key embryological concepts and review some general developmental molecular mechanisms. The phenomenon of *induction* occurs when a group of cells influences the fate of another. Signals emanating from an initial cell population can launch a developmental program in a secondary group and determine the latter's fate. Cells affected by an inducing signal become specified to a particular cell type; after a time, the targeted cells are unable to return to their initial state or differentiate into another cell type. An important corollary to induction is that the affected cells must be *competent* to respond to an inducing signal. Competence is often time dependent (i.e., cells from an earlier or later developmental stage do not react to an inducer). The competence of cells usually depends on previous inductive interactions. Induction is achieved primarily through short-range signaling molecules (discussed later). Without induction, increasing embryonic complexity is impossible.

Other important developmental concepts are *pattern formation* and *positional information* (Neumann and Cohen, 1997; Wolpert, 1978, 1996; Woychik et al., 1997). Pattern formation is the process by which an embryo is constructed in space; positional information directs this assembly. Positional information enables a cell to differentiate into its fated type based on its placement in a three-dimensional coordinate system; for example, positional information dictates which cell develops into a chondroblast of a developing vertebra and which develops into a myoblast of a developing erector spinae muscle.

Pattern formation, mediated through positional information, occurs in several steps (Wolpert, 1978). First, cells interpret their position relative to other cells within the embryo; that is, communication among cells allows each to "understand" exactly what portion of its genetic code it should express. That expression causes the cell to become a particular type. Cells receive information from other cells because either they express specific receptors for extracellular signaling molecules that they and other cells can synthesize and secrete or they can make bonds with one another and use these bonds as avenues of expression. These signaling molecules include members of the Hedgehog, Bmp, Wnt, Fgf, and Notch families, as well as retinoic acid.

Once their positional information is established, the cells then carry out specific programs of genetic expression by activating *transcription factors*. These are nuclear proteins that act upon their own DNA to cause production of other proteins, some of which may also be transcription factors. Obviously, the most fundamental transcription factors are those expressed earliest in development. In the development of the spine, one group of transcription factors of crucial importance are the *homeobox genes*.

Homeobox genes are found throughout the animal kingdom in organisms as diverse as fruit flies, chicks, and mice (Figure 3–6; Krumlauf, 1994). They specify much of the embryonic anteroposterior axis, as well as secondary axes such as those in the limbs. Their name derives from the *homeotic* genes of the fly—genes that, when mutated, replace one body part with another, a phenomenon called *homeosis*. One subset of these genes, the *Hox* genes, is essential to axis formation. All *Hox* genes contain a specific region of DNA, the *homeobox* (hence the name), which is highly conserved among diverse taxa. The homeobox is approximately 180 base pairs long and codes for a 60-amino acid region of the gene's protein product called the *homeodomain*. The homeodomain binds to specific regions of DNA to control its target gene's transcription, either negatively or positively (Duboule, 1994).

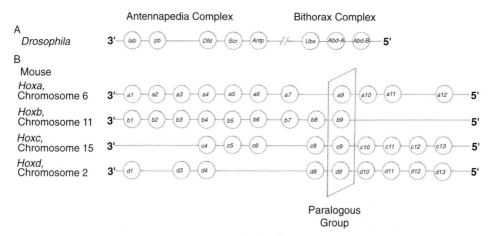

Figure 3–6   The mammalian *Hox* gene complex, homologous with (*A*) the fruit fly genes. (*B*) Each mammalian complex (*Hoxa, Hoxb, Hoxc, Hoxd*) is located on a different chromosome. Each cluster of genes is ordered sequentially, from *Hox1* to *Hox13*. *Hoxa9, Hoxb9, Hoxc9,* and *Hoxd9* are classified together as an example of a paralogous group. Note that no chromosome possesses the full complement of genes. The missing genes were deleted during evolution.

In fruit flies there is only one set of 8 homeobox genes, but in vertebrates there are four sets *(Hoxa, Hoxb, Hoxc, Hoxd),* each located on a different chromosome. The additional three sets in vertebrates have arisen by two duplications of the original set. Therefore, many *Hox* genes share sequence similarities with those in the other three complexes. These are called *paralogs.* As an example, *Hox12* paralogs share a degree of similarity not found in other paralogous groups (such as *Hox11* or *Hox13*). Although each chromosome possesses 13 possible slots, not every *Hox* complex contains all 13 genes (there are only 38 *Hox* genes out of a possible 52 [4 groups $\times$ 13 paralogous slots = 52 genes]). The missing genes have been lost during evolution.

Hox genes are ordered sequentially on a chromosome, with the group 1 paralogs located at the 3' area of the DNA master strand and the group 13 paralogs at the 5' region (Duboule, 1994). Genes located at the 3' end are expressed in more anterior parts of the embryo than those in the 5' end, which are expressed more posteriorly; for example, group 3 paralogs are expressed in the cervical region, whereas group 11 paralogs are expressed in the presumptive sacrum.

This correlation between a *Hox* gene's placement on the chromosome and its expression along the embryonic anteroposterior axis is termed *spatial colinearity.* Additionally, the 3' genes are expressed earlier in development than those in the 5' region, a phenomenon called *temporal colinearity.* If either spatial or temporal colinearity is disrupted during development, a partial or full homeosis (transformation into a vertebra of another type) may occur.

The upstream regulation of *Hox* expression is poorly understood. Data have been culled primarily from studies of *Hox*-related fruit fly genes and vertebrate brain development (Charité et al., 1998; Hanson et al., 1999; Manzanares et al., 1999). These studies identify the genes *cdx* and *kreisler* as important guides in assigning the positional information relevant to *Hox* expression in the developing brain and spinal cord (Subramanian et al., 1995). Several other genes have been found to affect *Hox* gene expression in the developing spinal column. They include *Mll* and *Bmi1*, which are related to the fruit fly gene families Trithorax and Polycomb-group (Hanson et al., 1999). Manipulations of these genes result in vertebral homeoses. Retinoic acid, a derivative of vitamin A (Durston et al., 1997; Marshall et al., 1996), is also a potent regulator of *Hox* expression (Kessel, 1992; Kessel and Gruss, 1991). A recent discovery is growth and differentiation factor 11 *(Gdf11). Gdf11* mutants show altered *Hox* expression that, as with retinoic acid, results in vertebral homeoses, indicating that it *may* be upstream of *Hox* (McPherron et al., 1999). Although these preliminary studies give us important clues as to the control of *Hox*, further work must be completed in the search of more universal regulators of *Hox* expression.

Although *Hox* genes are the primary regulators of embryonic patterning, other homeobox genes also contribute. *Pax* genes are another well-studied homeobox gene family (Dahl et al., 1997; Gruss and Walther, 1992). *Pax* genes also contain a highly conserved region of DNA, called the *paired box* (hence the name). Nine *Pax* genes are known, *Pax1* through *Pax9. Pax* genes have been implicated in many areas of development and are primarily, but not exclusively, expressed in such ectodermally derived structures as the eye and brain. Our interest lies in *Pax1, Pax3,* and *Pax9,* because their expression in the mesoderm is necessary for normal vertebral column development.

The signaling molecule *Hedgehog (Hh)* was also first discovered in the fruit fly. It is a secreted protein that mediates cell-to-cell interactions (Fietz et al., 1994). Its effect is exerted over a distance of only a few cell diameters (Hammerschmidt, 1997; Johnson and Tabin, 1995), and in fly development it helps determine cell polarity (i.e., resulting in a tissue axis) and fate. Genes related to *Hh* have been discovered in vertebrates and show high homology in both their genetic sequence and signaling pathways (Goodrich et al., 1996). Of the *Hh* homologues identified in vertebrates, the best known are *Sonic hedgehog (Shh), Indian hedgehog (Ihh),* and *Desert hedgehog (Dhh)* (Hammerschmidt, 1997). *Dhh* is involved in the development of the reproductive, nervous, and cardiovascular systems, whereas *Ihh* is involved in the digestive system and bone growth plates. *Shh* is integral to several key organizing centers of the embryo and is used several times in the developing vertebral column.

Among the most important discoveries is the fact that vertebrate *Hedgehog* genes are coexpressed with *bone morphogenetic protein (Bmp)* genes at different sites in the embryo, indicating that *Bmp*s may be downstream targets of *Hh* expression. This situation is analogous to that found in the fly, in which the *Bmp*-related gene *decapentaplegic* is a downstream target of *Hh* (Bitgood and McMahon, 1995).

*Bmp*s received their name because the first gene discovered in this family produced bone when it was applied experimentally to ectopic tissue sites. The name is misleading, however, because *Bmp*s are used in many situations that are unrelated to the development of the skeletal system. *Bmp*s are members of the larger Tgf-β (transforming growth factor-β) superfamily and, like *Hh,* are secreted proteins. With more than 20 members, *Bmp*s are involved in cell proliferation, differentiation, and determination (Hogan, 1996). *Bmp*s help control a variety of embryonic processes, such as mesoderm specification, neuronal patterning, bone development (including the vertebral column), and formation of several organs and organ systems (Hogan, 1996).

*Wnt*s (pronounced "wints") are yet another family of secreted cell-to-cell signaling molecules involved in many aspects of embryonic patterning (Cadigan and Nusse, 1997; Loureiro, 1999; Moon et al., 1997). Wnts are secreted glycoproteins, which, unlike Shh, can be found several cell diameters away from their initial source. Like *Bmp*s, *Wnt*s are involved in cell polarity and neuronal development, and they are found in a variety of adult tissues. Uncontrolled *Wnt* expression has been implicated in several cancers. As is the case for the other signaling molecules, *Wnt*s are also implicated in vertebral column morphogenesis.

Fibroblast growth factors (Fgfs) are a group of multifunctional secreted factors essential for proper embryonic and postembryonic development (Goldfarb, 1996). As in the other signaling molecules discussed here, *Fgf*s control the proper formation of the lungs, hair, and limbs. They have the ability to initiate the growth of entire structures, such as the limbs. They act by several mechanisms, primarily by inducing growth (hence the name *growth factor*). Alternately, they may prevent growth while inducing a cell lineage to differentiate. *Fgf*s and *Bmp*s are likely downstream targets of *Hox* genes.

The Notch signaling pathway is quite complex, and its importance in embryogenesis is confirmed by its ubiquitous presence in the animal kingdom (Artavanis-Tsakonas et al., 1999; Nye, 1999). First discovered in the fruit fly *Drosophila,* Notch proteins are cell receptors; cells communicate through the Notch pathway. Nye stated in 1999 that "[cells] that receive a Notch signal assume one cell fate, whereas those that do not receive it assume another fate." Many genes are involved in transducing the signal received by Notch cell receptors, including members of the Delta-like *(Dll)* family, *Jagged,* and *lunatic fringe.* The Notch pathway is used in a variety of developmental situations.

The interplay between *Hox* and *Pax* genes and the signaling molecules discussed here is quite complex. In the next section we find that these relationships are used repeatedly and in different combinations in forming a vertebra from undifferentiated paraxial mesoderm.

MOLECULAR CONTROL OF VERTEBRAL COLUMN FORMATION

A number of the genes previously described play fundamental roles in the development of the vertebral column. It is difficult to say that one is more important than another, because all must properly interact for normal formation to proceed. The effects of some gene mutants are very striking, however; for example, *Wnt3a* mutants form ectopic neural tubes and fail to show any paraxial mesodermal markers (Yoshikawa et al., 1997; for additional effects of *Wnt3a,* see also Ikeya and Takada, 2001).

Wnt3a guides paraxial mesoderm formation through its effect on the expression of the T-box gene *T (Brachyury)* and other T-box family genes, such as *Tbx6* (Chapman et al., 1996; Yamaguchi et al., 1999); mutations in these genes result in severe abnormalities. *Tbx6* mouse mutants show only a few irregularly shaped cervical somites, with numerous other malformations as well (Chapman and Papaioannou, 1998).

One of the most interesting problems in spinal development is the determination of segment number (Cooke, 1975; Cooke and Zeeman, 1976; Kerszberg and Wolpert, 2000; Schnell and Maini, 2000). How does an embryo determine the proper species-specific number of somites? When an embryo is experimentally reduced in size, it still forms the same number of somites as in a full-sized specimen. How is this accomplished? One proposal is called the clock-and-wavefront model. In this model, cells are assumed to have clocklike control devices that cause them to cycle at regular intervals until they receive a signal that leads to further differentiation. During spinal development that signal is sent down the column as a "wavefront" (Cooke, 1998).

The clock-and-wavefront theory had little supporting evidence before the analysis of the avian gene *c-hairy1,* which is related to a *Drosophila* segmentation gene (Palmeirim et al., 1997). The *c-hairy1* gene is expressed dynamically in the paraxial mesoderm of the chick, rising to high and then sinking to undetectable levels with regular periodicity.

The expression of another gene, called *lunatic fringe,* also regularly cycles in the paraxial mesoderm before somitogenesis, or somite formation, and may be a target of *c-hairy1* (Aulehla and Johnson, 1999; Dale and Pourquié, 2000; Forsberg et al., 1998; Holley et al., 2000; McGrew et al., 1998;). Mutants of *lunatic fringe* fail to form boundaries between and within somites, in addition to undergoing other changes. Several genes within the Notch pathway are also essential in border maintenance, as well as synchronization of the segmentation "clock" (Jiang et al., 2000; Jouve et al., 2000).

Notch1 mutants exhibit delayed and disorganized somitogenesis (Conlon et al., 1995). *Dll1* is required for normal polarity in somites (Beckers et al., 2000; Hrabe de Angelis et al., 1997), and *Dll3* mutants lack segment polarity because epithelialization fails to occur (Kusumi et al., 1998). In these mutants, the descendants of the somite, the sclerotome and dermamyotome, do form but are disorganized. Analysis of these and other genes has shown that segmentation and somitogenesis are different processes and that epithelial somites are required for the proper patterning of the sclerotome and dermamyotome.

Genes not directly involved with the Notch pathway also play a role in somite boundary formation. The gene *Paraxis* is a factor that controls epithelialization of somites (Barnes et al., 1997; Burgess et al., 1996; Correia and Conlon, 2000; Johnson et al., 2001; Sosic et al., 1997; see also Wilson-Rawls et al., 1999) and is required for the proper development and patterning of the body segments.

Mutations in other genes can also have dramatic effects on the formation of the spine. These genes, and the signals they convey, are expressed in two separate spinal organizing centers. The first such center is the notochord and the ventral part of the neural tube known as the floorplate. The second center is the dorsal part of the neural tube known as the roofplate and the adjoining lateral plate mesoderm. The first center primarily determines the dorsoventral patterning of the vertebral column; the second dictates mediolateral patterning. There is, however, interplay between these two centers. We examine dorsoventral patterning first.

If a notochord or a floorplate is experimentally moved to a site in the embryo where it is not normally found (e.g., dorsal to the neural tube), dramatic alterations occur in the adult form. The parts of the somite that normally form the dermamyotome instead take on the identity of a secondary sclerotome, resulting in a vertebral column with an excess of bone but a scarcity of muscle. Shh is produced by the notochord and floorplate (Chiang et al., 1996; Fan et al., 1995; Fan and Tessier-Lavigne, 1994; Johnson et al., 1994; Marcelle et al., 1999) and ultimately controls sclerotomic determination.

A downstream target of Shh is *Pax1* (Balling et al., 1996; Barnes et al., 1996a, 1996b; Ebensperger et al., 1995; Furumoto et al., 1999; Peters et al., 1999; Smith and Tuan, 1995). *Pax1* is expressed in the more ventral parts of the sclerotome, those parts that become the vertebral bodies, intervertebral discs, pedicles, and proximal ribs (Deutsch et al., 1988; Koseki et al., 1993; Wallin et al., 1994). Mutations in *Pax1*, which are known from the mouse mutant family *undulated* (Balling et al., 1988; Chalepakis et al., 1991; Deutsch et al., 1988; Dietrich and Gruss, 1995; Wallin et al., 1994), result in severe disorganization or lack of vertebral bodies and intervertebral discs. The neural arches remain relatively unaffected, whereas the proximal ribs are missing or deformed.

Although Shh controls much of the development of the bony parts of the vertebrae, other factors also come into play. Mutations in the gene *Uncx4.1* produce vertebrae that lack pedicles and transverse processes (Leitges et al., 2000; Mansouri et al., 2000). The gene *Bagpipe* appears to control proliferation of the sclerotome and its ability to interact with the notochord (Lettice et al., 1999; Tribioli and Lufkin, 1999). The development of the spinous process is controlled through local signaling by the roofplate and overlying ectoderm. These tissues express *Bmp4*. *Bmp4* in turn regulates the expression of the homeobox-containing genes *Msx1* and *Msx2*. Increased expression of these genes results in larger spinous processes, whereas their removal produces unfused neural arches lacking spinous processes, a condition resembling spina bifida (Monsoro-Burq et al., 1994, 1996).

Signals from the second organizing center, the roofplate, surface ectoderm, and lateral plate mesoderm, control dorsoventral patterning of the somite, often by counteracting the effects of one another. *Wnt1* and *Wnt3a* are expressed in the dorsal roofplate of the neural tube (Capdevila et al., 1998; Fan et al., 1997; Ikeya and Takada, 1998; Reshef et al., 1998; Stern et al., 1995). In this context, *Wnt*s participate in two processes.

First, *Wnt*s may prevent the dorsal expansion off Shh and therefore aid in forming the sclerotome (Borycki et al., 2000; Capdevila et al., 1998). Second, *Wnt1* and

Wnt3a regulate medial dermomyotome formation by counteracting the effect of the lateral plate, which produces *Bmp4* (Pourquié et al., 1996; Tonegawa et al., 1997). *Wnts* accomplish this by their production of a *Bmp* antagonist (a molecule that counteracts the effect of another molecule), *Noggin* (Hirsinger et al., 1997; Marcelle et al., 1997; McMahon et al., 1998). Correct specification of the mediolateral axis in the developing somite is consequently dependent on the proper interplay between *Wnts*, *Noggin,* and *Bmp4.*

A major target of Bmp4, which is produced in the lateral plate, is *Pax3. Pax3* is first expressed widely in presomitic tissues, but as the somite matures, its expression is restricted to the dermamyotome (Goulding et al., 1994; Maroto et al., 1997; Williams and Ordahl, 1994). *Pax3* regulates the onset of myogenesis, the formation of muscle tissue from more primitive cells. *Pax3* mutants lack ventral body wall musculature, indicating that the gene aids in the long-range migration of progenitor muscle cells (Tremblay et al., 1998). Mouse *splotch* mutants, who have a mutation in *Pax3,* show rib truncations, probably because of *Pax3*'s effect on intercostal muscles (Dickman et al., 1999; Henderson et al., 1999).

We should note that other axial structures have been implicated in the control and maintenance of myogenesis. These studies have implicated the notochord, floorplate, and roofplate (Buffinger and Stockdale, 1995; Münsterberg and Lassar, 1995; Pownall et al., 1996; Spence et al., 1996; Stern and Hauschka, 1995). The specific role of each of these structures in myogenesis is still debated.

The role of *Pax3* appears to be in its mediation of signals involved in the activation of myogenic differentiation factors, or Mdfs (Dietrich, 1999; Maroto et al., 1997). Myogenic differentiation factors include *myoD*, myogenin, *myf5,* and *mrf4.* They are expressed at different times and in different cell lineages (Currie and Ingham, 1998). Regardless, different members of this family share much functional redundancy, as evidenced by the fact that deletion of one gene often has no detectable phenotypic effect. Both *myoD* and *mrf4* have redundant functions (Rawls et al., 1998), as do *myf5* and myogenin (Wang and Jaenisch, 1997).

Although *myoD* and *myf5* appear necessary for initiation of muscle formation, downstream products such as *mrf4,* myogenin, and Mef2 (from another family of myogenic regulators) are required for maintenance of myogenesis (Brand-Saberi and Christ, 1999). *Growth and differentiation factor 8 (Gdf8),* also known as myostatin, determines muscle mass by regulating mitosis in myoblasts. Mutants of this gene produce double the muscle mass of the wildtype (McPherron et al., 1997), as seen most spectacularly in the double-muscled European cattle breeds Belgian Blue and Piedmontese (McPherron and Lee, 1997).

HOX CONTROL OF VERTEBRAL SPECIFICATION

Although we have thoroughly addressed the molecular processes in vertebral assembly, we have not yet discussed the molecular controls that determine vertebral identities. This role is clearly attributable to *Hox* genes. *Hox* genes encode positional information for vertebral identity before somitogenesis (Figure 3–7).

When presumptive thoracic paraxial mesoderm is transplanted ectopically to the cervical region, cervical vertebrae with ribs are formed (Kieny et al., 1972; for an update of this experiment, see Nowicki and Burke, 2000 and Burke and Nowicki, 2001). *Hox* genes obey spatial colinearity and are expressed in increasing numbers the

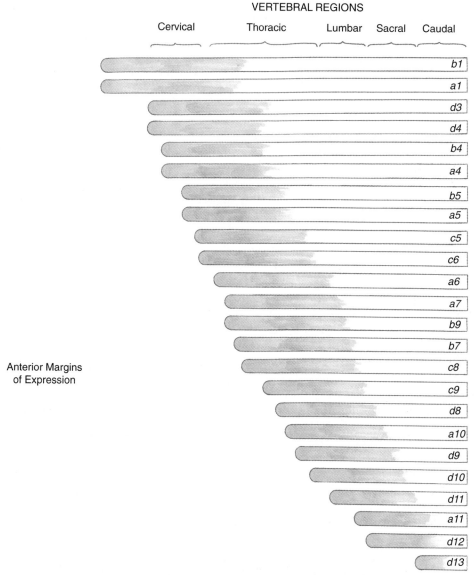

Figure 3–7 *Hox* gene expression along the developing spinal column. The darker banding indicates the strongest and most anterior limits of each gene's expression. The expression of each gene becomes weaker as the distance increases between the point of its initial expression and the most posterior extent of its domain.

farther caudally one moves down the vertebral column. Targeted gene deletions* have been instrumental in determining the functions of *Hox* genes in vertebral identity.

Both posterior and anterior vertebral transformations occur in mutants. Moreover, the severity of the mutant phenotype appears to be dose dependent; for example, *Hoxd3* mutants show anterior transformations of parts of the atlas into the oc-

---

*The literature of *Hox* mutants and the vertebral column is voluminous. References may be found in the categories that follow. *General:* Burke, 2000; Burke et al., 1995; Gaunt, 1991, 1994, 2000, 2001; Gaunt and Strachan, 1994; Gaunt et al.,1999; Kessel, 1992; Kessel and Gruss, 1990, 1991; Medina-Martínez et al., cipital bone and of the axis into atlaslike structures. With the addition of *Hoxa3* mutants, however, the dysmorphology increases. Double homozygous mutants for *Hoxa3* and *Hoxd3* show a complete loss of the atlas, with only a cartilage rudiment in its place (Condie and Capecchi, 1994). Furthermore, these studies show that paralogous genes may have redundant functions. The functional compensation of paralogous genes can rescue the loss of function of the targeted deletions and can hinder easy interpretation of results.

Kessel and Gruss (1991) proposed that individual vertebrae are specified by a particular combination of *Hox* genes expressed at a vertebral level—a *Hox* code. Duboule (1995) as well as Condie and Capecchi (1993, 1994) have suggested instead that combinations of *Hox* genes do not specify particular vertebrae but determine rates of proliferation in the mesenchymal vertebral precursors. Alterations in overall growth rates within different parts of a vertebra could explain the discrepancy in size and shape between cervical and lumbar vertebrae; for example, Condie and Capecchi (1994) suggest that the lack of an axis in *Hoxd3* and *Hoxa3* mutants results because the cell condensations forming this vertebra failed to proliferate.

Burke and colleagues (1995) proposed two equally possible mechanisms by which *Hox* genes specify vertebrae. First, *Hox* genes may score an invariant coordinate system along the craniocaudal axis that does not vary with respect to segment number. Changes in vertebral type would be specified by changes in the targets of *Hox*. There would be no correlation between the *Hox* position along the craniocaudal axis and a particular vertebral type.

Alternatively, vertebral morphology could change in concert with differences in *Hox* expression patterns up and down the body axis. *Hox* genes would therefore directly control changes in vertebral type. Differences in the timing and expression domains of *Hox* genes would cause shifts in type. Burke and colleagues (1995) and Belting and colleagues (1998) conclusively support the latter model. In a comparison of *Hox* expression between chicks and mice, these researchers found that specific genes are always associated with a change of one vertebral type to another. Important associations are found in *Hoxc5* and *Hoxc6*, which are connected to the cervicothoracic transition; *Hoxa9*, *Hoxb9*, and *Hoxc9*, which are associated with the end of the thoracic vertebrae; and *Hox10* paralogs, which are expressed in the first sacral vertebra.

Furthermore, Belting and colleagues (1998) noted a correlation between *Hoxc8* and the brachial plexus. They also found that the regulatory circuitry of this gene differed only very slightly between the mouse and the chick. Therefore, minor and subtle changes in the regulation of where and when *Hox* genes are expressed may have large downstream effects on adult morphology.

Finally, Chen and colleagues (1998) have noted that alterations caused by *Hox* mutants are often centered on transitional zones from one type of vertebra to another, even when the anterior limits of the affected genes do not correspond to these points. Transition zones appear to be more sensitive to *Hox* mutations than are vertebrae within a particular segmental zone.

2000; Richardson et al., 1998; Subramanian et al., 1995. *Hox3:* Condie and Capecchi, 1993, 1994; Manley and Capecchi, 1997. *Hox4:* Boulet and Capecchi, 1996; Folberg et al., 1999; Horan et al., 1994; Horan et al., 1995a, 1995b; Kostic and Capecchi, 1994; Ramírez-Solis et al., 1993; Saegusa et al., 1996. *Hox5:* Aubin et al., 1998; Jeannotte et al., 1993. *Hox6:* Jegalian and De Robertis, 1992. *Hox7:* Chen et al., 1998; Kessel et al., 1990. *Hox8:* Belting et al., 1998; Charité et al., 1994; Charité et al., 1995; Le Mouellic et al., 1992; Pollock et al., 1992; Shashikant and Ruddle, 1996; van den Akker et al., 2001. *Hox9:* Chen and Capecchi, 1997; de la Cruz et al., 1999; Fromental-Ramain et al., 1996; Suemori et al., 1995. *Hox10:* Rijli et al., 1995; Wahba et al., 2001. *Hox 11:* Beckers et al., 1996; Davis and Capecchi, 1994; Davis et al., 1995; Favier et al., 1995; Gérard et al., 1996; Hostikka and Capecchi, 1998; Small and Potter, 1993; Zákány et al., 1996.

Mutated genes with an anterior expression domain within a particular vertebral type often elicit their effects in the nearest caudal transition. This observation led the authors to suggest that "vertebral types are made in blocks and that the temporal phasing of these blocks is mediated by the ordered dosage of *Hox* gene expression within each region" (Chen et al., 1998, p. 55). Although this is an interesting hypothesis, further work is needed to support it.

Our understanding of vertebral column development has burgeoned considerably over the past decade. Progress has been made on many fronts, from the clarification of descriptive models of vertebral development, such as resegmentation, to the discovery of the genes that control the initiation, specification, and maintenance of vertebral morphogenesis. Future work will further expand our knowledge of the processes underlying the creation of the vertebral column.

References

Artavanis-Tsakonas, S, Rand, MD, and Lake, RJ (1999). Notch signaling: Cell fate control and signal integration in development. *Science, 284,* 770–776.

Aubin, J, Lemieux, M, Tremblay, M, Behringer, RR, and Jeannotte, L (1998). Transcriptional interferences at the *Hoxa4/Hoxa5* locus: Importance of correct *Hoxa5* expression for the proper specification of the axial skeleton. *Developmental Dynamics, 212,* 141–156.

Aulehla, A, and Johnson, RL (1999). Dynamic expression of *lunatic fringe* suggests a link between *notch* signaling and an autonomous cellular oscillator driving somite segmentation. *Developmental Biology, 207,* 49–61.

Bagnall, KM (1992a). Segmentation and compartments in the vertebrate embryo. In R Bellairs, EJ Sanders, and JW Lash (Eds), *Formation and Differentiation of Early Embryonic Mesoderm* (pp 133–147). Plenum Press, New York.

Bagnall, KM (1992b). The migration and distribution of somite cells after labelling with the carbocyanine dye, DiI: The relationship of this distribution to segmentation in the vertebrate body. *Anatomy and Embryology, 185,* 317–324.

Bagnall, KM, Higgins, SJ, and Sanders, EJ (1988). The contribution made by a single somite to the vertebral column: Experimental evidence in support of resegmentation using the chick-quail chimaera model. *Development, 103,* 69–85.

Bagnall, KM, Higgins, SJ, and Sanders, EJ (1989). The contribution made by cells from a single somite to tissues within a body segment and assessment of their integration with similar cells from adjacent segments. *Development, 107,* 931–943.

Bagnall, KM, Sanders, EJ, Higgins, SJ, and Leam, H (1988b). The effects of somite removal on vertebral formation in the chick. *Anatomy and Embryology, 178,* 183–190.

Balling, R, Deutsch, U, and Gruss, P (1988). *undulated,* a mutation affecting the development of the mouse skeleton, has a point mutation in the paired box of *Pax 1. Cell, 55,* 531–535.

Balling, R, Neubüser, A, and Christ, B (1996). *Pax* genes and sclerotome development. *Seminars in Cell and Developmental Biology, 7,* 129–136.

Barnes, GL, Alexander, PG, Hsu, CW, Mariani, BD, and Tuan, RS (1997). Cloning and characterization of chicken *Paraxis:* A regulator of paraxial mesoderm development and somite formation. *Developmental Biology, 189,* 95–111.

Barnes, GL, Hsu, CW, Mariani, BD, and Tuan, RS (1996a). Chicken *Pax-1* gene: Structure and expression during embryonic somite development. *Differentiation, 61,* 13–23.

Barnes, GL, Mariani, BD, and Tuan, RS (1996b). Valproic acid-induced somite teratogenesis in the chick embryo: Relationship with *Pax-1* gene expression. *Teratology, 54,* 93–102.

Beckers, J, Gérard, M, and Duboule, D (1996). Transgenic analysis of a potential *Hoxd-11* limb regulatory element present in tetrapods and fish. *Developmental Biology, 180,* 543–553.

Beckers, J, Schlautmann, N, and Gossler, A (2000). The mouse rib mutation disrupts anterior-posterior somite patterning and genetically interacts with a *Delta1* null allele. *Mechanisms of Development, 95,* 35–46.

Belting, HG, Shashikant, CS, and Ruddle, FH (1998). Modification of expression and *cis*-regulation of *Hoxc8* in the evolution of diverged axial morphology. *Proceedings of the National Academy of Sciences of the United States of America, 95,* 2355–2360.

Bitgood, MJ, and McMahon, AP (1995). *Hedgehog* and *Bmp* genes are co-expressed at many diverse sites of cell-cell interaction in the mouse embryo. *Developmental Biology, 172,* 126–138.

Borycki, AG, Brown, AMC, and Emerson, CP (2000). Shh and Wnt signaling pathways converge to control *Gli* gene activation in avian somites. *Development, 127,* 2075–2087.

Boulet, AM, and Capecchi, MR (1996). Targeted disruption of *hoxc-4* causes esophageal defects and vertebral transformations. *Developmental Biology, 177,* 232–249.

Brand-Saberi, B, and Christ, B (1999). Genetic and epigenetic control of muscle development in vertebrates. *Cell and Tissue Research, 296,* 199–212.

Buffinger, N, and Stockdale, FE (1995). Myogenic specification of somites is mediated by diffusible factors. *Developmental Biology, 169,* 96–108.

Bundy, J, Rogers, R, Hoffman, S, and Conway, SJ (1998). Segmental expression of aggrecan in the nonsegmented perinotochordal sheath underlies normal segmentation of the vertebral column. *Mechanisms of Development, 79,* 213–217.

Burgess, R, Rawls, A, Brown, D, Bradley, A, and Olson, EN (1996). Requirement of the *Paraxis* gene for somite formation and musculoskeletal patterning. *Nature, 384,* 570–573.

Burke, AC (2000). *Hox* genes and the global patterning of the somitic mesoderm. *Current Topics in Developmental Biology, 47,* 155–181.

Burke, AC, Nelson, CE, Morgan, BA, and Tabin, C (1995). *Hox* genes and the evolution of vertebrate axial morphology. *Development, 121,* 333–346.

Burke, AC, and Nowicki, JL (2001). *Hox* genes and axial specification in vertebrates. *American Zoologist, 41,* 687–697.

Cadigan, KM, and Nusse, R (1997). Wnt signaling: A common theme in animal development. *Genes and Development, 11,* 3286–3305.

Capdevila, J, Tabin, C, and Johnson, RL (1998). Control of dorsoventral somite patterning by Wnt-1 and β-catenin. *Developmental Biology, 193,* 182–194.

Chalepakis, G, Fritsch, R, Fickenscher, H, Deutsch, U, Goulding, M, and Gruss, P (1991). The molecular basis of the *undulated/Pax-1* mutation. *Cell, 66,* 873–884.

Chapman, DL, Agulnik, I, Hancock, S, Silver, LM, and Papaioannou, VE (1996). *Tbx6*, a mouse T-box gene implicated in paraxial mesoderm formation at gastrulation. *Developmental Biology, 180,* 534–542.

Chapman, DL, and Papaioannou, VE (1998). Three neural tubes in mouse embryos with mutations in the T-box gene *Tbx6. Nature, 391,* 695–697.

Charité, J, de Graaff, W, Consten, D, Reijnen, MJ, Korving, J, and Deschamps, J (1998). Transducing positional information to the *Hox* genes: Critical interaction of *cdx* gene products with position-sensitive regulatory elements. *Development, 125,* 4349–4358.

Charité, J, de Graaff, W, and Deschamps, J (1995). Specification of multiple vertebral identities by ectopically expressed *Hoxb-8. Developmental Dynamics, 204,* 13–21.

Charité, J, de Graaff, W, Shen, S, and Deschamps, J (1994). Ectopic expression of *Hoxb-8* causes duplication of the ZPA in the forelimb and homeotic transformation of axial structures. *Cell, 78,* 589–601.

Chen, F, and Capecchi, MR (1997). Targeted mutations in *hoxa-9* and *hoxb-9* reveal synergistic interactions. *Developmental Biology, 181,* 186–196.

Chen, F, Greer, J, and Capecchi, MR (1998). Analysis of *Hoxa7/Hoxb7* mutants suggests periodicity in the generation of the different sets of vertebrae. *Mechanisms of Development, 77,* 49–57.

Chevallier, A (1978). Etude de la migration des cellules somitiques dans le mésoderme somatopleural de l'ébauche de l'aile. *Wilhelm Roux's Archives, 184,* 57–73.

Chevallier, A, Kieny, M, and Mauger, A (1977). Limb-somite relationship: Origin of the limb musculature. *Journal of Embryology and Experimental Morphology, 41,* 245–258.

Chiang, C, Litingtung, Y, Lee, E, Young, KE, Corden, JL, Westphal, H, and Beachy, PA (1996). Cyclopia and defective axial patterning in mice lacking *Sonic hedgehog* gene function. *Nature, 383,* 407–413.

Christ, B, Huang, R, and Wilting, J (2000). The development of the avian vertebral column. *Anatomy and Embryology, 202,* 179–194.

Christ, B, and Ordahl, CP (1995). Early stages of chick somite development. *Anatomy and Embryology, 191,* 381–396.

Christ, B, Schmidt, C, Huang, R, Wilting, J, and Brand-Saberi, B (1998). Segmentation of the vertebrate body. *Anatomy and Embryology, 197,* 18.

Christ, B, and Wilting, J (1992). From somites to vertebral column. *Annals of Anatomy, 174,* 23–32.

Condie, BG, and Capecchi, MR (1993). Mice homozygous for a targeted disruption of *Hoxd-3 (Hox-4.1)* exhibit anterior transformations of the first and second cervical vertebrae, the atlas and axis. *Development, 119,* 579–595.

Condie, BG, and Capecchi, MR (1994). Mice with targeted disruptions in the paralogous genes *hoxa-3* and *hoxd-3* reveal synergistic interactions. *Nature, 370,* 304–307.

Conlon, RA, Reaume, AG, and Rossant, J (1995). *Notch1* is required for the coordinate segmentation of somites. *Development, 121,* 1533–1545.

Cooke, J (1975). Control of somite number during morphogenesis of a vertebrate, *Xenopus laevis. Nature, 254,* 196–199.

Cooke, J (1998). A gene that resuscitates a theory—Somitogenesis and a molecular oscillator. *Trends in Genetics, 14,* 85–88.

Cooke, J, and Zeeman, EC (1976). A clock and wavefront model for control of the number of repeated structures during animal morphogenesis. *Journal of Theoretical Biology, 58,* 455–476.

Correia, KM, and Conlon, RA (2000). Surface ectoderm is necessary for the morphogenesis of somites. *Mechanisms of Development, 91,* 19–30.

Currie, PD, and Ingham, PW (1998). The generation and interpretation of positional information within the vertebrate myotome. *Mechanisms of Development, 73,* 321.

Dahl, E, Koseki, H, and Balling, R (1997). *Pax* genes and organogenesis. *Bioessays, 19,* 755–765.

Dale, KJ, and Pourquié, O (2000). A clock-work somite. *BioEssays, 22,* 72–83.

Davis, AP, and Capecchi, MR (1994). Axial homeosis and appendicular skeleton defects in mice with targeted disruption of *hoxd-11. Development, 120,* 2187–2198.

Davis, AP, Witte, DP, Hsieh-Li, HM, Potter, SS, and Capecchi, MR (1995). Absence of radius and ulna in mice lacking *hoxa-11* and *hoxd-11. Nature, 375,* 791–795.

de la Cruz, CC, Der-Avakian, A, Spyropoulos, DD, Tieu, DD, and Carpenter, EM (1999). Targeted disruption of *Hoxd9* and *Hoxd10* alters locomotor behavior, vertebral identity, and peripheral nervous system development. *Developmental Biology, 216,* 595–610.

Denetclaw, WF, and Ordahl, CP (2000). The growth of the dermomyotome and formation of early myotome lineages in thoracolumbar somites of chicken embryos. *Development, 127,* 893–905.

Deutsch, U, Dressler, GR, and Gruss, P (1988). *Pax 1,* a member of a paired box homologous murine gene family, is expressed in segmented structures during development. *Cell, 53,* 617–625.

Dickman, ED, Rogers, R, and Conway, SJ (1999). Abnormal skeletogenesis occurs coincident with increased apoptosis in the *Splotch (Sp^{2H})* mutant: Putative roles for *Pax3* and *PDGFR* in rib patterning. *Anatomical Record, 255,* 353–361.

Dietrich, S (1999). Regulation of hypaxial muscle development. *Cell and Tissue Research*, *296*, 175–182.

Dietrich, S, and Gruss, P (1995). *undulated* phenotypes suggest a role of *Pax-1* for the development of vertebral and extravertebral structures. *Developmental Biology, 167*, 529–548.

Duboule, D (Ed) (1994). *Guidebook to the Homeobox Genes.* Oxford University Press, Oxford.

Duboule, D (1995). Vertebrate *Hox* genes and proliferation: An alternative pathway to homeosis? *Current Opinion in Genetics and Development, 5*, 525–528.

Durston, AJ, van der Wees, J, Pijnappel, WWM, Shilthuis, JG, and Godsave, SF (1997). Retinoid signaling and axial patterning during early vertebrate embryogenesis. *Cellular and Molecular Life Sciences, 53*, 339–349.

Ebensperger, C, Wilting, J, Brand-Saberi, B, Mizutani, Y, Christ, B, Balling, R, and Koseki, H (1995). *Pax-1*, a regulator of sclerotome development, is induced by notochord and floor plate signals in avian embryos. *Anatomy and Embryology, 191*, 297–310.

Ewan, KBR, and Everett, AW (1992). Evidence for resegmentation in the formation of the vertebral column using the novel approach of retroviral-mediated gene transfer. *Experimental Cell Research, 198*, 315–320.

Fan, CM, Lee, CS, and Tessier-Lavigne, M (1997). A role for WNT proteins in induction of dermomyotome. *Developmental Biology, 191*, 160–165.

Fan, CM, Porter, JA, Chiang, C, Chang, DT, Beachy, PA, and Tessier-Lavigne, M (1995). Long-range sclerotome induction by Sonic hedgehog: Direct role of the amino-terminal cleavage product and modulation of the cyclic AMP signalling pathway. *Cell, 81*, 457–465.

Fan, CM, and Tessier-Lavigne, M (1994). Patterning of mammalian somites by surface ectoderm and notochord: Evidence for sclerotome induction by a hedgehog homolog. *Cell, 79*, 1175–1186.

Favier, B, Le Meur, M, Chambon, P, and Dollé, P (1995). Axial skeleton homeosis and forelimb malformations in *Hoxd-11* mutant mice. *Proceedings of the National Academy of Sciences of the United States of America, 92*, 310–314.

Fietz, MJ, Concordet, JP, Barbosa, R, Johnson, R, Krauss, S, McMahon, AP, Tabin, C, and Ingham, PW (1994). The *hedgehog* gene family in *Drosophila* and vertebrate development. *Development Supplement*, 43–51.

Folberg, A, Kovács, EN, Huang, H, Houle, M, Lohnes, D, and Featherstone, MS (1999). *Hoxd4* and *Rarg* interact synergistically in the specification of the cervical vertebrae. *Mechanisms of Development*, *89*, 65–74.

Forsberg, H, Crozet, F, and Brown, NA (1998). Waves of mouse *Lunatic fringe* expression, in four-hour cycles at two-hour intervals, precede somite boundary formation. *Current Biology, 8*, 1027–1030.

Fromental-Ramain, C, Warot, X, Lakkaraju, S, Favier, B, Haack, H, Birling, C, Dierich, A, Dollé, P, and Chambon, P (1996). Specific and redundant functions of the paralogous *Hoxa-9* and *Hoxd-9* genes in forelimb and axial skeleton patterning. *Development, 122*, 461–472.

Furumoto, T, Miura, N, Akasaka, T, Mizutani-Koseki, Y, Sudo, H, Fukuda, K, Maekawa, M, Yuasa, S, Fu, Y, Moriya, H, Taniguchi, M, Imai, K, Dahl, E, Balling, R, Pavlova, M, Gossler, A, and Koseki, H (1999). Notochord-dependent expression of MFH1 and PAX1 cooperates to maintain the proliferation of sclerotome cells during vertebral column development. *Developmental Biology, 210*, 15–29.

Gaunt, SJ (1991). Expression patterns of mouse Hox genes: Clues to an understanding of developmental and evolutionary strategies. *BioEssays, 13*, 505–513.

Gaunt, SJ (1994). Conservation in the Hox code during morphological evolution. *International Journal of Developmental Biology, 38*, 549–552.

Gaunt, SJ (2000). Evolutionary shifts of vertebrate structures and *Hox* expression up and down the axial series of segments: A consideration of possible mechanisms. *International Journal of Developmental Biology, 44*, 109–117.

Gaunt, SJ (2001). Gradients and forward spreading of vertebrate Hox gene expression detected by using a *Hox/lacZ* transgene. *Developmental Dynamics, 221,* 26–36.

Gaunt, SJ, Dean, W, Sang, H, and Burton, RD (1999). Evidence that Hoxa expression domains are evolutionary transposed in spinal ganglia, and are established by forward spreading in paraxial mesoderm. *Mechanisms of Development, 82,* 109–118.

Gaunt, SJ, and Strachan L (1994). Forward spreading in the establishment of a vertebrate Hox expression boundary: The expression domain separates into anterior and posterior zones, and the spread occurs across implanted glass barriers. *Developmental Dynamics, 199,* 229–240.

Gérard, M, Chen, JY, Gronemeyer, H, Chambon, P, Duboule, D, and Zákány, J (1996). In vivo targeted mutagenesis of a regulatory element required for positioning the *Hoxd-11* and *Hoxd-10* expression boundaries. *Genes and Development, 10,* 2326–2334.

Goldfarb, M (1996). Functions of fibroblast growth factors in vertebrate development. *Cytokine and Growth Factor Reviews, 7,* 311–325.

Goodrich, LV, Johnson, RL, Milenkovic, L, McMahon, JA, and Scott, MP (1996). Conservation of the *hedgehog/patched* signaling pathway from flies to mice: Induction of a mouse *patched* gene by Hedgehog. *Genes and Development, 10,* 301–312.

Gossler, A, and Hrabe de Angelis, M (1998). Somitogenesis. *Current Topics in Developmental Biology, 38,* 225–287.

Goulding, M, Lumsden, A, and Paquette, AJ (1994). Regulation of *Pax-3* expression in the dermomyotome and its role in muscle development. *Development, 120,* 957–971.

Gruss, P, and Walther, C (1992). Pax in development. *Cell, 69,* 719–722.

Hall, BK (1977). Chondrogenesis of the somitic mesoderm. *Advances in Anatomy, Embryology and Cell Biology, 53,* 1–50.

Hammerschmidt, M (1997). The world according to *hedgehog*. *Trends in Genetics, 13,* 14–21.

Hanson, RD, Hess, JL, Yu, BD, Ernst, P, van Lohuizen, M, Berns, A, van der Lugt, NMT, Shashikant, CS, Ruddle, FH, Seto, M, and Korsmeyer, SJ (1999). Mammalian Trithorax and polycomb-group homologues are antagonistic regulators of homeotic development. *Proceedings of the National Academy of Sciences of the United States of America, 96,* 14372–14377.

Henderson, DJ, Conway, SJ, and Copp, AJ (1999). Rib truncations and fusions in the Sp^{2H} mouse reveal a role for Pax3 in specification of the ventrolateral and posterior parts of the somite. *Developmental Biology, 209,* 143–158.

Hirsinger, E, Duprez, D, Jouve, C, Malapert, P, Cooke, J, and Pourquié, O (1997). Noggin acts downstream of Wnt and Sonic hedgehog to antagonize BMP4 in avian somite patterning. *Development, 124,* 4605–4614.

Hogan, BLM (1996). Bone morphogenetic proteins: Multifunctional regulators of vertebrate development. *Genes and Development, 10,* 1580–1594.

Holley, SA, Geisler, R, and Nüsslein-Volhard, C (2000). Control of *her1* expression during zebrafish somitogenesis by a *Delta*-dependent oscillator and an independent wavefront activity. *Genes and Development, 14,* 1678–1690.

Horan, GSB, Kovacs, EN, Behringer, RR, and Featherstone, MS (1995a). Mutations in paralogous *Hox* genes result in overlapping homeotic transformations of the axial skeleton: Evidence for unique and redundant function. *Developmental Biology, 169,* 359–372.

Horan, GSB, Ramírez-Solis, R, Featherstone, MS, Wolgemuth, DJ, Bradley, A, and Behringer, RR (1995b). Compound mutants for the paralogous *hoxa-4, hoxb-4,* and *hoxd-4* genes show more complete homeotic transformations and a dose-dependent increase in the number of vertebrae transformed. *Genes and Development, 9,* 1667–1677.

Horan, GSB, Wu, K, Wolgemuth, DJ, and Behringer, RR (1994). Homeotic transformation of cervical vertebrae in *Hoxa-4* mutant mice. *Proceedings of the National Academy of Sciences of the United States of America, 91,* 12644–12648.

Horikawa, K, Radice, G, Takeichi, M, and Chisaka, O (1999). Adhesive subdivisions intrinsic to the epithelial somites. *Developmental Biology, 215,* 182–189.

Hostikka, SL, and Capecchi, MR (1998). The mouse *Hoxc-11* gene: Genomic structure and expression pattern. *Mechanisms of Development, 70,* 133–145.

Hrabe de Angelis, M, McIntyre, J, and Gossler, A (1997). Maintenance of somite borders in mice requires the Delta homologue *Dll1. Nature, 386,* 717–721.

Huang, R, Zhi, Q, Brand-Saberi, B, and Christ, B (2000a). New experimental evidence for somite resegmentation. *Anatomy and Embryology, 202,* 195–200.

Huang, R, Zhi, G, Neubüser, A, Müller, TS, Brand-Saberi, B, Christ, B, and Wilting, J (1996). Function of somite and somitocoele cells in the formation of the vertebral motion segment in avian embryos. *Acta Anatomica, 155,* 231–241.

Huang, R, Zhi, Q, Schmidt, C, Wilting, J, Brand-Saberi, B, and Christ, B (2000b). Sclerotomal origin of the ribs. *Development, 127,* 527–532.

Huang, R, Zhi, Q, Wilting, J, and Christ, B (1994). The fate of somitocoele cells in avian embryos. *Anatomy and Embryology, 190,* 243–250.

Ikeya, M, and Takada, S (1998). Wnt signaling from the dorsal neural tube is required for the formation of the medial dermomyotome. *Development, 125,* 4969–4976.

Ikeya, M, and Takada, S (2001). Wnt-3a is required for somite specification along the anteroposterior axis of the mouse embryo and for regulation of *cdx-1* expression. *Mechanisms of Development, 103,* 27–33.

Jeannotte, L, Lemieux, M, Charron, J, Poirier, F, and Robertson, EJ (1993). Specification of axial identity in the mouse: Role of the *Hoxa-5 (Hox1.3)* gene. *Genes and Development, 7,* 2085–2096.

Jegalian, BG, and De Robertis, EM (1992). Homeotic transformations in the mouse induced by overexpression of a human *Hox3.3* transgene. *Cell, 71,* 901–910.

Jiang, YJ, Aerne, B, Smithers, L, Haddon, C, Ish-Horowicz, D, and Lewis, J (2000). Notch signalling and the synchronization of the somite segmentation clock. *Nature, 408,* 475–479.

Johnson, J, Rhee, J, Parsons, SM, Brown, D, Olson, EN, and Rawls, A (2001). The anterior/posterior polarity of somites is disrupted in Paraxis-deficient mice. *Developmental Biology, 229,* 176–187.

Johnson, RL, Laufer, E, Riddle, RD, and Tabin, C (1994). Ectopic expression of *Sonic hedgehog* alters dorsal-ventral patterning of somites. *Cell, 79,* 1165–1173.

Johnson, RL, and Tabin, C (1995). The long and short of *hedgehog* signaling. *Cell, 81,* 313–316.

Jouve, C, Palmeirim, I, Henrique, D, Becker, J, Gossler, A, Ish-Horowicz, D, and Pourquié, O (2000). Notch signalling is required for cyclic expression of the hair-like gene *HES1* in the presomitic mesoderm. *Development, 127,* 1421–1429.

Kalcheim, C, Cinnamon, Y, and Kahane, N (1999). Myotome formation: A multistage process. *Cell and Tissue Research, 296,* 161–173.

Kant, R, and Goldstein, RS (1999). Plasticity of axial identity among somites: Cranial somites can generate vertebrae without expressing *Hox* genes appropriate to the trunk. *Developmental Biology, 216,* 507–520.

Kerszberg, M, and Wolpert, L (2000). A clock and trail model for somite formation, specialization and polarization. *Journal of Theoretical Biology, 205,* 505–510.

Kessel, M (1992). Respecification of vertebral identities by retinoic acid. *Development, 115,* 487–501.

Kessel, M, Balling, R, and Gruss, P (1990). Variations of cervical vertebrae after expression of a *Hox-1.1* transgene in mice. *Cell, 61,* 301–308.

Kessel, M, and Gruss, P (1990). Murine developmental control genes. *Science, 249,* 374–379.

Kessel, M, and Gruss, P (1991). Homeotic transformations of murine vertebrae and concomitant alteration of *Hox* codes induced by retinoic acid. *Cell, 67,* 89–104.

Kieny, M, Mauger, A, and Sengel, P (1972). Early regionalization of the somitic mesoderm as studied by the development of the axial skeleton of the chick embryo. *Developmental Biology, 28,* 142–161.

Koseki, H, Wallin, J, Wilting, J, Mizutani, Y, Kispert, A, Ebensperger, E, Herrmann, BG, Christ, B, and Balling, R (1993). A role for *Pax-1* as a mediator of notochordal signals during the dorsoventral specification of vertebrae. *Development, 119,* 649–660.

Kostic, D, and Capecchi, MR (1994). Targeted disruptions of the murine *Hoxa-4* and *Hoxa-6* genes result in homeotic transformation of components of the vertebral column. *Mechanisms of Development, 46,* 231–257.

Krumlauf, R (1994). *Hox* genes in vertebrate development. *Cell, 78,* 191–201.

Kusumi, K, Sun, ES, Kerrebrock, AW, Bronson, RT, Chi, DC, Bulotsky, MS, Spencer, JB, Birren, BW, Frankel, WN, and Lander, ES (1998). The mouse pudgy mutation disrupts *Delta* homologue *Dll3* and initiation of early somite boundaries. *Nature Genetics, 19,* 274–278.

Lash, JW, Seitz, AW, Cheney, CM, and Ostrovsky, D (1984). On the role of fibronectin during the compaction stage of somitogenesis in the chick embryo. *Journal of Experimental Zoology, 232,* 197–206.

Leitges, M, Neidhardt, L, Haenig, B, Herrmann, BG, and Kispert, A (2000). The paired homeobox gene *Uncx4.1* specifies pedicles, transverse processes and proximal ribs of the vertebral column. *Development, 127,* 2259–2267.

Le Mouellic, H, Lallemand, Y, and Brulet, P (1992). Homeosis in the mouse induced by a null mutation in the *Hox-3.1* gene. *Cell, 69,* 251–264.

Lettice, LA, Purdie, LA, Carlson, GJ, Kilanowski, F, Dorn, J, and Hill, RE (1999). The mouse bagpipe gene controls development of the axial skeleton, skull, and spleen. *Proceedings of the National Academy of Sciences of the United States of America, 96,* 9695–9700.

Linask, KK, Ludwig, C, Han, MD, Liu, X, Radice, GL, and Knudsen, KA (1998). N-cadherin/catenin-mediated morphoregulation of somite formation. *Developmental Biology 202,* 85–102.

Loureiro, JJ (1999). The Wnts. *Current Biology, 9,* R4.

Manley, NR, and Capecchi, MR (1997). Hox group 3 paralogous genes act synergistically in the formation of somitic and neural crest-derived structures. *Developmental Biology, 192,* 274–288.

Mansouri, A, Voss, AK, Thomas, T, Yokota, Y, and Gruss, P (2000). *Uncx4.1* is required in the formation of the pedicles and proximal ribs and acts upstream of *Pax9. Development, 127,* 2251–2258.

Manzanares, M, Trainor, PA, Nonchev, S, Ariza-McNaughton, L, Brodie, J, Gould, A, Marshall, H, Morrison, A, Kwan, CT, Sham, MH, Wilkinson, DG, and Krumlauf, R (1999). The role of *kreisler* in segmentation during hindbrain development. *Developmental Biology, 211,* 220–237.

Marcelle, C, Ahlgren, S, and Bronner-Fraser, M (1999). *In vivo* regulation of somite differentiation and proliferation by Sonic Hedgehog. *Developmental Biology, 214,* 277–287.

Marcelle, C, Stark, MR, and Bronner-Fraser, M (1997). Coordinate action of BMPs, Wnts, Shh and Noggin mediate patterning of the dorsal somite. *Development, 124,* 3955–3963.

Maroto, M, Reshef, R, Münsterberg, AE, Koester, S, Goulding, M, and Lassar, AB (1997). Ectopic *Pax-3* activates *MyoD* and *Myf-5* expression in embryonic mesoderm and neural tissue. *Cell, 89,* 139–148.

Marshall, H, Morrison, A, Studer, M, Pöpperl, H, and Krumlauf, R (1996). Retinoids and *Hox* genes. *FASEB Journal, 10,* 969–978.

McGrew, MJ, Dale, JK, Fraboulet, S, and Pourquié, O (1998). The *lunatic fringe* gene is a target of the molecular clock linked to somite segmentation in avian embryos. *Current Biology, 8,* 979–982.

McGrew, MJ, and Pourquié, O (1998). Somitogenesis: Segmenting a vertebrate. *Current Opinion in Genetics and Development, 8,* 487–493.

McMahon, JA, Takada, S, Zimmerman, LB, Fan, CM, Harland, RM, and McMahon, AP (1998). Noggin-mediated antagonism of BMP signalling is required for growth and patterning of the neural tube and somite. *Genes and Development, 12,* 1438–1452.

McPherron, AC, Lawler, AM, and Lee, SJ (1997). Regulation of skeletal muscle mass in mice by a new TGF- superfamily gene. *Nature, 387,* 83–90.

McPherron, AC, Lawler, AM, and Lee, SJ (1999). Regulation of anterior/posterior patterning of the axial skeleton by growth/differentiation factor 11. *Nature Genetics, 22,* 260–264.

McPherron, AC, and Lee, SJ (1997). Double muscling in cattle due to mutations in the myostatin gene. *Proceedings of the National Academy of Sciences of the United States of America, 94,* 12457–12461.

Medina-Martínez, O, Bradley, A, and Ramírez-Solis, R (2000). A large targeted deletion of *Hoxb1-Hoxb9* produces a series of single-segment anterior homeotic transformations. *Developmental Biology, 222,* 71–83.

Meier, S (1979). Development of the chick embryo mesoblast: Formation of the embryonic axis and establishment of the metameric pattern. *Developmental Biology, 73,* 25–45.

Monsoro-Burq, AH, Bontoux, M, Teillet, MA, and Le Douarin, NM (1994). Heterogeneity in the development of the vertebra. *Proceedings of the National Academy of Sciences of the United States of America, 91,* 10435–10439.

Monsoro-Burq, AH, Duprez, D, Watanabe, Y, Bontoux, M, Vincent, C, Brickell, P, and Le Douarin, N (1996). The role of bone morphogenetic proteins in vertebral development. *Development, 122,* 3607–3616.

Moon, RT, Brown, JD, and Torres, M (1997). WNTs modulate cell fate and behavior during vertebrate development. *Trends in Genetics, 13,* 157–162.

Münsterberg, AE, and Lassar, AB (1995). Combinatorial signals from the neural tube, floor plate and notochord induce myogenic bHLH gene expression in the somite. *Development, 121,* 651–660.

Neumann, C, and Cohen, S (1997). Morphogens and pattern formation. *Bioessays, 19,* 721–729.

Nowicki, JL, and Burke, AC (2000). *Hox* genes and morphological identity: Axial versus lateral patterning in the vertebrate mesoderm. *Development, 127,* 4265–4275.

Nye, JS (1999). The Notch proteins. *Current Biology, 9,* R118.

Ordahl, CP (1993). Myogenic lineages within the developing somite. In M. Bernfield (Ed), *Molecular Basis of Morphogenesis* (pp 165–176). Wiley-Liss, New York.

Ordahl, CP, and Le Douarin, NM (1992). Two myogenic lineages within the developing somite. *Development, 114,* 339–353.

Palmeirim, I, Henrique, D, Ish-Horowicz, D, and Pourquié, O (1997). Avian *hairy* gene expression identifies a molecular clock linked to vertebrate segmentation and somitogenesis. *Cell, 91,* 639–648.

Peters, H, Wilm, B, Sakai, N, Imai, K, Maas, K, and Balling, R (1999). Pax1 and Pax9 synergistically regulate vertebral column development. *Development, 126,* 5399–5408.

Pollock, RA, Jay, G, and Bieberich, CJ (1992). Altering the boundaries of *Hox3.1* expression: Evidence for antipodal gene regulation. *Cell, 71,* 911–923.

Pourquié, O, Fan, CM, Coltey, M, Hirsinger, E, Watanabe, Y, Bréant, C, FrancisWest, P, Brickell, P, Tessier-Lavigne, M, and Le Douarin, NM (1996). Lateral and axial signals involved in avian somite patterning: A role for BMP4. *Cell, 84,* 461–471.

Pownall, ME, Strunk, KE, and Emerson, CP (1996). Notochord signals control the transcriptional cascade of myogenic bHLH genes in somites of quail embryos. *Development, 122,* 1475–1488.

Ramírez-Solis, R, Zheng, H, Whiting, J, Krumlauf, R, and Bradley, A (1993). *Hoxb-4 (Hox-2.6)* mutant mice show homeotic transformation of a cervical vertebra and defects in the closure of the sternal rudiments. *Cell, 73,* 279–294.

Rawls, A, Valdez, MR, Zhang, W, Richardson, J, Klein, WH, and Olson, EN (1998). Overlapping functions of the myogenic bHLH genes *MRF4* and *MyoD* in double mutant mice. *Development, 125,* 2349–2358.

Reshef, R, Maroto, M, and Lassar, AB (1998). Regulation of dorsal somitic cell fates: BMPs and Noggin control the timing and pattern of myogenetic regulator expression. *Genes and Development, 12,* 290–303.

Richardson, MK, Allen, SP, Wright, GM, Raynaud, A, and Hanken, J (1998). Somite number and vertebrate evolution. *Development, 125,* 151–160.

Rijli, FM, Matyas, R, Pellegrini, M, Dierich, A, Gruss, P, Dollé, P, and Chambon, P (1995). Cryptorchidism and homeotic transformations of spinal nerves and vertebrae in *Hoxa-10* mutant mice. *Proceedings of the National Academy of Sciences of the United States of America, 92,* 8185–8189.

Saegusa, H, Takahashi, N, Noguchi, S, and Suemori, H (1996). Targeted disruption in the mouse *Hoxc-4* locus results in axial skeleton homeosis and malformation of the xiphoid process. *Developmental Biology, 174,* 55–64.

Schnell, S, and Maini, PK (2000). Clock and induction model for somitogenesis. *Developmental Dynamics, 217,* 415–420.

Shashikant, CS, and Ruddle, FH (1996). Combinations of closely situated *cis*-acting elements determine tissue-specific patterns and anterior extent of early *Hoxc8* expression. *Proceedings of the National Academy of Sciences of the United States of America, 93,* 12364–12369.

Small, KM, and Potter, SS (1993). Homeotic transformations and limb defects in *Hox A11* mutant mice. *Genes and Development, 7,* 2318–2328.

Smith, CA, and Tuan, RS (1995). Functional involvement of *Pax-1* in somite development: Somite dysmorphogenesis in chick embryos treated with *Pax-1* paired-box antisense oligodeoxynucleotide. *Teratology, 52,* 333–345.

Solursh, M, Fisher, M, Meier, S, and Singley, CT (1979). The role of extracellular matrix in the formation of the sclerotome. *Journal of Embryology and Experimental Morphology, 54,* 75–98.

Sosic, D, Brand-Saberi, B, Schmidt, C, Christ, B, and Olson, EN (1997). Regulation of *paraxis* expression and somite formation by ectoderm and neural tube-derived signals. *Developmental Biology, 185,* 229–243.

Spence, MS, Yip, J, and Erickson, CA (1996). The dorsal neural tube organizes the dermomyotome and induces axial myocytes in the avian embryo. *Development, 122,* 231–241.

Stern, CD, and Keynes, RJ (1987). Interactions between somite cells: The formation and maintenance of segment boundaries in the chick embryo. *Development, 99,* 261–272.

Stern, HM, Brown, AM, and Hauschka, SD (1995). Myogenesis in paraxial mesoderm: Preferential induction by dorsal neural tube and by cells expressing *Wnt-1*. *Development, 121,* 3675–3686.

Stern, HM, and Hauschka, SD (1995). Neural tube and notochord promote *in vitro* myogenesis in single somite explants. *Developmental Biology, 167,* 87–103.

Subramanian, V, Meyer, BI, and Gruss, P (1995). Disruption of the murine homeobox gene *Cdx1* affects axial skeletal identities by altering the mesodermal expression domains of *Hox* genes. *Cell, 83,* 641–653.

Suemori, H, Takahashi, N, and Noguchi, S (1995). *Hoxc-9* mutant mice show anterior transformation of the vertebrae and malformation of the sternum and ribs. *Mechanisms of Development, 51,* 265–273.

Tam, PPL, and Trainor, PA (1994). Specification and segmentation of the paraxial mesoderm. *Anatomy and Embryology, 189,* 275–305.

Tonegawa, A, Funayama, N, Ueno, N, and Takahashi, Y (1997). Mesodermal subdivision along the mediolateral axis in chicken controlled by different concentrations of BMP-4. *Development, 124,* 1975–1984.

Tremblay, P, Dietrich, S, Mericskay, M, Shubert, FR, Li, Z, and Paulin, D (1998). A crucial role for *Pax3* in the development of the hypaxial musculature and the long-range migration of muscle precursors. *Developmental Biology, 203,* 49–61.

Tribioli, C, and Lufkin, T (1999). The murine *Bapx1* homeobox gene plays a critical role in embryonic development of the axial skeleton and spleen. *Development, 126,* 5699–5711.

van den Akker, E, Fromental-Ramain, C, de Graaf, W, Le Mouellic, H, Brulet, P, Chambon, P, and Deschamps, J (2001). Axial skeletal patterning in mice lacking all paralogous group 8 *Hox* genes. *Development, 128,* 1911–1921.

Venters, SJ, Thorsteinsdóttir, S, and Duxson, MJ (1999). Early development of the myotome in the mouse. *Developmental Dynamics, 216,* 219–232.

Verbout, AJ (1976). A critical review of the "Neugliederung" concept in relation to the development of the vertebral column. *Acta Biotheoretica, 25,* 219–258.

Verbout, AJ (1985). The development of the vertebral column. *Advances in Anatomy, Embryology and Cell Biology, 90,* 11–19.

Wahba, GM, Hostikka, SL, and Carpenter, EM (2001). The paralogous *Hox* genes *Hoxa10* and *Hoxd10* interact to pattern the mouse hindlimb peripheral nervous system and skeleton. *Developmental Biology, 231,* 87–102.

Wallin, J, Wilting, J, Koseki, H, Fritsch, R, Christ, B, and Balling, R (1994). The role of *Pax-1* in axial skeleton development. *Development, 120,* 1109–1121.

Walmsley, R (1953). The development and growth of the intervertebral disc. *Edinburgh Medical Journal, 60,* 341–364.

Wang, Y, and Jaenisch, R (1997). Myogenin can substitute for Myf5 in promoting myogenesis but less efficiently. *Development, 124,* 2507–2513.

Williams, BA, and Ordahl, CP (1994). *Pax-3* expression in segmental mesoderm marks early stages in myogenic cell specification. *Development, 120,* 785–796.

Williams, BA, and Ordahl, CP (1997). Emergence of determined myotome precursor cells in the somite. *Development, 124,* 4983–4997.

Wilson-Rawls, J, Hurt, CR, Parsons, SM, and Rawls, A (1999). Differential regulation of epaxial and hypaxial muscle development by Paraxis. *Development, 126,* 5217–5229.

Wolpert, L (1978). Pattern formation in biological development. *Scientific American, 239,* 154–164.

Wolpert, L (1996). One hundred years of positional information. *Trends in Genetics, 12,* 359–364.

Woychik, R, Hogan, B, Bryant, S, Eichele, G, Kimelman, D, Noden, D, Shoenwolf, G, and Wright, C (1997). Pattern formation. *Reproductive Toxicology, 11,* 339–344.

Yamaguchi, TP, Takada, S, Yoshikawa, Y, Wu, N, and McMahon, AP (1999). *T* (Brachyury) is a direct target of Wnt3a during paraxial mesoderm specification. *Genes and Development, 13,* 3185–3190.

Yoshikawa, Y, Fujimori, T, McMahon, AP, and Takada, S (1997). Evidence that absence of *Wnt-3a* signalling promotes neuralization instead of paraxial mesoderm development in the mouse. *Developmental Biology, 183,* 234–242.

Zákány, J, Gérard, M, Favier, B, Potter, SS, and Duboule, D (1996). Functional equivalence and rescue among group 11 *Hox* gene products in vertebral patterning. *Developmental Biology, 176,* 325–328.

Chapter 4

Bones of the Postcranial Skeleton: The Vertebral Column

The adult human skeleton (Figure 4–1) is composed of 206 bones that can be divided into an axial and an appendicular skeleton. The *axial skeleton* consists of the cranium (or skull), the vertebrae, and associated structures:

Cranium	28 bones
Hyoid	1 bone
Vertebral column	26 bones
Ribs	24 bones
Sternum	1 bone

The *appendicular skeleton* consists of the bones of the upper and lower limbs, including the *pectoral* and *pelvic girdles*:

Upper limbs	60 bones
Pectoral girdle	4 bones
Lower limbs	60 bones
Pelvic girdle	2 bones

This chapter considers the osteology and articulations of the vertebral column. Chapter 5 covers the ribs and sternum. Chapters 6 and 7 discuss the appendicular skeleton, and Chapter 8 is devoted to the cranium.

(*Text continues on page 85*)

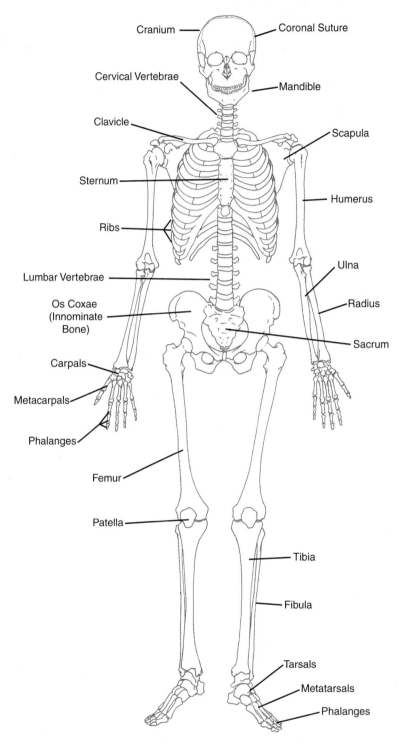

Figure 4-1   The human skeleton: (A) anterior.

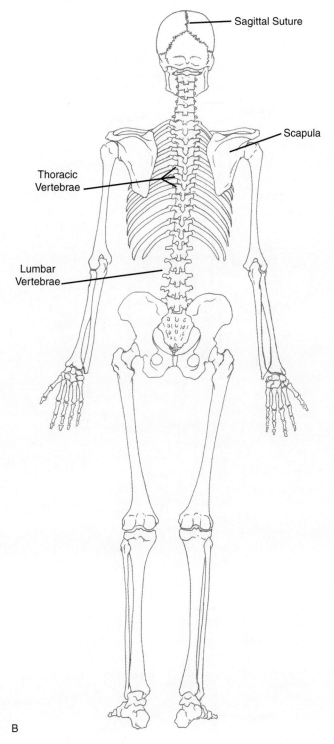

B

Figure 4-1 *(Continued)* *(B)* posterior.

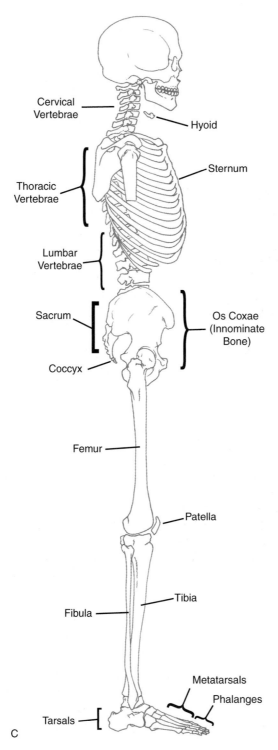

C

Figure 4-1 *(Continued)* *(C)* lateral.

BONES OF THE VERTEBRAL COLUMN
The Vertebral Column in General

The human *vertebral column* is composed of 33 segments, or *vertebrae*. Some are fused in adult life, so that the total number of individual bones is only 26. Between each vertebral segment is a fibrocartilaginous *intervertebral disc*. The 33 vertebral segments and their associated intervertebral discs taken together constitute the vertebral column.

The vertebrae may be broken into five groups, cranially to caudally (Figure 4–2):

Cervical	7 bones
Thoracic	12 bones
Lumbar	5 bones
Sacral	5 segments fused into one bone
Coccygeal	4 segments typically fused into one bone

It should be noted that these are the most typical numbers of vertebrae in each group but that there can be some variation. There is rarely (in fact, virtually never) any variation in the number of cervical vertebrae, but it is fairly common to find one segment more or one segment fewer in the lumbar, sacral, and coccygeal segments of the vertebral column. The probability of encountering an atypical number of vertebrae increases caudally.

The vertebral column serves three primary functions: (1) to support the trunk and transmit its weight to the pelvis and lower limb, (2) to house and protect the spinal cord and its membranes, and (3) to provide a central axis for the thorax (each rib articulates with a vertebra, and coordinated motion of the ribs is a critical aspect of normal breathing) and protect its contents (the thorax is also the attachment point of the forelimbs). All vertebrae are formed along a common plan but vary according to their positions and functions in the spinal column. These parts may be examined in a typical vertebra.

Regions of the Vertebral Column

As mentioned, the vertebral column can be divided into five groups or regions: cervical (C1–C7), thoracic (T1–T12), lumbar (L1–L5), sacral (S1–S5), and coccygeal (no individual designation). Vertebrae of each region demonstrate specific characteristics diagnostic for that region.

In humans, the vertebral column demonstrates a series of curvatures associated with these regions (see Fig. 4–2). The human vertebral column has four curvatures: the *cervical curvature,* the *thoracic curvature,* the *lumbar curvature,* and the *sacral curvature.* The curve of the coccyx continues along the sacral curvature. In most terrestrial vertebrates, the vertebral column demonstrates a single horizontal arc that is convex dorsally and is supported cranially and caudally by the pectoral and pelvic limbs. As humans, however, we are unique in our bipedal form of walking in that we habitually balance all the weight of the trunk over the pelvic limb and girdle alone, with the vertebral column held more or less vertically over the sacrum.

Embryologically, a single dorsoconvex arc is present in the human vertebral column, just as is true of other terrestrial vertebrates. The thoracic and sacral curvatures of the human adult vertebral column are convex dorsally. They are called

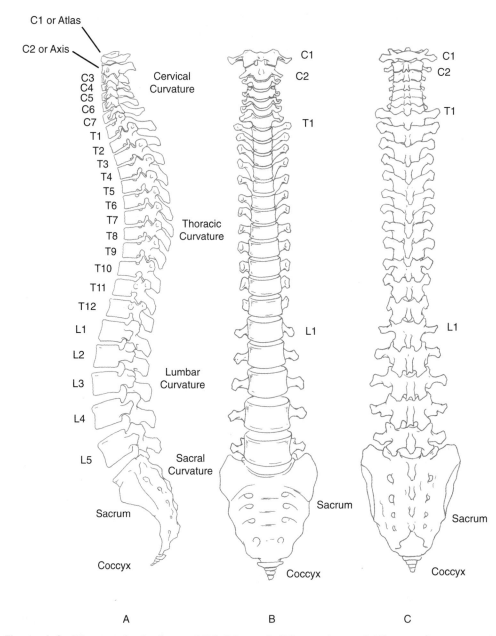

Figure 4-2　The vertebral column: (A) left lateral, (B) anterior, and (C) posterior aspects.

primary curvatures because they were present embryologically and are the adult remnants of this embryological curvature. The cervical and lumbar curvatures begin to appear before birth but are not obvious until later. They are referred to as *secondary curvatures*. The cervical curvature becomes apparent when the infant begins to hold its head up. This curvature can be obliterated by flexing the neck, but it is present in normal standing, sitting, and walking. The thoracic curvature is formed by the articulation of the 12 thoracic vertebrae. It is permanent. The lumbar curvature, which becomes pronounced as a child begins to walk, is generally greater in women than in men, whereas the sacral curvature is generally slightly greater in men than in women, although this feature has a great deal of gender overlap.

Osteological Features of Vertebrae in General

As examples of typical vertebrae, Figure 4–3A illustrates a thoracic vertebra viewed superiorly and Figure 4–3B, a lumbar vertebra viewed laterally. The most anterior portion of a typical vertebra is the *body,* which is the largest portion of a vertebra and approximately cylindrical in shape. Its *cranial (superior)* and *caudal (inferior) surfaces* are roughened and give attachment to the intervertebral discs. The circumferences of the cranial and caudal surfaces of the body contain slightly elevated rims. The diameters of the cranial and caudal surfaces of the vertebral bodies are somewhat greater than the diameter of the center portion of the body, making it appear constricted, or "waisted."

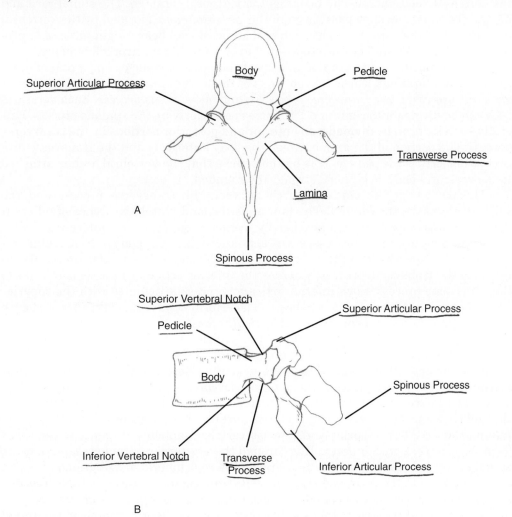

Figure 4-3   Features of typical vertebrae: (*A*) superior view of a midthoracic vertebra, and (*B*) left lateral view of a lumbar vertebra.

The posterior surface of the body faces the *vertebral foramen,* an opening for the spinal cord, and contains one or more large, irregular openings, the *foramina vasculare (basivertebral foramina),* for the passage of the basivertebral veins draining from the interior of the vertebral bodies to the internal vertebral plexus, a venous plexus that surrounds the spinal cord and receives venous drainage from both the vertebral column and spinal cord.

The bodies of the vertebrae transmit the weight of a person's body as well as muscular and other compressive forces (e.g., reaction forces from walking, running, jumping, etc.). The vertebrae are separated from one another by fibrocartilaginous intervertebral discs, which transmit forces from one vertebra to the next. Posterior to the vertebral body is the *vertebral arch*, formed by the pedicles and laminae (see Fig. 4–3A).

The *neural arch* is the developmental structure contributing to both the vertebral arch and part of the vertebral body. It is sometimes used, incorrectly, as a synonym for the vertebral arch. The vertebral arch, along with the posterior surface of the vertebral body, encloses an opening, the vertebral foramen. The spinal cord and its associated membranes pass through the *vertebral canal*, formed by the vertebral foramina of all the vertebrae. The vertebral arches do not bear weight but rather protect the spinal column. They are connected to one another by strong ligaments.

As mentioned, the vertebral arch consists of a pair of pedicles and a pair of laminae (singular: *lamina*). These two portions of the arch support seven processes: four *articular processes,* two *transverse processes,* and one *spinous process*. Each vertebral arch can be divided into right and left halves posteriorly by the spinous process. Laterally, each half can be divided into anterior and posterior portions by the transverse process. The portion of the arch between the body anteriorly and the transverse process posteriorly is the *pedicle*. It is by the pedicle that the vertebral arch is attached to the vertebral body. It is short, strong, and rounded.

The portion of the vertebral arch between the transverse process and the spinous process is the *lamina*. The lamina is flat and platelike. Arches of adjacent vertebrae articulate with one another by means of superior and inferior articular processes. The articular processes are also known as *zygapophyses* (singular: *zygapophysis*). On each side of the vertebral arch, the superior articular process is superior to the transverse process, whereas the inferior articular process is inferior to the transverse process. Each inferior articular process articulates with the superior articular process of the vertebra below it. These form small synovial joints, and each articular process bears a small, smooth *articular facet*.

Because the craniocaudal height of the pedicles is less than the height of the bodies of the vertebrae to which they are attached, "notches," or depressions, exist on the superior and inferior surfaces of the pedicles. These are the *superior vertebral notches* above the pedicles and the *inferior vertebral notches* below them (see Fig. 4–3B). The inferior vertebral notch is much deeper than the superior notch because the pedicle attaches nearer to the superior surface of the vertebral body than to its inferior surface. The superior and inferior vertebral notches of adjacent vertebrae form the *intervertebral foramen*. It is through these intervertebral foramina that the spinal nerves exit the spinal column to reach their peripheral distributions.

In addition to the body, pedicles, laminae, transverse processes, spinous process, and articular processes associated with each vertebra, there is a *costal element* (Figure 4–4). The costal element takes a different form in different regions of the spinal column. *Costal* means "rib" (Latin: *costa*). In the thoracic region, the costal element is not a part of the thoracic vertebrae but is present as a separate bone, the *rib*. In cervical, lumbar, and sacral vertebrae, the costal element is incorporated into the vertebrae. In cervical vertebrae, the costal element is present as the *anterior* and *posterior costal tubercles,* the *anterior costal bar,* and the *costal lamella* (described in detail with the cervical vertebrae in the next section), all parts of the transverse process. These structures define the anterior and lateral borders of the characteristic *transverse foramen* of cervical vertebrae.

In lumbar vertebrae, the costal element also forms the bulk of the transverse process, the "true" transverse process being represented by the *accessory process,* a posterior protrusion that serves as a muscle attachment. The accessory process of the lumbar region is homologous to the transverse process of the thoracic region. In the sacral vertebrae the costal elements become incorporated into the lateral masses of the sacrum. The coccygeal vertebrae consist primarily of degenerate bodies and lack costal elements. The specific details of each type of vertebra are discussed in the following sections.

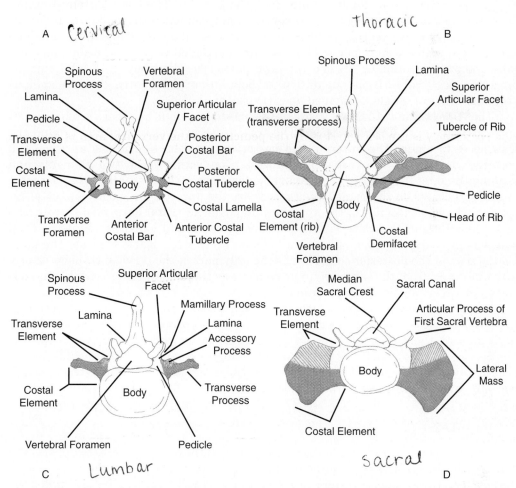

Figure 4-4 *Costal elements* (stippled) and *transverse elements* (hatched) of vertebrae: (*A*) cervical, (*B*) thoracic, (*C*) lumbar, and (*D*) sacral vertebrae, diagrammatic representations, superior views.

Regional Osteology of the Vertebral Column

The Cervical Vertebrae

There are seven cervical vertebrae (C1–C7). They are located in the neck between the base of the skull and the thoracic vertebrae. The identifying characteristic of cervical vertebrae is the presence of the transverse foramen in the transverse process. The transverse foramina of the first six cervical vertebrae transmit the paired vertebral arteries and their accompanying venous and sympathetic plexuses to the head. The vertebral arteries do not pass through the transverse foramina of the seventh cervical vertebra. The third through sixth cervical vertebrae share a common morphological pattern (Figure 4–5), whereas the first, second, and seventh possess unique morphological details. These three vertebrae also have unique names. The first is the atlas, the second is the axis, and the seventh is the vertebra prominens.

A typical cervical vertebra (see Fig. 4–5) has a small but relatively broad body. The vertebral foramen is large and triangular. The pedicles project dorsolaterally. The laminae then curve dorsomedially from the pedicles. The large vertebral foramina of the cervical vertebrae house the cervical enlargement of the spinal cord. The superior and inferior vertebral notches are of almost equal depth. The laminae are long and narrow, with a thin upper border, and are roughened ventrally. The spinous process is short and bifid, or divided into two parts. The distribution of bifid spinous processes is variable from population to population; frequently, cervical spinous processes end in a single, undivided apex (Duray et al., 1999).

The superior and inferior articular processes of a single cervical vertebra are at opposite ends of an *articular pillar.* The transverse process is centered around the transverse foramen. The anterior and posterior costal bars form the anterior and posterior margins of the transverse process. Connecting these two elements and forming the lateral border of the transverse foramen is the costal lamella. The most lateral structures on the transverse process are the anterior and posterior costal tubercles, which are the tips of the anterior and posterior costal bars, respectively. The costal lamella and the more lateral portions of the costal bars represent the final morphology of the developmental costal element of the cervical vertebrae. The more medial part of the posterior costal bar is the only part of the cervical transverse process that arose from the same origin or element as the transverse process of thoracic vertebrae (developmental transverse process).

Occasionally *cervical ribs*, which are separate costal elements, may be present in the lower cervical vertebrae. Cervical ribs are not a normal condition; when such a rib is present, there is no transverse foramen associated with the transverse process. The cervical rib may compress the roots of the nerves composing the brachial plexus, leading to potential neurological problems in the upper limb and other structures innervated by branches of the brachial plexus.

THE ATLAS

The first cervical vertebra (Figure 4–6) is called the *atlas* because it supports the globe of the head. It is the widest of the cervical vertebrae, with the exception of the seventh. It is a unique vertebra in that it lacks a body. Its body instead takes the unique form of the dens, a "process" or projection of the second cervical vertebra, around which the atlas rotates. The atlas also lacks a spinous process and consists

Figure 4-5   Features of cervical vertebrae 3 through 6: (*A*) superior view, (*B*) lateral view, (*C*) anterior view showing the uncinate processes.

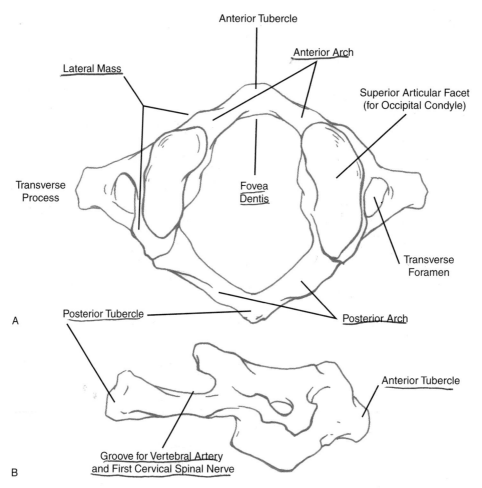

Figure 4-6   The atlas (first cervical vertebra): (*A*) superior view, (*B*) right lateral view.

primarily of two lateral masses connected by a short anterior arch and a longer, more curved posterior arch.

The *anterior arch* comprises about one-fifth of the circumference of the ring of the atlas. On the ventral surface of the anterior arch is a swelling called the *anterior tubercle.* On the dorsal surface of the anterior arch is a small articular facet, the *fovea dentis.* The dens of the axis articulates here.

The *posterior arch* forms about two-fifths of the ring of the atlas. On the dorsal surface of the posterior arch is the *posterior tubercle* of the atlas; the posterior tubercle represents the spinous process of the atlas. On the cranial surface of the posterior arch, between the posterior tubercle and the lateral masses, are the grooves for the vertebral artery and first cervical spinal nerve. One of these grooves may occasionally be converted to a foramen called the *arcuate foramen.* This occurs by the formation of a bony strut called the *posterior ponticle* passing over the nerve and artery. Inferiorly are the shallow inferior vertebral notches.

The *lateral masses* (see Fig. 4–6*B*) are masses of bone on the lateral aspects of the atlas that bear the superior and inferior articular facets. The superior articular facets are large and ovoid. They articulate with the occipital condyles of the skull. On the medial surfaces of the masses are tubercles for the attachment of the transverse atlantal ligament. The inferior articular facets project posteriorly and slightly medially. They are almost circular and slightly concave. They articulate with the superior articular facets of the axis. The transverse processes project laterally and inferiorly from the lateral masses and are very long. Each transverse process ends in a single tubercle homologous to the posterior costal tubercle of other cervical vertebrae. A very small vestigial anterior tubercle may occasionally be present on the lateral mass. The transverse foramen is oval.

The first cervical spinal nerve emerges from the spinal cord within the vertebral canal to exit between the skull and the atlas. Note that this is not a true intervertebral foramen because it is not formed between two vertebrae. The boundaries of the passage for the first cervical spinal nerve are as follows:

Anterior: Lateral mass
Posterior: The posterior atlanto-occipital membrane (described later)
Superior: The edges of an opening in the posterior atlanto-occipital
               membrane
Inferior: The groove for the vertebral artery and first cervical spinal nerve

THE AXIS

The second cervical vertebra (Figure 4–7) is called the *axis* (or *epistropheus*) because it forms the pivot upon which the atlas, carrying the head, rotates. Its characteristic feature is the *dens* (or *odontoid process*), a superior projection of the body that articulates with the anterior arch of the atlas. The dens has a slight constriction, or neck, where it joins the body of the axis. It was at one time considered to be the displaced body of the first cervical vertebra, but more recent research does not entirely support this view. The dens has an anterior articular facet for articulation with the anterior arch of the atlas. There is a groove on the posterior aspect for the transverse atlantal ligament. This ligament keeps the dens applied to the anterior arch of the atlas.

The body of the axis is small and continuous with the dens. The vertebral foramen is triangular. It is large, but it is smaller than the vertebral foramen of the atlas. The transverse processes are smaller and shorter than those of the atlas. The transverse processes are anterior to the inferior articular processes. They each end in a single posterior costal tubercle; there is no anterior tubercle on the axis. The pedicles are broad and strong. They are covered cranially by the superior articular facets. The laminae are thick and strong as well.

The superior vertebral notches are shallow and lie dorsal to the articular processes. The inferior vertebral notches lie ventral to the articular processes, as in other cervical vertebrae. The spinous process is large and bifid. The superior articular facets are round, slightly convex, directed cranially and laterally, and supported by the body, the pedicles, and the transverse processes. The inferior articular facets face ventrally, similar to those in other cervical vertebrae. The intervertebral foramen between the atlas and the axis is not well defined. It allows the exit of the second cervical spinal nerve. Its boundaries are as follows:

Anterior: Lateral atlantoaxial joint capsule (described later)
Posterior: Posterior atlantoaxial ligament (described later)
Superior: Inferior vertebral notch of the posterior arch of the atlas
Inferior: Superior surface of the lamina of the axis

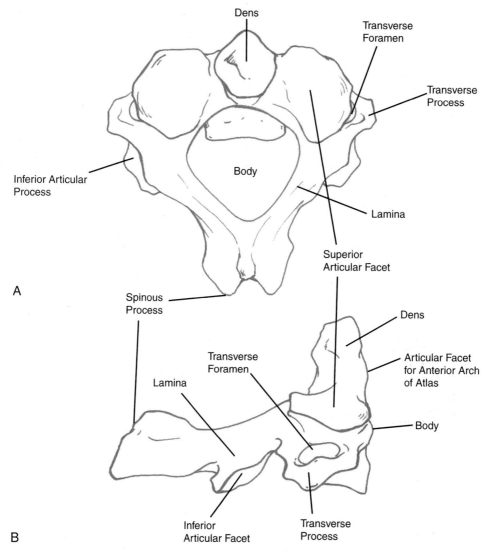

Figure 4-7   The axis (second cervical vertebra): (*A*) superior view, (*B*) right lateral view.

THE THIRD THROUGH SIXTH CERVICAL VERTEBRAE

The third through sixth cervical vertebrae (see Fig. 4–5) are morphologically similar and exhibit the typical features of cervical vertebrae. Their bodies are oval, broader mediolaterally than anteroposteriorly, and uniform in height posteriorly and anteriorly. The pedicles are short, and the laminae are thin and long. The spinous process is short and bifid, and the two divisions are often unequal in size. The superior and inferior articular processes are fused to form an articular pillar.

The superior articular facets are directed superiorly and dorsally, at about a 45-degree angle to the horizontal plane. The inferior articular facets are directed inferiorly and ventrally. The superior and inferior vertebral notches are formed by constrictions of the pedicles. The anterior tubercle of the sixth cervical vertebra is relatively large and is known as the *carotid tubercle;* it is so called because it is possible for the common carotid artery to be compressed between this tubercle and the body of the vertebra.

A specialization of the vertebral bodies of the caudal five cervical and the first, and sometimes second, thoracic vertebrae is the *uncinate process,* or *lip of Luschka* (see Fig. 4–5C), a liplike projection on the superior lateral surface of the vertebral bodies. This uncinate process articulates with a beveled surface on the lateral aspect of the inferior surface of the vertebra above it. This beveled surface is found on the second through seventh cervical vertebrae and sometimes on the first thoracic vertebra. The articulation of the uncinate process with the beveled surface on the vertebra above it is the *uncovertebral joint,* or *joint of Luschka.*

The intervertebral foramina are formed similarly among the lower cervical vertebrae. The boundaries of each intervertebral foramen among these vertebrae are as follows:

Superior:	Inferior vertebral notch of the cranial vertebra
Inferior:	Superior vertebral notch of the caudal vertebra
Posterior:	Joint capsule of the articular processes
Anterior:	Uncovertebral joint (joint of Luschka)

THE SEVENTH CERVICAL VERTEBRA

The seventh cervical vertebra (Figure 4–8) is also called the *vertebra prominens* (literally, "the most prominent vertebra"). It is a typical cervical vertebra, but it is unique in one feature: The spinous process is very long and prominent, and its tip is not bifid, as is usually the case in the other cervical vertebrae. The palpable prominence of the spinous process of the seventh cervical vertebra makes it a useful landmark for counting vertebral levels. The transverse process of C7 usually has a prominent posterior costal tubercle, but the anterior costal tubercle is rudimentary. In addition, the transverse foramen may be small, double, or even absent. As mentioned before, the transverse foramen of the seventh cervical vertebra does not transmit the vertebral artery.

The Thoracic Vertebrae

There are 12 thoracic vertebrae (T1–T12; refer to Figures 4–9 and 4–10 throughout the discussion of the thoracic vertebrae). They are of intermediate size and located between the cervical and lumbar vertebrae. The thoracic vertebrae are unique in that they articulate with the ribs. They are easily distinguished by the presence of costal facets on the sides of the bodies for articulation with the heads of the ribs and by facets on their transverse processes for articulation with the tubercles of the ribs. Some of the thoracic vertebrae bear complete, rounded costal facets (T1 and T10–T12), by which a rib articulates with a single vertebral body.

In most of the thoracic vertebrae (inferior portion of T1, T2–T8, and superior portion of T9), each side of the body bears both a superior and an inferior semicircular costal facet called a *demifacet.* The inferior demifacets of the more cranial vertebrae combine with the superior demifacets of the adjacent caudal vertebrae to form a cuplike cavity that receives the head of the rib. The articulations between the heads of the ribs and the costal facets form the *costovertebral joints.* The *costotransverse joints* are formed by the articulation of the tubercles of the ribs with the transverse processes of the thoracic vertebrae.

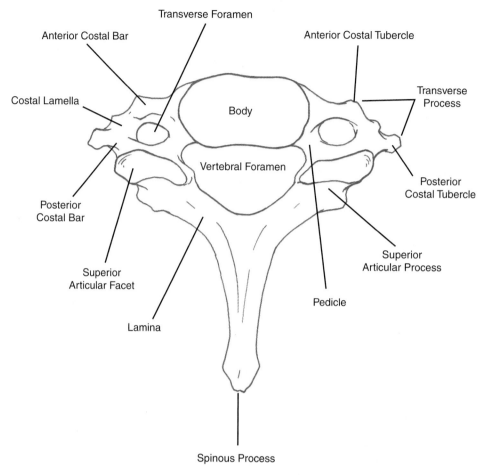

Figure 4-8   The vertebra prominens (seventh cervical vertebra): superior view.

The bodies of the thoracic vertebrae, in the midthoracic region, are heart-shaped and as broad anteroposteriorly as mediolaterally. The body is slightly thicker dorsally than ventrally, contributing to the thoracic curvature of the spine. The superior demifacets are slightly anterior to the pedicles, whereas the inferior demifacets are slightly anterior to the inferior vertebral notch. The pedicles are directed slightly cranially. The superior vertebral notches are very shallow and barely recognizable. The inferior vertebral notches are large and deeper than in other regions of the spine. The laminae are broad and thick and, unlike other regions of the column, overlap those of the inferior vertebrae. The vertebral foramen is small and circular.

The spinous processes of thoracic vertebrae are long and directed obliquely inferior. The thoracic spinous processes end in a single tubercle. In T1 and T2, the process is more horizontal and the interspinous spaces are large. In T3 and T4, the processes are more oblique but the interspinous spaces are still large. The spinous processes of T5 through T8 are very oblique and overlap to a greater extent than do the spinous processes of more cranial vertebrae; the interspinous spaces become smaller. The processes of T9 and T10 are oblique with small interspinous spaces, whereas those of T11 and T12, like those of the lumbar vertebrae, are horizontal.

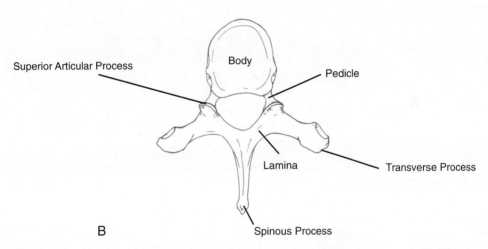

Figure 4-9   Features of a typical thoracic vertebra: (*A*) right lateral view and (*B*) superior view.

The superior articular processes are thin and platelike, projecting up from the junctions of the pedicles and laminae. The articular facets are practically flat and face dorsally and laterally. The inferior articular processes are fused to a considerable extent with the laminae, appearing to lie on the anterior surface of the laminae and projecting only slightly beyond the laminae's inferior borders. The inferior articular facets are oriented at nearly 90 degrees to the horizontal and are angled to the coronal plane such that they face slightly medially.

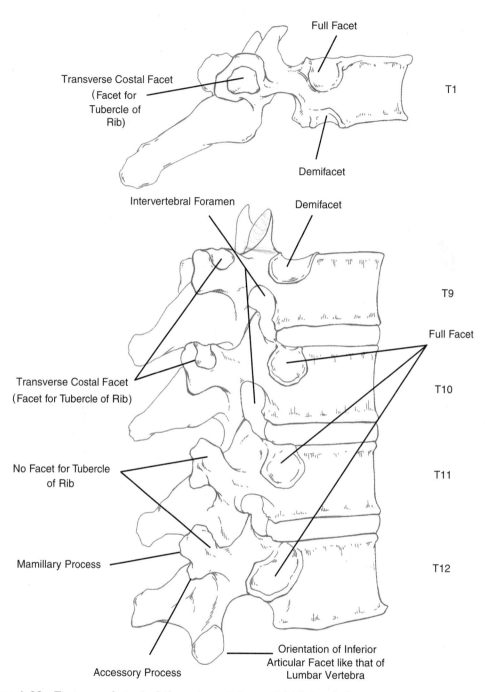

Full Facet

Transverse Costal Facet
(Facet for
Tubercle of
Rib)

T1

Demifacet

Intervertebral Foramen

Demifacet

T9

Full Facet

Transverse Costal Facet
(Facet for Tubercle of Rib)

T10

No Facet for Tubercle
of Rib

T11

Mamillary Process

T12

Accessory Process

Orientation of Inferior
Articular Facet like that of
Lumbar Vertebra

Figure 4-10   Features of atypical thoracic vertebrae, right lateral view.

The transverse processes arise from the vertebral arch just posterior to the superior articular processes and pedicles. They are long, thick, and strong, with an obliquely posterior and lateral direction. On the ventral surface of the lateral extremity of the transverse process is the *transverse costal facet,* the facet for articulation with the tubercle of the rib.

In general, the body of the first thoracic vertebra bears an entire costal facet for the first rib and an inferior demifacet for the superior portion of the head of the second rib. The body of the first thoracic vertebra is transversely broad, like a cervical vertebra. The spinous process is long, thick, and almost horizontal.

The second through eighth thoracic vertebrae are the most typical. They bear two demifacets on each side, a superior and an inferior.

The ninth thoracic vertebra usually bears only a superior demifacet and no inferior demifacet. In some persons, however, it may bear both a superior and a small inferior demifacet.

The 10th thoracic vertebra usually bears one large circular articular facet on each side, placed partly on the pedicle and partly on the body.

The 11th thoracic vertebra approaches the lumbar vertebrae in size and form. On each side it bears only a single costal facet, which is large and placed upon the lateral aspect of the pedicle. The pedicles are thicker and stronger in the 11th and 12th thoracic vertebrae than in any other part of the column. In both the 11th and 12th thoracic vertebrae, transverse processes are short and bear *no* transverse costal facets.

The 12th thoracic vertebra is very similar to the 11th. It may be distinguished, however, by its inferior articular facets. They are convex and directed laterally, like those of the lumbar vertebrae. As noted, the 12th thoracic vertebra bears no transverse costal facets on its transverse processes. In many ways, it is a transitional vertebra between the thoracic and lumbar regions, just as the first represents a transition between the cervical and thoracic regions. T12 exhibits accessory processes that are very small, rough elevations on the inferolateral surfaces of the transverse processes. They are also found occasionally on T11 and T10. The *mamillary processes* are small, round enlargements on the superior aspect of the transverse processes of T12 and possibly T11 and T10. Both accessory and mamillary processes are characteristic of lumbar vertebrae, although their locations are slightly different, probably because of the developmental origins of thoracic and lumbar transverse processes from transverse and costal elements, respectively.

The intervertebral foramina in the thoracic region have the following borders:

Superior:	Inferior vertebral notch of the cranial vertebra
Inferior:	Superior vertebral notch of the caudal vertebra
Posterior:	Joint capsule of the articular process
Anterior:	Body of the cranial vertebra, articular capsule of the costovertebral joint

The Lumbar Vertebrae

There are normally five lumbar vertebrae (Figure 4–11). Aside from the fused upper sacral segments, the lumbar vertebrae are the largest. They are characterized by large bodies, the presence of mamillary processes and accessory processes, and a *lack of* transverse costal facets or transverse foramina.

The body is large, wider transversely, and a little thicker ventrally. It is flattened or slightly concave superiorly and inferiorly. The sides of the body are concave. The vertebral foramen is triangular but smaller than in the cervical region. The transverse processes are anterior to the articular processes instead of posterior to them, as in the thoracic vertebrae, and posterior to the inferior vertebral notch. They are

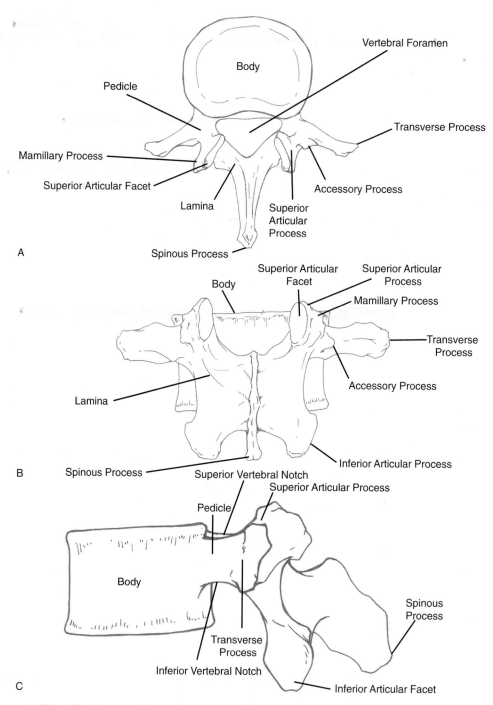

Figure 4-11   A lumbar vertebra: (*A*) superior, (*B*) posterior, and (*C*) left lateral views.

long, slender, and horizontal in the cranial three lumbar vertebrae, whereas they incline a little caudally in the caudal two. The accessory processes are small, rough elevations on the dorsal surfaces at the bases of the transverse processes.

The spinous process is thick, broad, and quadrilateral. It is thickest caudally. The spinous process of the fifth lumbar vertebrae is small for the lumbosacral angle.

The superior articular processes possess slightly concave, vertical facets that face medially and dorsally. On the posterolateral borders of the superior articular processes are round enlargements, the mamillary processes. The inferior articular processes possess convex, vertical facets that face laterally and ventrally.

The pedicles unite with the cranial part of the body; as a result, the inferior vertebral notches are very deep, whereas the superior vertebral notches are shallow. The laminae are tall superoinferiorly, narrow mediolaterally, and robust.

The intervertebral foramina allow the passage of lumbar spinal nerves to exit the vertebral canal. In the lumbar region, the borders of the foramina are as follows:

Superior:	Inferior vertebral notch of the cranial vertebrae
Inferior:	Superior vertebral notch of the caudal vertebrae
Posterior:	Zygapophyseal joint capsule
Anterior:	Bodies of the cranial and caudal vertebrae and their intervertebral disc

The Sacrum

The sacrum (S1–S5; refer to Figures 4–12 through 4–15 throughout the discussion of the sacrum) is a large triangular mass formed by the fusion of five vertebrae. It forms the posterosuperior wall of the pelvic cavity, being wedged between the auricular surfaces of the two ossa coxae. It presents for examination a base, a pelvic (ventral) surface, a dorsal surface, two lateral surfaces, and an apex. The base of the sacrum is superior and articulates with the fifth lumbar vertebra, whereas its apex is inferior and articulates with the coccyx. Because the sacrum is formed by the fusion of five (on average) separate vertebrae, all the typical features of a vertebra are present in the sacrum, but in modified form.

The *base* is the superior surface of the body of the first sacral vertebral segment. It projects ventrally to form the lumbosacral angle. The *promontory* is the ventral border of the superior surface of the body of S1. It is the most ventral portion of the sacrum and helps define the border of the pelvic inlet. The *sacral canal* is formed by the five vertebral foramina of the sacral vertebrae. The *alae* (Latin: "wings"; singular: *ala*) are the lateral processes extending from the bodies of S1 and S2. They are formed by the fusion of the costal elements of the sacral vertebrae and support the auricular surfaces. The superior articular processes of the sacrum articulate with the inferior articular facets of the fifth lumbar vertebra. The articular facets face dorsomedially.

The *pelvic surface* is concave and characterized by four *transverse ridges* that indicate the site of fusion of the five sacral vertebrae. Also on the pelvic surface are four pairs of *anterior sacral foramina*. They communicate with the sacral canal by means of the intervertebral foramina and allow the passage of the ventral rami of the first four sacral nerves as well as the lateral sacral arteries and veins.

The posterior (dorsal) surface is convex and narrower than the pelvic surface. In the midline, the *median sacral crest* is surmounted by three or four tubercles, the rudimentary spinous processes of the first three or four sacral segments. The *sacral*

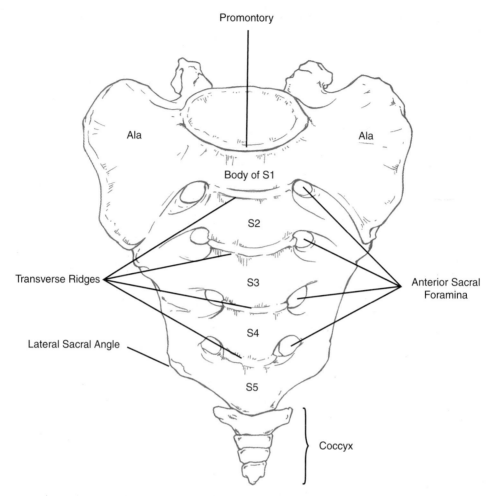

Figure 4-12   The sacrum and coccyx, anterior view (pelvic surface).

groove is a shallow groove on either side of the median sacral crest. It is formed by the union of the laminae of the sacral vertebrae. The *sacral hiatus* is a defect in the floor of the sacral groove inferiorly. It is caused by the nonfusion of the laminae of S5 with those of S4.

On either side of the dorsal surface, on the lateral aspect of the sacral groove, is the *intermediate sacral crest*. It is a linear series of tubercles produced by the fusion of the articular processes of the sacral vertebrae. At the distal ends of the intermediate crests are the two *sacral cornua*. These are the inferior articular processes of S5; they articulate with the coccyx via ligaments. The *lateral sacral crest* is formed by the fusion of three or four transverse tubercles, rudimentary transverse processes of the sacral vertebrae. There are four *posterior sacral foramina* between the intermediate and lateral sacral crests. These allow the exit of the dorsal rami of the sacral spinal nerves from the sacral canal.

The lateral surface of the sacrum is dominated by the *auricular surface*. This surface articulates with the similarly shaped auricular surface of the ilium. The

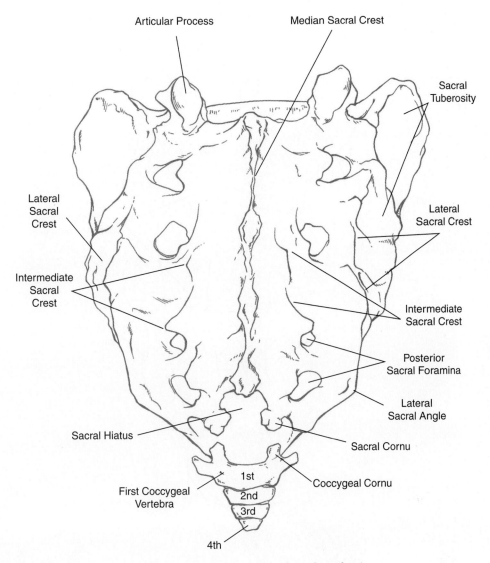

Figure 4-13   The sacrum and coccyx, posterior view (dorsal surface).

sacral tuberosity is the rough area between the auricular surface and the lateral sacral crest. It has deep impressions for the attachment of the interosseous sacroiliac ligament. Caudal to the auricular surface, the lateral surface is nonarticular. More caudally the lateral surface curves medially to the body of the fifth sacral vertebra at the *lateral sacral angle*.

The *apex* of the sacrum is its caudal end; it presents a *facet* for articulation with the coccyx. This is the inferior surface of the body of the fifth sacral vertebra.

To have the ability of increasing the size of the pelvic cavity for childbirth, the female sacrum is wider and relatively shorter, and its pelvic surface faces more caudally than the male's because of the specialized growth of the ilium, which decreases the acuity of the greater sciatic notch.

Figure 4-14   The sacrum and coccyx, median section, left lateral view.

The Coccyx

The coccyx (refer to Figs. 4–12 through 4–15 throughout the discussion of the coccyx) is the most caudal portion of the vertebral column. It is formed by the fusion of (usually) four rudimentary vertebral bodies. As a rule, only the first coccygeal vertebra possesses rudiments of transverse processes and superior articular processes.

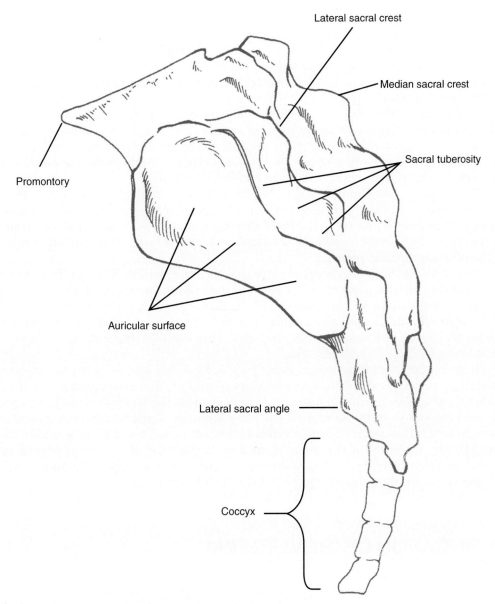

Figure 4-15 The sacrum and coccyx, left lateral view.

These articular processes are termed the *cornua* of the coccyx. The coccyx is a site of muscle attachment for the pelvic floor.

LANDMARKS OF THE VERTEBRAL COLUMN

Specific landmarks of the vertebral column and back may be projected to the surface of the body and palpated. Such landmarks are important in recognizing the vertebral level of interest in a living person.

The *external occipital protuberance* (see Chap. 8, Fig. 8–19) is the prominence on the back of the cranium that marks the superior attachment of the ligamentum nuchae (the ligamentous structure that passively supports the head) and the cervical musculature. If the finger is drawn down the midline of the neck from the external occipital protuberance, the first bony structure that can be felt is the spinous process of the second cervical vertebra. The posterior tubercle of the atlas is not palpable.

At the base of the neck, inferior to the external occipital protuberance, is the vertebra prominens. We have already referred to this structure. This is the spinous process of the seventh cervical vertebra. It projects considerably farther posteriorly than the spinous processes of the upper six cervical vertebrae and marks the junction of the cervical and thoracic portions of the vertebral column.

The *scapulae* (see Chap. 6, Fig. 6–14) are important guides to vertebral levels as well. In a person in the anatomical position, the *spines of the scapulae* lie in the same plane as the spinous process of the third thoracic vertebra. Similarly, in the anatomical position, the *inferior angles of the scapulae* lie at the level of the spinous process of the seventh thoracic vertebra.

Points on the bony pelvis serve as guides to lower vertebral levels. The *crest of the ilium* (the highest point of the *os coxae*, or *innominate bone*; see Chap. 7, Fig. 7–2) lies at the level of the spinous process of the fourth lumbar vertebra. The *posterior superior iliac spine* (a posterior projection of the os coxae, or innominate bone) is at the same level as the second sacral vertebra. This level corresponds to the obvious *sacral dimples* on the overlying skin.

Bony landmarks of the thorax (see Chap. 5, Figs. 5–1 and 5–5) can be projected posteriorly to vertebral levels. Anteriorly, the *sternal angle* marks the junction of the manubrium and the body of the sternum. It also marks the location of the *junction of the costal cartilage of the second rib with the sternum.* Projected directly posterior, this marks the location of the *intervertebral disc between T4 and T5* in a supine person. The *jugular notch* of the manubrium lies at the level of the lower part of the second thoracic vertebra. The *xiphisternal junction* between the body and xiphoid process of the sternum lies at the level of the 10th thoracic vertebra.

OSSIFICATION OF THE VERTEBRAL COLUMN

A typical vertebra has three primary centers of ossification and five secondary centers. The vertebral body represents one of the primary centers (the *centrum;* plural: *centra*), whereas the neural (vertebral) arch is formed by two primary centers that fuse in the midline to form the spinous process and fuse anteriorly with the body (Figure 4–16A). In addition, a typical vertebra has secondary centers at the tips of each transverse process, one at the tip of the spinous process and two ring-shaped annular epiphyses capping the top and bottom of the cylinder of the vertebral body, for a total of five secondary centers. Each secondary center is separated from the primary centers by an epiphyseal growth plate.

The primary centers for the centra appear first in the lower thoracic and upper lumbar regions at 9 or 10 weeks in utero and proceed cranially and caudally. At the eighth or ninth week in utero, the centers for the neural arches appear in the cervical region and upper two thoracic segments, T1 and T2, ossifying before some of the cervical levels; ossification then proceeds caudally.

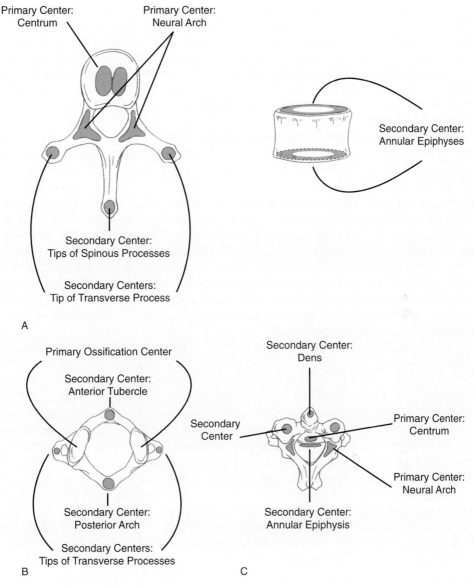

Figure 4-16   Centers of ossification of vertebrae: (A) the three primary centers and five secondary centers of a typical vertebra, (B) centers of ossification in the atlas, and (C) centers of ossification in the axis.

At birth all three primary centers for each vertebra are still distinct but are joined by cartilage. The halves of the neural arches fuse with each other during the first year, starting in the lumbar region. Following the same pattern, the arches then fuse with the bodies of the vertebrae a few years later. The costal element of the vertebra articulates with the primary center for the neural arch, not the primary center for the body. Thus, the centrum is not strictly synonymous with the body of the vertebra; for example, in thoracic vertebrae, the costal demifacets are described as part of the body of the vertebrae, but developmentally they are part of the primary center of ossification for the neural arch.

The five secondary centers appear after puberty and fuse with the primary centers by the age of 21 (Breathnach, 1965; Gray, 1985, 1995). In U.S. males, the superior and inferior annular epiphyses of the centrum fuse at 17 or 18 at the earliest and are always completed by age 25 (McKern and Stewart, 1957). The presacral vertebral column is completely ossified by the 25th year, with T4 and T5 representing the final elements to complete ossification. The sacrum is complete by age 23, although there may be a gap between the centra of S1 and S2 as late as age 32 (Krogman, 1962; McKern and Stewart, 1957). Some individual vertebrae or vertebral segments exhibit some differences from this general arrangement.

The Atlas

The atlas (see Fig. 4–16*B*), or first cervical vertebra, differs from other vertebrae in its lack of a body or spinous process and its possession of anterior and posterior arches. These differences are reflected in its pattern of ossification. It has two primary ossification centers, a left and a right, from which the bulk of the posterior arch and lateral mass of each side develops. The two halves of the posterior arch fuse at about 4 years of age, whereas the anterior arch forms and joins the two lateral masses between ages 5 and 9. Secondary centers have been noted at the tips of the transverse processes, for the posterior tubercle and for the anterior tubercle (Breathnach, 1965; Gray, 1985, 1995).

Axis

The axis (Fig. 4–16*C*) has all the typical centers noted for other vertebrae, plus two for the dens, which some ascribe to being the displaced body of the atlas. The centrum begins to ossify in the third or fourth month in utero, with the centers for the dens appearing in the fourth or fifth month in utero. The axis has two centers of ossification, placed laterally, which unite before birth (Breathnach, 1965; Gray, 1985, 1995). The centers for the neural arch appear by the ninth week in utero. The bone consists of four centers at birth: the dens, the true centrum, and each half of the neural arch. By 6 or 7 years of age the primary centers have fused, but the center of the union between the dens and the centrum may remain cartilaginous until middle age. An annular epiphysis for the inferior surface of the body appears at about puberty (Breathnach, 1965; Gray, 1985, 1995).

The Sacrum

The body of each sacral verteba develops from a primary center for the centrum and from secondary centers in epiphyses on the superior and inferior surfaces of each centrum. The vertebral arches form from the typical two primary centers of ossification as elsewhere in the vertebral column. Two additional ossification centers appear laterally for each of the upper three or four sacral segments for the costal elements. On each lateral surface of the sacrum, two secondary centers of ossification develop, one for the auricular surface and another for the lower, thinner part of the lateral edge of the bone. At 8 or 9 weeks in utero, the body of the first segment begins to ossify. The bodies of the second and third segments follow rapidly, but those of the fourth and fifth segments do not ossify until between 5 and 8 fetal months.

Between 6 and 8 months in utero, the centers for the costal elements and the centers for the neural arches begin to appear. Between the second year and the fifth or sixth year, the neural arches join with the bodies of the sacral vertebrae, the lower segments fusing first and the upper segments fusing last. Around age 16 the annular epiphyses for the bodies appear; the lateral epiphyses appear at about age 18 to 20.

Intervertebral discs separate the sacral vertebral bodies, but synostosis begins at about age 18 between S4 and S5 and then proceeds cranially so that by age 25 to 30, all sacral segments are fused solidly together (Breathnach, 1965; Gray, 1985, 1995). McKern and Stewart (1957) found that, among U.S. Army males killed in the Korean War, by age 24 all but the disc between S1 and S2 had synostosed, and by age 33, S1 and S2 had synostosed in all cases.

The Coccyx

The coccyx has four primary centers of ossification, one for each segment. Embryos show the rudiments of at least six coccygeal segments, but the distal ones fuse, so that only four cartilaginous segments remain at birth. The primary ossification center for the first segment appears soon after birth; for the second segment, it appears between ages 5 and 10. The third segment ossifies between ages 10 and 15, and the fourth ossifies after puberty, between ages 14 and 20. With age, there is a tendency for the segments to fuse with one another, occurring after age 25 or 30 for the first and second segments and later for the others. The coccyx has a tendency to fuse with the sacrum, especially among women (Breathnach, 1965: Gray, 1985, 1995).

ARTICULATIONS OF THE VERTEBRAL COLUMN

Any joint between two bones is known as an *articulation* or *arthrosis*. The study of the joints is the science of *arthrology. Joints,* or arthroses, are defined as junctions between bones. They may take a number of forms, based on the types of connective tissue that join the bones together and the shapes of the surfaces of the articulating bones. In some instances joints provide mobility between body segments, as in the joints of the limb. In other instances they stabilize and unify bony elements, as, for example, at the cranial sutures. Throughout the following descriptions of the elements of the skeleton, we make frequent reference to the joints of the body; therefore, we offer a short introduction to the descriptive terminology of the joints.

Joints or articulations may be defined in a number of ways. One of the most useful schemes for joint classification is according to the manner in which the involved bones are joined to one another. Broadly they can be divided into diarthroses (synovial joints) and synarthroses. Synarthroses may be subdivided into fibrous joints and cartilaginous joints.

Diarthroses

Diarthroses, or *synovial joints,* are usually very movable. They are characterized by opposing articular surfaces covered in hyaline articular cartilage with a synovial cavity between them. They are also characterized by the presence of an articular capsule composed of an outer fibrous layer and an inner synovial membrane surrounding the joint. Synovial joints are commonly categorized by the shapes of the articular surfaces and the motions allowed. One common schema lists the synovial joints according to the following classifications:

PLANE SYNOVIAL JOINT: A plane synovial joint, or gliding joint, is characterized by opposition of almost flat surfaces with pure translatory (gliding) motion. Examples include zygapophyseal joints and joints between carpal bones. In many instances, the surfaces of plane joints may have a small degree of curvature. This is true of the articular surfaces of zygapophyseal joints, as well as the joints between carpal bones and the joints between tarsal bones.

GINGLYMUS JOINT: A ginglymus, or hinge, joint is uniaxial; that is, it has 1 degree of freedom of motion. It is usually not pure hinge motion but more often is coupled with a slight degree of rotation. An example is the humeroulnar (elbow) joint.

TROCHOID JOINT: A trochoid, or pivot, joint is uniaxial. It is an osseous pivot in which one bone rotates about an axis. In the vertebral column, the joint between the dens of the axis and the anterior arch of the atlas is an example of a trochoid joint: As the head turns, the atlas rotates relative to the fixed dens of the axis. Another good example of a trochoid joint is the proximal radioulnar joint: The round head of the radius is bound to the ulna by the annular ligament, which forms a "collar" around the head of the radius. In pronation and supination of the forearm, the radial head spins within the circular confines formed by the annular ligament and radial notch of the ulna.

BICONDYLAR JOINT: A bicondylar, or condyloid, joint, is largely uniaxial, with some rotatory movement. It consists of two convex condyles rigidly fixed to the same bone and articulating with two concave joint surfaces. Examples include the joint between the femoral condyles and the tibial plateau (knee joint), the temporomandibular joint, and the atlanto-occipital joints.

ELLIPSOID JOINT: An ellipsoid joint is biaxial; an oval convex surface articulates with an oval concave surface. It allows movement on two orthogonal axes (i.e., flexion/extension in one axis and abduction/adduction in the other). The best example is the joint occuring between the distal end of the radius and the scaphoid and lunate.

SELLAR JOINT: A sellar, or saddle, joint is multiaxial. Two concavoconvex (saddle-shaped) surfaces articulate with one another. Examples include the pollical carpometacarpal joint between the base of the thumb and the carpal bones, as well as the sternoclavicular joint.

SPHEROIDAL JOINT: A spheroidal joint, or ball-and-socket joint, is multiaxial. It allows 3 degrees of freedom of motion. The only examples in the human skeleton are the glenohumeral (shoulder) joint and the hip joint (between the acetabulum and the head of the femur).

Synarthroses

Synarthroses are usually categorized by the types of materials joining the involved bones. Movements at synarthroses are usually more restricted than those at synovial joints. They are described next.

Fibrous Joints

Fibrous joints are characterized by a union of the bones involved by fibrous connective tissue.

SUTURES

Sutures are joints between bones of the cranium. The bones are joined at the sutures by short, strong, collagenous *intersutural ligaments.* For all practical mechanical purposes, these ligaments effectively block motion at the sutures and unify the cranium into a rigid structural unit that protects the delicate brain. There is a school of thought in chiropractic and osteopathic medicine that physiologically important amounts of motion continue at the sutures and that adjustment of the sutures can affect cerebrospinal fluid (Adams et al., 1992; Heisey and Adams, 1993). See Rogers and Witt (1997) for a contrary view.

GOMPHOSES

Gomphoses (singular: *gomphosis*) are joints between the teeth and alveolar processes of the mandible and maxilla. Gomphoses are unusual in that bone is present on one side of the joint only. In a gomphosis, the bone of the alveolar process of the maxilla or mandible is joined to the cementum (a bonelike substance) of the tooth's root by a short, strong *periodontal ligament.* Teeth are composed of three types of calcified tissue: the cementum of the root, the enamel of the external surface of the tooth crown, and the dentin at the core of the crown and root. Like bone, they are calcified connective tissue, but they differ from bone in their microscopic structure and material properties. (For more information about teeth, see Ash, 1984; Bhaskar, 1990.)

SYNDESMOSES

Syndesmoses (singular: *syndesmosis*) are characterized by the bonding of bones by collagenous (and sometimes elastic) interosseous ligaments, cords, or membranes.

Cartilaginous Joints

Cartilaginous joints are characterized by the presence of hyaline cartilage or fibrocartilage between the opposing joint surfaces.

SYNCHONDROSES

Synchondroses (singular: *synchondrosis*) are characterized by the presence of hyaline cartilage. Epiphyseal plates in growing long bones are synchondroses, as are the costal cartilages.

SYMPHYSES

In *symphyses* (singular: *symphysis*), both joint surfaces are encased in hyaline cartilage and joined by an intervening fibrocartilaginous disc. All symphyses are median. The intervertebral discs represent symphyses between the vertebral bodies.

The Vertebral Column

Joints between the vertebral bodies consist of the inferior surface of the body of the more cranial vertebra, the fibrocartilaginous intervertebral disc (refer to Figures 4–17 through 4–19 throughout the discussion of the intervertebral discs), and the su-

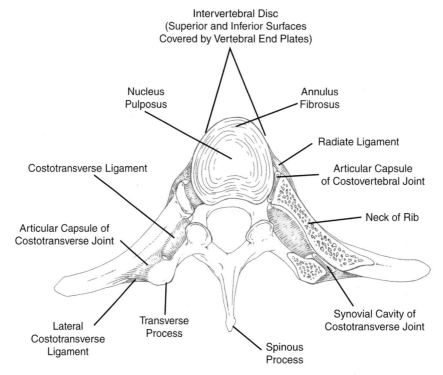

Figure 4-17   Ligaments of the ribs and the intervertebral disc, left superior view.

perior surface of the more caudal vertebra. These joints are stabilized by the *anterior* and *posterior longitudinal ligaments*.

The joints between vertebral arches are the articulations between the inferior articular facets of the more cranial vertebra with the superior articular facets of the more caudal vertebra, as well as the ligaments running between laminae, transverse processes, and spinous processes of adjacent vertebrae.

The Intervertebral Disc

The *intervertebral discs* constitute a specific type of synarthrodial joint, a symphysis. They adhere to the superior and inferior surfaces of the adjacent vertebrae by thin layers of hyaline cartilage called *vertebral end plates*, which are considered to be an integral part of the disc (Bogduk, 1986). Each disc consists of the vertebral end plates, an outer laminated *annulus fibrosus*, and an inner *nucleus pulposus*. The annulus fibrosus is fibrocartilage, whereas the nucleus pulposus (better developed in cervical and lumbar regions) is made up at birth of soft, gelatinous mucoid material and a few multinucleated notochordal cells. Notochordal cells disappear in the first decade of life, and the substance of the nucleus pulposus is replaced gradually by fibrocartilage; with maturity, the nucleus pulposus becomes less distinct from the rest of the disc.

Intervertebral discs are present between vertebral bodies from C2 to the sacrum, and a degenerate disc is present between S5 and the coccyx. They are generally thicker anteriorly than posteriorly in the cervical and lumbar regions, which creates the spinal curvatures in these regions. The intervertebral discs are nearly flat in

Figure 4–18   Articulations of the ribs and thoracic vertebrae, right lateral view.

the thoracic spine. They are thinnest in the upper thoracic spine and thickest in the lumbar spine. The outer annulus fibrosus has a narrow outer collagenous zone and a wider inner fibrocartilaginous zone. The annulus fibrosus consists of a number of laminae, with fibers of adjacent laminae set obliquely to one another and at a 30-degree angle relative to the horizontal.

Recent studies suggest that this is not the case in the cervical region. Mercer and Bogduk (1999) report that the cervical annulus fibrosus has a structure unlike that generally reported for the lumbar region. They note that cervical annuli are crescent-shaped and deficient posteriorly and that they do not consist of concentric lamellae of collagen fibers. Instead, cervical intervertebral discs take the form of a crescentic mass of collagen anteriorly and laterally and are deficient posteriorly, where the deficiency is covered by the posterior longitudinal ligament. The researchers conclude that "the three dimensional architecture of the cervical annulus

Post.

Ant.

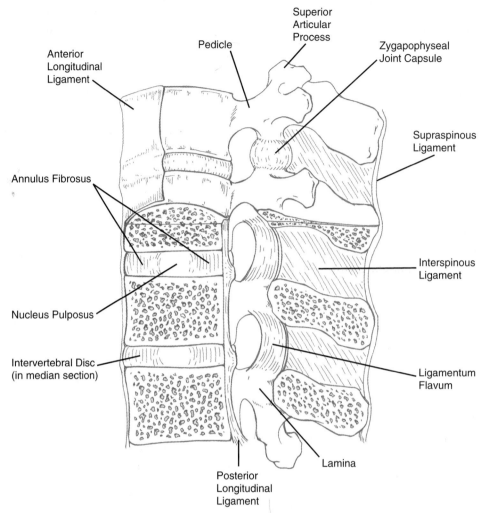

Figure 4-19   Joints between the vertebral arches, the anterior and posterior longitudinal ligaments, and the intervertebral disc, left lateral view.

fibrosus is more like a crescentic anterior interosseous ligament than a ring of fibers surrounding the nucleus pulposus" (Mercer and Bogduk, 1999, p. 619).

The oblique arrangement of fibers in adjacent laminae, as found in the lumbar region, imparts great torsional strength to the disc. Additionally, the outer laminae bulge externally, whereas the inner laminae bulge internally toward the nucleus pulposus. The annulus fibrosus is thickest anteriorly and thinnest posteriorly. The functions of the annulus fibrosus are to enclose and retain the nucleus pulposus, absorb compressive shocks, form a structural unit between vertebral bodies, and allow restricted motion between adjacent vertebral segments.

The inner nucleus pulposus accounts for 40 percent of the bulk of the disc. The nucleus pulposus contains the remains of the notochord and has a high water content. Notochordal cells disappear during the first decade of life and are replaced eventually by fibrocartilage. The nucleus pulposus is relatively larger at birth but decreases in relative size as it dehydrates with age. The nucleus pulposus is better developed in the cervical and lumbar regions than in the thoracic region and lies nearer the posterior part of the disc than the anterior. The nucleus pulposus provides a resilient spacer, allowing motion between vertebral segments, and distributes compressive forces, even though the nuclei are noncompressible, although deformable, themselves.

The vertebral end plates help prevent the vertebral body from suffering damage from pressure, and they contain the annulus fibrosus and nucleus pulposus within their normal borders. A rupture of the nucleus pulposus through the end plate is known as a *Schmorl's node*. When the nucleus herniates through the end plate, it allows the bodies of adjacent vertebrae to move closer together and can cause degenerative joint disease in the affected area of the vertebral column.

Intervertebral discs are avascular structures, but they do have vasculature surrounding their peripheries. They are attached to the anterior and posterior longitudinal ligaments and to the heads of the ribs by the intra-articular ligaments. They contribute about one-fifth of the total height of the vertebral column and are relatively thicker in the lumbar and cervical regions, thus contributing to greater mobility in these regions. They are thinnest, and essentially flat, anteroposteriorly in the thoracic region. Also, the discs are thicker anteriorly than posteriorly in the lumbar and cervical regions, helping to create the lumbar and cervical curvatures.

The functions of the intervertebral discs are to bear weight (with bodies of vertebrae), distribute loads, and dissipate shock (acting as "shock absorbers"). High water content aids this function. With age, the discs become less capable of holding water, because the nucleus becomes progressively replaced by fibrocartilage. They also have a higher water content in the morning than later in the day. The intervertebral discs also act as a flexible buffer between rigid vertebrae and permit adequate motion at low loads while providing stability at higher loads. When a disc is healthy, it is more likely that vertebrae will be damaged before disc damage occurs.

The intervertebral disc is innervated by the recurrent meningeal nerve (sinuvertebral nerve) posteriorly, the ventral rami and gray rami communicantes posterolaterally, and the gray rami communicantes and branches of the sympathetic trunk anterolaterally.

The Anterior Longitudinal Ligament

The *anterior longitudinal ligament* (Figure 4–20; see also Figs. 4–18 and 4–19 throughout the discussion of the anterior longitudinal ligament) is a strong band of fibers forming a syndesmosis that extends along the anterior surface of the bodies of the vertebrae from the occipital bone to the sacrum. It is composed of superficial, intermediate, and deep fibers. The superficial fibers are the longest and extend over four to five vertebrae. Intermediate fibers extend two to three vertebral levels, whereas the deep fibers are shorter, crossing between adjacent vertebrae only. This ligament is specialized in the region of the atlas and axis. From its lateral aspects, fibers spread out to form the anterior atlantoaxial ligament between the atlas and axis and the anterior atlanto-occipital membrane between the atlas and the occipital bone.

Its morphology is more typical in lower cervical vertebrae and the rest of the column. In the cervical area it is thin and narrow, and in general it is *narrow cranially* and *wider caudally*. It is thicker in the thoracic than in the lumbar or cervical regions. It is also somewhat thicker over the vertebral bodies than over the intervertebral discs. It attaches to the basilar portion of the occipital bone, the anterior tubercle of the atlas, the body of the axis, and the vertebral bodies and intervertebral discs

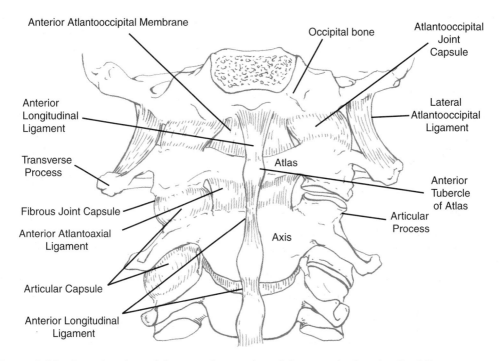

Figure 4-20   Anterior view of the superior portion of the anterior longitudinal ligament, anterior connections between the atlas, the axis and occiput, and the zygaphophyseal joint capsules of the cervical region.

down to the superior part of the anterior surface of the sacrum. The anterior longitudinal ligament functions to limit extension of the vertebral column.

The Posterior Longitudinal Ligament

The *posterior longitudinal ligament* (Figure 4–21; see also Fig. 4–19 throughout the discussion of the posterior longitudinal ligament) forms another vertebral syndesmosis and attaches to the dorsal surfaces of the bodies of the vertebrae within the vertebral canal. The portion of the posterior longitudinal ligament superior to the axis is specialized as the tectorial membrane. The posterior longitudinal ligament extends from the axis to the sacrum and lies within the sacral canal. It consists of superficial and deep layers of fibers. The superficial fibers cross three to four vertebrae, whereas the deep fibers run between adjacent vertebral bodies. This ligament is not firmly attached to vertebral bodies because the basivertebral veins and the vertebral venous plexus are situated between the ligament and the vertebral bodies. The posterior longitudinal ligament is *broad cranially* and *narrow caudally*. In the lower thoracic region and lumbar region it is denticulated, being broad over the intervertebral discs and narrow over the vertebral bodies. It limits flexion of the vertebral column.

Zygapophyseal Joints and Joints of the Vertebral Arches

The synovial joints between articular processes of the vertebrae are of the plane synovial type and are known as *zygapophyseal joints* (also referred to as the *posterior*

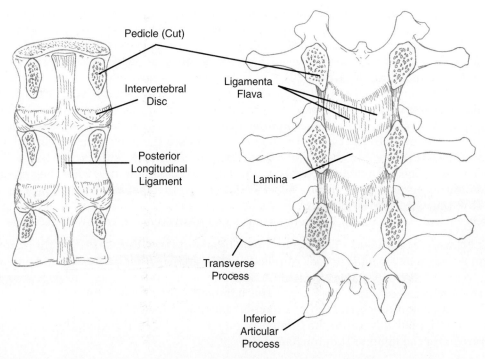

Figure 4-21   The posterior longitudinal ligament and the ligamenta flava in the lumbar region.

joints, facet joints, or *apophyseal joints*). The fibrous articular capsules of the zygapophyseal joints (see Figs. 4–19 and 4–20) surround the margins of the articular processes. They are thin and loose, being longer and looser in the cervical region than elsewhere. The size, shape, and movements of the zygapophyseal joints vary from one vertebral level to another. These joints may contain fat pads or fibroadipose menisci (articular discs), especially in the lumbar region. They are innervated by medial branches of dorsal rami of spinal nerves, both the ascending branch of the dorsal ramus below the joint and the descending branch of the dorsal ramus above the joint.

The vertebral arches are also connected to one another by the following ligaments:

- The supraspinous ligament
- The ligamentum nuchae
- The ligamentum flavum (plural: *ligamenta flava*)
- The interspinous ligament
- The intertransverse ligament

The latter three ligaments (ligamentum flavum, interspinous ligament, and intertransverse ligament) constitute the *intervertebral syndesmosis.*

INTERVERTEBRAL, OR SEGMENTAL, SYNDESMOSES

LIGAMENTA FLAVA: The ligamenta flava (singular: *ligamentum flavum*; see Figs. 4–19 and 4–21) are segmental syndesmoses connecting the laminae of adjacent vertebrae from the axis to the first segment of the sacrum. They are specialized as the *posterior atlantoaxial ligament* or *membrane,* which is between the posterior arch of the atlas and the laminae of the axis, and the *posterior atlanto-occipital membrane,* which is between the posterior arch of the atlas and the posterior margin of the foramen magnum (Figure 4–22).

The ligamenta flava consist of two lateral portions that begin posterior to the articular processes and extend posteriorly to the point where the laminae meet to form the spinous process. They are composed primarily of yellow elastic tissue (Latin: *flavum* = "yellow"). In the cervical region the ligamenta flava are thin, but broad and long. They are thickest in the lumbar region and of intermediate thickness in the thoracic region. There is one pair between adjacent vertebrae, running from the anterior and inferior surfaces of the more superior lamina to the posterior and superior surfaces of the more inferior lamina. They stop the separation of the laminae in flexion of the vertebral column. Elastin fibers permit them to stretch and regain their shapes.

INTERSPINOUS LIGAMENTS: The interspinous ligaments (see Fig. 4–19) are thin, membranous segmental syndesmoses connecting adjoining spinous processes and extending from the root to the apex of each process. The interspinous ligaments limit flexion of the vertebral column. They meet the ligamenta flava ventrally and the supraspinous ligament dorsally. They are narrow and elongated in the thoracic region and thicker and quadrilateral in the lumbar region. In the cervical region, they are incorporated into the ligamentum nuchae.

INTERTRANSVERSE LIGAMENTS: The intertransverse ligaments (see Fig. 4–18) are segmental syndesmoses connecting the transverse processes of adjacent vertebrae. They limit lateral flexion of the vertebral column. In the cervical region they are represented by only a few irregular fibers and are largely replaced by the intertransverse

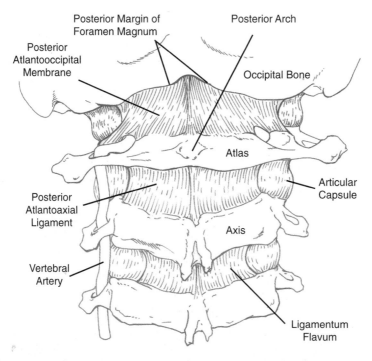

Figure 4-22   Posterior ligaments connecting the atlas, axis, and occiput.

muscles. In the thoracic region they are well-developed cords blended intimately with adjacent muscles, whereas in the lumbar region they are thin and membranous.

CONTINUOUS, OR NONSEGMENTAL, SYNDESMOSES

SUPRASPINOUS LIGAMENT: The supraspinous ligament (see Fig. 4–19), a nonsegmental syndesmosis, is a strong fibrous cord connecting the apices of the spinous processes from the seventh cervical vertebra to the sacrum. It has superficial, intermediate, and deep fibers. The superficial fibers span three to four vertebrae, the intermediate fibers span two to three, and the deep fibers run between adjacent vertebrae. It is thicker and broader in the lumbar region than in the thoracic, where it is relatively thin. In the cervical region above C7, the supraspinous and interspinous ligaments are specialized as the ligamentum nuchae (Figure 4–23).

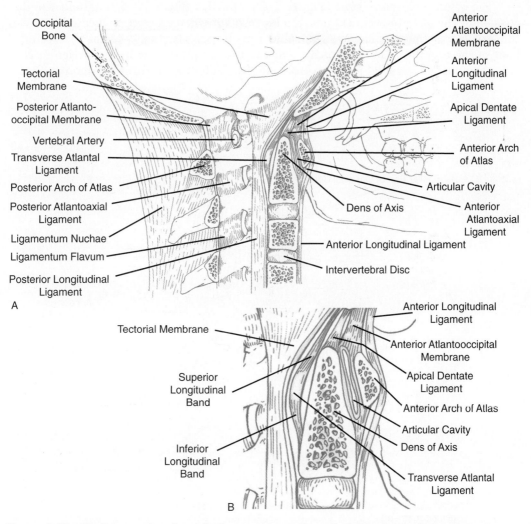

Figure 4–23   Median section through the cranium and cervical vertebral column, demonstrating the ligamentum nuchae, ligaments between the vertebral arches, anterior and posterior longitudinal ligaments, and ligaments of the atlantoaxial and atlanto-occipital joints. (A) Overview of median structures. (B) Close-up of the median atlantoaxial joint region.

LIGAMENTUM NUCHAE: **Above C7 the interspinous ligaments along with the supraspinous ligament are replaced by the more specialized *ligamentum nuchae*, a nonsegmental syndesmosis. The ligamentum nuchae extends from the external occipital protuberance, external occipital crest, posterior tubercle of the atlas, and spines of the cervical vertebrae to the spinous process of C7. The ligamentum nuchae comprises fibers that are developmentally homologous with the interspinous and supraspinous ligaments of lower vertebral levels. These fibers exist as a pair of dense, bilateral fibroelastic laminae separated by a layer of areolar tissue. The two laminae blend at the free dorsal border. This structure passively supports the head. It is relatively much reduced in humans, being much larger in quadrupedal mammals.**

Craniovertebral Joints

THE ATLANTO-OCCIPITAL JOINT

The *atlanto-occipital joint* (Figure 4–24; see also Fig. 4–23 throughout the discussion of the atlanto-occipital joint), a *bicondylar synovial joint,* is located between the superior articular facets of the atlas and the occipital condyles of the occipital bone of the cranium. The atlas is attached to the occipital bone by the articular capsules around the synovial joint surfaces and by the following three ligaments:

Figure 4-24 The cruciform ligament and associated structures, posterior view. A cervical laminectomy has been performed to expose the anterior view of the vertebral canal.

- The anterior atlanto-occipital membrane
- The posterior atlanto-occipital membrane
- The two lateral atlanto-occipital ligaments

The fibrous joint capsules (see Fig. 4–20) are thickened posterolaterally but are thin medially, and they sometimes communicate medially with a bursa between the dens and the transverse atlantal ligament. The capsules surround the occipital condyles and the superior articular facets of the atlas. The *anterior atlanto-occipital membrane* (see Fig. 4–20) forms a syndesmosis anteriorly, extending from the anterior margins of the foramen magnum to the cranial border of the anterior arch of the atlas. The *posterior atlanto-occipital membrane* (see Fig. 4–22) forms a syndesmosis posteriorly and extends from the posterior margin of the posterior arch of the atlas to that of the foramen magnum. It is has an opening over the groove for the vertebral artery to allow the vertebral artery to enter the vertebral canal and the first cervical spinal nerve to exit. The *lateral atlanto-occipital ligaments* are lateral thickenings of the articular capsules. They run from the *jugular processes* of the occipital bone to the transverse processes of the atlas (see Fig. 4–20).

THE ATLANTOAXIAL JOINTS

There are two sets of articulations between the atlas and axis: the lateral atlantoaxial joints and the median atlantoaxial joint. The *lateral atlantoaxial joints* are between the lateral masses of the atlas and the superior articular facets of the axis, whereas the *median atlantoaxial joint* is between the dens and the anterior arch of the atlas.

Ligaments associated with these joints are as follows:

- The accessory atlantoaxial ligaments
- The anterior atlantoaxial ligament
- The posterior atlantoaxial ligament
- The cruciform ligament, consisting of:
  - The transverse atlantal ligament
  - The superior and inferior longitudinal bands

The lateral atlantoaxial joints (Figure 4–25) are between the inferior articular facets of the atlas and the superior articular facets of the axis. This is a plane synovial joint capable of translational (gliding) movement. The articular capsule surrounds the margins of the inferior articular facets of the atlas and the superior articular facets of the axis. The fibrous part is thin and loose but is strengthened at its posterior and medial aspects by an *accessory atlantoaxial ligament* (see Fig. 4–24), which is attached to the body of the axis near the base of the dens and to the lateral mass of the atlas near the transverse ligament.

The *anterior atlantoaxial ligament* (see Fig. 4–20) extends from the inferior border of the anterior arch of the atlas to the ventral surface of the body of the axis. It is an expansion of the cranial extension of the anterior longitudinal ligament (see Fig. 4–20), a sheet of dense regular connective tissue running the length of the vertebral column and attached to the ventral aspects of the vertebral bodies and the intervening intervertebral discs.

A

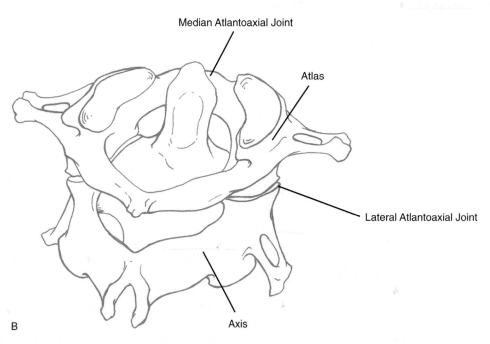

B

Figure 4–25   The median atlantoaxial joint: (A) superior view, (B) three-quarter view from lateral superoposterior angles, demonstrating the lateral atlantoaxial joints.

The *posterior atlantoaxial ligament* (see Fig. 4–22) extends from the inferior border of the posterior arch of the atlas to the superior edges of the laminae of the axis. It is homologous with the *ligamentum flavum,* which runs between the adjacent laminae of all other vertebrae.

The *median atlantoaxial joint* (refer to Figs. 4–23 through 4–25 throughout the discussion of the median atlantoaxial joint) is located between the anterior articular facet of the dens and the fovea dentis of the anterior arch of the atlas. This is a *trochoid*, or pivot, joint. The dens is held against the anterior arch of the atlas by the *transverse atlantal ligament.* Two synovial cavities are related to the dens, one between the dens and the anterior arch of the atlas and the other between the dens and the transverse atlantal ligament. This ligament attaches to small tubercles on the medial surfaces of the lateral masses of the atlas; the fibers pass transversely posterior to the dens to help hold the dens in place.

As the transverse atlantal ligament crosses the dens posteriorly, a small fasciculus extends superiorly and another inferiorly to form the *superior* and *inferior longitudinal bands* of the *cruciform ligament.* The superior band attaches to the internal aspect of the basilar part (or clivus) of the occipital bone deep to the tectorial membrane, whereas the inferior band attaches to the body of the axis deep to the tectorial membrane. The transverse atlantal ligament together with the longitudinal bands forms the cruciform ligament.

LIGAMENTS ATTACHING THE AXIS TO THE OCCIPITAL BONE

The axis not only articulates with the atlas, but it is also connected to the occipital bone by ligaments and membranes (refer to Figs. 4–23 and 4–24 throughout the discussion of these structures). Movements occurring between the axis and the occipital bone are flexion, extension, and slight lateral tilting. There are three primary attachments between the axis and the occipital bone. They are the following:

- The tectorial membrane
- The two alar ligaments
- The apical ligament of the dens (apical dentate ligament)

The *tectorial membrane* extends from the dorsal surface of the body of the axis to the clivus, the internal aspect of the basilar portion of the occipital bone. It attaches along the anterior border of the foramen magnum and blends with the periosteal layer of the cranial dura mater surrounding the brain. It expands to cover the dens and its ligaments posteriorly within the vertebral canal. The tectorial membrane is the continuation of the posterior longitudinal ligament above the second cervical vertebra. The two *alar ligaments* extend from each side of the cranial part of the dens to rough depressions on the medial sides of the occipital condyles.

The alar ligaments are also known as the *check ligaments* because they limit or "check" the rotation of the cranium to the contralateral side on the vertebral column. They also tighten with head flexion but are relaxed during head extension. The *apical ligament of the dens* extends from the tip of the dens to the anterior margin of the foramen magnum between the alar ligaments. It is intimately blended with the deep portion of the anterior atlanto-occipital membrane anteriorly and the superior longitudinal band of the cruciform ligament posteriorly. It is believed to be the developmental core of the *proatlas* and contains some notochordal cells. The proatlas is a transitional structure that normally does not form a bone in humans but has formed a separate bone between the atlas and occipital bone in experimental mice (Carlsen, 1994).

Innervation of Intervertebral Joints

All intervertebral joints are segmentally innervated by the adjoining spinal nerves.

Lumbosacral Articulation

Lumbar vertebrae are joined with the sacrum and pelvis via the anterior and posterior longitudinal ligaments, the intervertebral disc between L5 and S1, the ligamenta flava, the interspinous and supraspinous ligaments, and the articular capsules of the zygapophyseal joints. Additionally, the fifth lumbar vertebra, and occasionally the fourth, is joined with the pelvis via one additional ligament on each side, the iliolumbar ligaments (Figures 4–26 and 4–27). The *iliolumbar ligament* consists of a superior band and an inferior band, which is also known as the *lumbosacral ligament*. Both bands attach medially to the transverse process of L5. The superior band runs from the transverse process of L5 to the crest of the ilium immediately ventral to the sacroiliac articulation. The inferior band runs from the transverse process of L5 to the base of the sacrum, where it blends with the *anterior sacroiliac ligament*. These two bands limit lateral flexion of the lumbar spine.

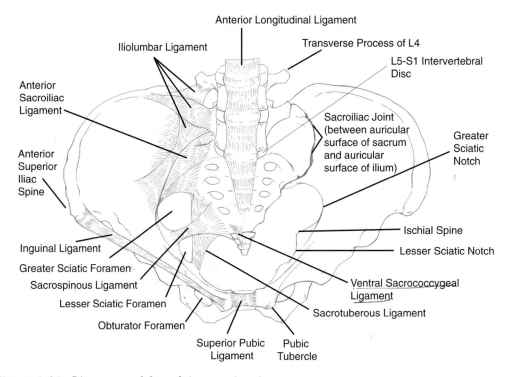

Figure 4-26   Ligaments of the pelvis, anterior view.

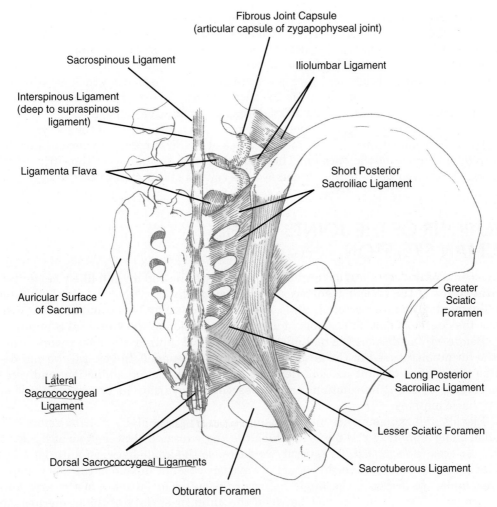

Figure 4-27   Ligaments of the pelvis, posterior view.

Sacrococcygeal Joint

The *sacrococcygeal joint* (refer to Figs. 4–26 and 4–27 throughout the discussion of the sacrococcygeal joint) is a slightly movable joint between the first coccygeal vertebra and the fifth sacral vertebra. A small intervertebral disc is present between these two vertebral bodies. The following ligaments strengthen this joint:

- The ventral sacrococcygeal ligament
- The superficial dorsal sacrococcygeal ligament
- The deep dorsal sacrococcygeal ligament
- The lateral sacrococcygeal ligaments
- The intercornual (interarticular) ligaments

The *ventral sacrococcygeal ligament* consists of a few irregular fibers running from the ventral surface of the sacrum to the ventral surface of the coccyx that blend with the periosteum. The *superficial dorsal sacrococcygeal ligament* runs from the free margin of the sacral hiatus and attaches to the dorsal surface of the coccyx. It closes the posterior aspect of the most distal part of the sacral canal and corresponds to the ligamenta flava. The *deep dorsal sacrococcygeal ligament* corresponds to the posterior longitudinal ligament and is a flat band that arises from the posterior aspect of the fifth sacral segment inside the sacral canal and attaches to the dorsal surface of the coccyx deep to the superficial dorsal sacrococcygeal ligament.

The *lateral sacrococcygeal ligaments* are present on either side of the coccyx. They run from the rudimentary transverse processes of the first coccygeal vertebra to the lower lateral angle of the sacrum. They complete the foramina for the fifth sacral nerves. The *intercornual ligaments* connect the cornua of the sacrum and coccyx.

MOTIONS OF THE JOINTS OF THE HUMAN SKELETON

Movements of the vertebral column are in large part allowed by, and likewise limited by, the forms of the articular surfaces of the zygapophyses. Other factors, including the ligaments, the intervertebral discs, and the surrounding bones and muscles, also affect the degree of motion possible in a particular region of the vertebral column.

Before we can discuss the motions of the vertebral column, we must review some of the terminology used in the description of joint movement. In general, we can describe three types of joint motion: flexion/extension, abduction/adduction, and rotation (Figure 4–28). Other motions can be described as variations or combinations of these basic motions.

Flexion and extension are motions along a parasagittal plane. *Flexion* refers to a motion along a parasagittal plane in which the angle formed between two designated body surfaces is *decreased*. In general, we decrease the angle between anterior body surfaces in flexion, although this is not always the case. In flexion of the elbow joint, for example, we decrease the angle between the anterior surfaces of the arm and forearm, or, in osteological terms, between the anterior surface of the humerus (the bone of the arm) and the anterior surfaces of the radius and ulna (the bones of the forearm); the upper limb is bent at the elbow, as in lifting a cup of coffee to the mouth. In the case of the knee, however, flexion brings the posterior surfaces of the tibia (a bone of the leg) and femur (the bone of the thigh) closer together.

Extension refers to a motion along a parasagittal plane in which the angle formed between two designated body surfaces is *increased*. To return to our example of the elbow joint, in extension the angle between the anterior surfaces of the humerus superiorly and the radius and ulna inferiorly is *increased* (the upper limb is straightened at the elbow).

Abduction and adduction are motions along a coronal plane. They are carried out at a 90-degree angle to flexion and extension. In *abduction,* a body part is moved *away* from the midline of the body. Conversely, in *adduction,* a body part is moved *toward* the midline of the body. An easy way to remember the difference is that in abduction, a body part is taken away from the midline just as an *abducted* child is taken away from its parents; in adduction, a body part is *added* to the midline of the body. Let us again turn to an example from the upper limb. In the anatomical position, the upper limb is in the adducted position. When the upper limb is raised away from the side of the body in a coronal plane, it is abducted. When the fingers are spread apart, they are abducted. When they are brought back together, they are adducted.

A   Flexion   Anatomical Position   Extension

B   Abduction (right arm)   C   Circumduction
      Adduction (left arm)

Figure 4-28   (*A*) Flexion/extension of the body. (*B*) Abduction/adduction of the arm and leg, with the broken lines indicating the anatomical position. The solid lines on the right side of the subject indicate abduction of the arm and leg; the solid lines on the left side demonstrate adduction of the arm and leg. (*C*) Circumduction of the arm.   (*Continues on next page*)

Right Rotation

Supination

Anatomical Position

D   Pronation   E   Left Rotation   F

Figure 4-28   (*Continued*)   (*D*) Supination/pronation of the forearm. (*E*) Rotation of the head.
(*F*) Right lateral flexion of the vertebral column, posterior view.

Rotation, as the name implies, is a turning of a body part about a longitudinal axis. *Supination* is the turning of the forearm such that the palm faces forward (supination is the anatomical position). *Pronation* is the turning of the forearm such that the palm faces backward. If the upper limb is extended with the palm facing upward, such as in holding a bowl of soup, the forearm is supinated. If the upper limb is extended and the palm now faces downward, with the soup spilled on the floor, the forearm is now pronated. In supination and pronation, the radius rotates about an axis that passes through the proximal radius and the distal ulna.

Circumduction is a motion that combines elements of flexion, abduction, extension, and adduction. In circumduction, a body part describes a cone of motion. One end of the concerned body part is more fixed, whereas the other end is more free to move. Using another example from the upper limb, think of this: if the entire upper limb is circumducted, the shoulder joint and head of the humerus constitute the more fixed end and the tips of the fingers constitute the freer end.

In circumduction of the upper limb, the shoulder joint is flexed, abducted, extended, then adducted (or the order is reversed). During this movement, the tips of the fingers roughly describe a circle in space, while the proximal humerus remains relatively fixed at the shoulder joint. The motion of the upper limb in circumduction thus describes a cone in which the shoulder represents the apex and the motion of the tips of the fingers describes its base. It is perhaps easier to explain these motions with respect to the limb bones than to those of the vertebral column; however, now that we have defined the basic terms of motion as they apply to the limbs, we turn to the motions of the vertebral column.

MOVEMENTS OF THE VERTEBRAL COLUMN

Movements of the vertebral column may involve the entire column or only a part of the column. In bending over to touch your toes, for example, the entire vertebral column is flexed. Bowing from the waist involves flexion of the lumbar column only. If you bend your head forward so that your chin rests on your chest, you have flexed only the cervical vertebral column. As we shall see, the degree of flexion and extension allowed varies throughout the vertebral column.

Also, the range of movements of the vertebral column is restricted by the intervertebral disc. These joints at the discs are slightly movable, allowing flexion, extension, and lateral flexion, a movement of the vertebral column in the coronal plane. In general, only small movements occur between adjacent vertebrae, but the cumulative range is great. When discussing motions of the vertebral column, it is also important to consider the occipital bone of the cranium as well (discussed in Chap. 8). In a sense, we can think of the occipital bone and its condyles as cervical vertebra 0.

Now we can consider the individual motions of the vertebral column.

Flexion of the Vertebral Column

In flexion of the vertebral column, the angle between the anterior surfaces of the abdomen and thorax and the anterior surfaces of the thighs is decreased, as in bending forward. During flexion, the inferior articular processes of the more superior vertebrae glide superiorly relative to the superior articular processes of the lower vertebrae. The fibrous joint capsules of the zygapophyseal joint capsules become taut. When the vertebral column is flexed, the anterior longitudinal ligament becomes relaxed; the intervertebral discs are compressed anteriorly; the laminae and spinous processes spread apart; and the posterior longitudinal ligament, ligamentum flavum, interspinous and supraspinous ligaments, and posterior fibers of the intervertebral discs are all tensed. The vertebral extensor muscles resist and help control flexion of the vertebral column.

Extension of the Vertebral Column

Extension of the vertebral column increases the angle between the anterior surfaces of the thighs and the anterior surfaces of the thorax and abdomen, as in straightening up or even bending backward. Events that occur during extension are opposite those that occur during flexion. The anterior longitudinal ligament and anterior fibers of the annulus fibrosus tense, the intervertebral discs are compressed posteriorly, and the spinous processes and zygapophyses are approximated.

Rotation of the Vertebral Column

Rotation of a vertebra involves the turning of the vertebra about its superoinferior axis relative to adjacent vertebrae. Rotation of a vertebra upon another results in torsional deformation of the intervertebral discs. In any given vertebra, the axis of rotation lies somewhere between the anterior aspect of the body and the posterior tip of the spinous process. Rotation is defined according to the motion of the anterior aspect of the vertebral body. In *left rotation* of a vertebra, any given point on the anterior surface of the body of that vertebra moves toward the left, whereas the tip of the spinous process of that vertebra moves toward the right. In *right rotation,* the opposite events occur: the anterior surface of the vertebral body turns to the right whereas the tip of the spinous process moves to the left.

Lateral Flexion of the Vertebral Column

A special motion of the vertebral column is *lateral flexion.* Lateral flexion of the vertebral column corresponds to abduction and adduction of the limbs. It is a motion primarily in the coronal plane, as in leaning to one side from the waist. As with flexion and extension, we can laterally flex a portion of the vertebral column or the entire column. If we keep the trunk still but bend the head in a coronal plane toward the left shoulder, we are laterally flexing the cervical vertebral column to the left.

The opposite motion is lateral flexion to the right. Because of the forms of the zygapophyses, lateral flexion always involves some degree of rotation. This rotation can be either *ipsilateral* (to the same side) or *contralateral* (to the opposite side), depending on the region of the column; for example, lateral flexion of the cervical vertebral column is accompanied by ipsilateral rotation, meaning that when we flex the cervical vertebral column to the left, the cervical vertebrae undergo left rotation. During lateral flexion, the intervertebral discs are compressed on the side flexed to and they are tensed on the contralateral side.

Circumduction of the Vertebral Column

Circumduction of the vertebral column combines elements of vertebral flexion, lateral flexion, extension, and rotation. Circumduction may involve only a part of the column, such as the cervical region, or it may involve the entire vertebral column above the sacrum. In the case of circumduction of the cervical vertebral column, for example, the top of the head is the free point describing the base of our cone of motion, and the top of the first thoracic vertebral body represents the apex of the cone.

Regional Differences in Motion of the Vertebral Column

The extent of all motions of the vertebral column is largely a result of the shape of the zygapophyseal joints, which vary from region to region. In the cervical region, the orientation of superior articular facets from anterosuperior to posteroinferior (facing dorsally and superiorly) facilitates flexion and extension. The relatively thick intervertebral discs in the cervical region also contribute to greater flexion and extension in this region. Between adjacent cervical vertebrae, on average 15 degrees of flexion/extension takes place. There is moderate rotation in the cervical region, except between C1 and C2, where rotation is considerable.

The cervical vertebral column shows the greatest degree of lateral flexion of the vertebral regions. Between adjacent cervical vertebrae, approximately 10 degrees of lateral flexion is possible. Lateral flexion in this region is coupled with ipsilateral rotation of vertebral bodies. The articular facets slope downward laterally and posteriorly, guiding the superior vertebra into ipsilateral rotation during lateral flexion.

In the thoracic region, the vertical orientation of the articular facets limits flexion, and overlapping laminae and spinous processes limit extension. The thin intervertebral discs in the thoracic region also limit flexion and extension. An average of 6 degrees of flexion/extension occurs in the thoracic region, varying from the top to the bottom of the thoracic column, with 4 degrees allowed in the upper thorax and 12 degrees possible in the lower thorax. The articular facets lie along a horizontal arc, permitting considerable rotation. The greatest rotation is in the upper thoracic region. Lateral flexion of thoracic vertebrae is about 6 degrees between adjacent vertebrae; this motion is restricted by the ribs. In the upper thoracic region, lateral flexion is coupled with ipsilateral rotation of vertebral bodies. In the lower thoracic region, it is coupled with contralateral rotation of vertebral bodies.

In the lumbar region, flexion, extension, and lateral flexion occur freely. Approximately 15 degrees of flexion/extension takes place between adjacent vertebrae in the lumbar region. The greater thickness of the intervertebral disc in the lumbar region increases the allowable range of movement here. When the vertebral column as a whole is flexed (as in touching the toes) and extended, about 75 percent of this motion is movements of the lumbar region. Rotation is most restricted in the lumbar region because the articular facets are oriented along parasagittal planes. Lateral flexion is about 6 degrees between adjacent lumbar vertebrae, as in the thoracic region, and it is coupled with contralateral rotation of the vertebral bodies.

It is especially interesting, considering the effects of the zygapophyseal joints in restricting flexion and extension, that these joints in the lumbar region of humans are unlike those of other primates. To obtain and maintain an erect trunk position, humans, as well as other primates, must ensure that their center of mass falls on a vertical line that intersects some portion of their foot. If that line falls forward of the foot, they fall forward; if the line falls behind the foot, they fall backward (this assumes that they are standing still—in motion this is not true because of the effects of inertia).

But positioning the center of mass over the foot in the erect stance is virtually impossible for other primates because the inferior zygapophyseal joints of each lumbar vertebra are in the same position as the superior ones in the subjacent vertebra. This prevents any signifiant lordosis, forcing primates such as chimpanzees to adopt a bent-hipped, bent-kneed posture to position their center of mass over the ground contact points of their feet. In humans, the progressive widening of each pair of inferior zygapophyseal joints in the lumbar column allows considerably more imbrication (sliding). This in turn permits significant lordosis and a fully erect stance without flexion at either the hip or the knee.

DISORDERS OF THE VERTEBRAL COLUMN

The vertebral column has many anomalies. Only a few are discussed here, most of which can be attributed to abnormal vertebral column development.

Variation in Numbers of Vertebral Segments

One of the most common anomalies of the vertebral column is a variation in the numbers of vertebral segments. Variation occurs either in the total number of segments in the column—that is, more or fewer than 33—or in the numbers of vertebrae found in the different regions even though the total number of segments remains 33. In the latter case, 1 vertebra is usually "shifted" from one region to an adjacent region; for example, the lumbar region may have 4 vertebrae and the sacrum may have 6. Variation in the number of cervical vertebrae is rare but may occur in pathological conditions such as Klippel-Feil syndrome, in which there is often fusion and a reduced number of cervical vertebrae, among other anomalies.

Curvatures

As described earlier, four curvatures to the vertebral column are considered normal: cervical, thoracic, lumbar, and sacral (which includes the coccyx). The thoracic and sacral curvatures develop first (primary curvatures) and are convex posteriorly. The cervical and lumbar curvatures develop somewhat later and are convex anteriorly.

Any of these curvatures can become pathologically exaggerated. When a curvature is abnormally convex posteriorly, it is called a *kyphosis* (or hyperkyphosis) (Figure 4–29). This is most frequently seen in the thorax and is often associated with osteoporosis in elderly women ("dowager's hump"). It also develops in adolescents with *Scheuermann's disease,* in which the anterior parts of the annular epiphyses do not develop properly.

If a curvature is abnormally convex anteriorly, it is a *lordosis* (or hyperlordosis). This condition is most often seen in the lumbar region. It occurs often with obesity or temporarily with pregnancy, both of which place the body's center of gravity farther forward than normally seen. The lumbar lordosis increases to move the center of gravity of the body back over the pelvis.

NOTE: Anatomists usually refer to normal curvatures and reserve the terms *kyphosis* and *lordosis* for pathological curvatures. Some clinicians use *kyphosis* and *lordosis* to refer to normal curvatures and qualify them as *hyperkyphosis* or *hyperlordosis* to indicate a pathological condition.

Figure 4-29   Kyphosis of the thoracic region.

Another pathological curvature is *scoliosis* (Figure 4–30), a mediolateral curvature of the vertebral column. This condition has a frequency of about 1 in 200 and is more often seen in females than in males. It may have different causes, such as a muscular weakness on one side ("myopathic") or the presence of a hemivertebra (Figure 4–31). In the case of a hemivertebra, only one side of a vertebral body develops, causing the column above it to tilt, or curve, to the side. In other cases, the cause of scoliosis is unknown ("idiopathic").

Herniated Discs

A *herniated disc* involves a defect in the annulus fibrosus of an intervertebral disc, through either degeneration (which occurs after the second decade of life) or trauma, and protrusion of the nucleus pulposus through this defect. This most commonly occurs in the lumbar region, with 95 percent of herniations occurring at the level of L4-L5 or L5-S1. The herniation is usually to the posterolateral aspect of the disc, where the annulus fibrosus is thin and unprotected by the posterior longitudinal ligament. The nucleus pulposus thus tends to herniate into the intervertebral foramen,

Figure 4-30   Scoliosis.

compressing the spinal nerve roots. At the lower lumbar levels, this often results in *sciatica,* or severe pain in the leg along the course of the sciatic nerve. This nerve is a branch of the lumbosacral plexus and receives contributions from spinal nerves L4 through S3.

Spondylolysis

In *spondylolysis,* the spinous processes, laminae, and inferior articular processes are not attached to the body of the vertebra. This can be unilateral or bilateral and most often occurs at L5. It is found in about 5 to 10 percent of people. Although the cause is unknown, it is thought that it may be congenital and/or caused by trauma or stress fractures. It is not seen in newborns, but the frequency increases with age up to 20 years. If congenital, it may result from a failure of the vertebral arch(es) to fuse with the body during development.

Spondylolisthesis

Spondylolisthesis is an anterior displacement of the vertebral column; it usually occurs at the lumbosacral joint. It may have several causes, including bilateral spondy-

Figure 4-31   Hemivertebra on the right side, with ankylosis to the inferior vertebra, posterior view.

lolysis at L5, fracture of the pedicles or inferior articular processes of L5, fracture of the superior articular processes of the sacrum, or congenital abnormalities of the zygapophyseal joints or vertebral arches. If both vertebral arches are not attached to the vertebral body, the entire body's center of gravity (located just anterior to the lumbosacral joint) causes L5 to slip forward on the sacrum. Spondylolisthesis at the lumbosacral joint usually results in compression of spinal nerves S1 and S2, producing symptoms of sciatica.

Spina Bifida

Spina bifida results from the failure of the two halves of the neural arch to fuse during development, leaving a defect in the arch. Next to variation in segment numbers, this is the most frequent congenital anomaly of the vertebral column. Spina bifida can be classified into two types: spina bifida occulta and spina bifida cystica. In *spina bifida occulta* (Figure 4–32), the laminae fail to fully develop and fuse. It may occur in only one or two vertebrae and does not involve herniation of the spinal cord or meninges. It is usually asymptomatic but may occasionally be associated with some neurological disturbances. About 2 percent of people have spina bifida occulta of L5.

Spina bifida cystica (spina bifida vara) is a much more severe condition. It involves a cystlike herniation of the spinal cord and/or meninges through a defect in the vertebral arch. There are three types of spina bifida cystica: *Spina bifida cystica with meningocele* occurs when there is herniation of the meninges but not of the spinal cord itself. When both the spinal cord and the meninges are included in the herniation, it is called *spina bifida cystica with meningomyelocele.* The most severe form is *spina bifida cystica with myeloschisis.* In this condition, there is not only herniation of the spinal cord and meninges but also malformation and flattening of the spinal cord because of the failure of the neural tube to close during early development of the central nervous system. Spina bifida cystica occurs about once in every

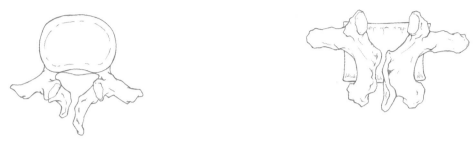

Figure 4–32   Spina bifida occulta of a lumbar vertebra.

1000 births and usually involves meningomyelocele. It is often associated with other defects, such as clubfoot and hydrocephaly, and can be fatal to an infant. Infants that survive often show evidence of damage to the nervous system, such as paralysis of the limbs and disturbances in bladder and bowel control.

Whiplash

Whiplash is a soft tissue injury of the cervical spine. It is commonly caused by automobile accidents. The term *whiplash* is descriptive of the motions of the cervical spine that cause the injury. It is generally induced in persons in a stationary automobile that is struck in the rear by a moving vehicle. The person's body and automobile seat are driven forward by the impact, but the head does not move with the body; as a result, the cervical spine is thrown into hyperextension. The anterior cervical muscles are severely stretched and, as a consequence, they contract and throw the head forward by flexion of the cervical vertebral column. As the car stops, the body stops as well, but the head continues moving forward. Motion is stopped posteriorly as the occiput hits the back and stopped anteriorly as the chin strikes the sternum. This is referred to as an "acceleration injury."

A "deceleration injury" can result when the driver of a moving vehicle strikes a stationary vehicle. The opposite motions occur in this instance, with flexion followed by hyperextension. It is more appropriate to describe whiplash as musculoligamentous sprain or strain of the cervical spine (Edwardson, 1995; Hirsch et al., 1988).

In the *extension phase* of whiplash, damage can occur to the prevertebral muscles, the anterior longitudinal ligament, the intervertebral discs, the odontoid process, the zygapophyseal joints, the spinous processes, the temporomandibular joints, the frontal and temporal lobes of the brain, and the esophagus. In the *flexion phase,* the vertebral bodies, the intervertebral discs, the interspinous ligaments, the zygapophyseal joints, the ligamentum nuchae, and the posterior neck muscles can all be damaged (Bogduk, 1986; Edwardson, 1995). Additionally, nerve root compression has been identified as a result of whiplash (Downs and Twomey, 1979; Edwardson, 1995). See Edwardson (1995) for a more complete discussion of the clinical manifestations of whiplash.

Degenerative Joint Disease

The vertebral column in whole or in part may be affected by degenerative joint diseases. Osteoarthritis is a common affliction of the vertebral column. Substantial lipping of the vertebral bodies can occur. Likewise, the zygapophyseal joints may be affected as well. *Cervical spondylosis* (*spondylosis* = breakdown of vertebral structures) affects up to 40 percent of the population. It can be asymptomatic or may cause compression of cervical spinal nerves. It can affect the intervertebral discs, the vertebral bodies, the zygapophyseal joints, the uncovertebral joints (of Luschka), and the ligaments. It is most frequent at C5-C6 and then C6-C7 (Edwardson, 1995, and references therein).

References

Adams, T, Heisey, RS, Smith, MC, and Briner, BJ (1992). Parietal bone mobility in the anesthetized cat. *Journal of the American Osteopathic Association, 92,* 599–600, 603–610, 615–622.

Ash, MM (1984). *Wheeler's Dental Anatomy, Physiology, and Occlusion.* WB Saunders, Philadelphia.

Bhaskar, SN (1990). *Orban's Oral Histology and Embryology* (11th ed). Mosby-Yearbook Publishers, Chicago.

Bogduk, N (1986). The anatomy and physiology of whiplash. *Clinical Biomechanics, 1,* 92–101.

Breathnach, AS (Ed) (1965). *Frazer's Anatomy of the Human Skeleton* (6th ed). J and A Churchill, London.

Carlsen, BM (1994). *Human Embryology and Developmental Biology.* Mosby, St Louis.

Downs, J, and Twomey, L (1979). The whiplash syndrome. *Australian Journal of Physiotherapy, 25,* 233–241.

Duray, SM, Morter, HB, and Smith, FJ (1999). Morphological variation in cervical spinous processes: Potential applications in forensic identification of race from the skeleton. *Journal of Forensic Sciences, 44,* 937–944.

Edwardson, BM (1995). *Musculoskeletal Disorders: Common Problems.* Singular Publishing Group, San Diego.

Gray, H (1985). *Gray's Anatomy* (30th Am ed). CD Clemente (Ed). Lea and Febiger, Philadelphia.

Gray, H (1995). *Gray's Anatomy* (38th Brit ed). PL Williams, LH Bannister, MM Berry, P Collins, M Dyson, JE Dussek, and MWJ Ferguson (Eds). Churchill Livingstone, New York.

Heisey, SR, and Adams, T (1993). Role of cranial bone mobility in cranial compliance. *Neurosurgery, 33,* 869–877.

Hirsch, SA, Hirsch, PJ, Hiramoto, H, and Weiss, A (1988). Whiplash syndrome: Fact or fiction? *The Orthopedic Clinics of North America, 19,* 791–795.

Krogman, WM (1962). *The Human Skeleton in Forensic Medicine.* Charles C Thomas, Springfield, IL.

McKern, TW, and Stewart, TD (1957). *Skeletal Age Changes in Young American Males* (Technical Report EP-45). US Army Quartermaster Research and Development Center, Natick, MA.

Mercer, S, and Bogduk, N (1999). The ligaments and anulus fibrosus of human adult cervical intervertebral discs. *Spine, 24,* 619–628.

Rogers, JS, and Witt, PL (1997). The controversy of cranial bone motion. *Journal of Orthopaedic and Sports Physical Therapy, 26,* 95–103.

Chapter 5

Bones of the Postcranial Skeleton: The Ribs and Sternum

THE RIBS

The *ribs* are elastic arches of bone that, together with the thoracic vertebrae, the sternum, and the costal cartilages, form the skeleton of the thorax (Figure 5–1). There are 12 pairs of ribs. The first 7 pairs articulate posteriorly with the bodies and transverse processes of the thoracic vertebrae; anteriorly, they articulate with the sternum via their costal cartilages. The costal cartilages are composed of hyaline cartilage. Their dorsal ends articulate with the ventral extremities of ribs 1 through 10. Their ventral ends articulate either with the sternum (ribs 1 through 7) or with the costal cartilage of the rib above them (ribs 8 through 10).

Ribs 1 through 7 are referred to as the *true* or *vertebrosternal ribs*. The remaining five pairs are referred to as the *false ribs*. The costal cartilages of pairs 8 through 10 attach to the costal cartilage of the rib above. They are known as the *vertebrochondral ribs*. Pairs 11 and 12 are known as the *floating ribs*. Their extremities are embedded in the musculature of the posterior thoracic wall. They are tipped with hyaline cartilage but do not articulate with the sternum or other costal cartilages. Furthermore, unlike the cranial 10 pairs of ribs, the 11th and 12th pairs do not articulate with the transverse processes of their corresponding vertebrae.

The description that follows applies to the more typical *3rd through 9th ribs* (Figure 5–2). The 1st and 2nd ribs and the 10th, 11th, and 12th ribs present unique features that diverge from this common pattern.

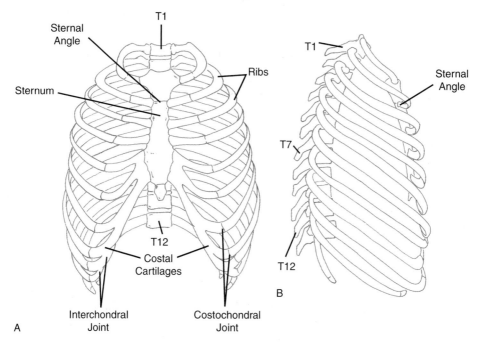

Figure 5-1   The bony thorax: (A) anterior view and (B) lateral view.

Each rib has two extremities, a *dorsal,* or *vertebral, extremity* and a *ventral,* or *sternal, extremity.* The intervening portion of the rib is the *body,* or *shaft.* The dorsal extremity bears a *head,* a *neck,* and a *tubercle* (refer to Fig. 5–2 throughout the discussion of a typical rib).

The *head* bears a kidney-shaped *articular facet* divided into superior and inferior *demifacets* by a horizontal *interarticular crest* (crest of the head). The superior portion of this articular facet is for articulation with the inferior demifacet of a thoracic vertebra, whereas the inferior portion is for articulation with the superior demifacet of the vertebra below. These demifacets on the heads of the ribs vary in their configurations in the same manner as do the costal facets and demifacets of the thoracic vertebrae.

The *neck* is a flattened portion of the rib extending laterally from the head. The ventral surface of the neck is flat and smooth, whereas the dorsal surface is roughened for attachments of various ligaments. It has a cranial and a caudal border. The cranial border bears a rough *crest of the neck* for the attachment of the anterior layer of the superior costotransverse ligament. The caudal border is rounded.

The *tubercle* of the rib is a raised area on the posterior surface of the dorsal extremity at the junction of the neck and the body. It consists of an *articular portion* and a *nonarticular portion.* The articular portion is more caudal and medial; it bears a small oval facet for articulation with the transverse process of the more caudal of the two vertebrae with which the head articulates. The lateral nonarticular portion is roughened and receives the attachment of the lateral costotransverse ligament.

The body of the rib is thin and flat, with an *external* and an *internal surface.* The body has a rounded *superior border* and a sharp *inferior border.* A little beyond the tubercle, the body is marked by a prominent line that gives attachment to a tendon of

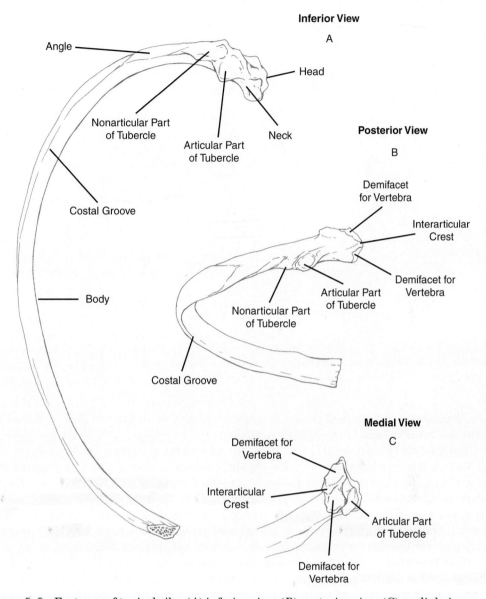

Figure 5-2   Features of typical ribs: (A) inferior view, (B) posterior view, (C) medial view.

the iliocostalis muscle. This is the *angle* of the rib. At the angle of the rib, the shaft turns anteromedially. The distance between the tubercle and the angle progressively increases from the 2nd to the 10th ribs. Along the inferior margin of the internal surface of the rib is the *costal groove*. This groove is on the inferior border of the rib dorsally; just ventral to the angle, it comes to lie on the internal surface of the rib. The superior edge of the groove is rounded and gives attachment to the internal intercostal muscle. The inferior border of the groove, which is also the inferior border of the body of the rib, is sharp. The groove houses the intercostal nerve, artery, and

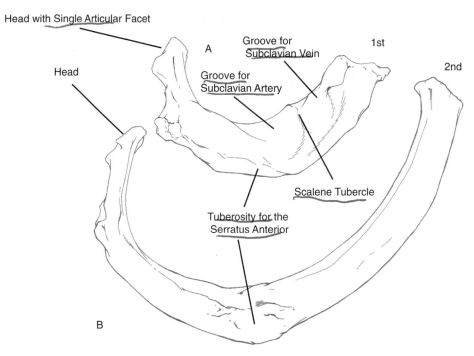

Figure 5-3   (A) The first rib and (B) the second rib, superior view.

vein. The *sternal extremity* of the body is flattened and presents a hollow oval that receives the rounded end of the costal cartilage.

The *first rib* (Figure 5–3) is the most curved and the shortest. It has no angle and the body is flattened horizontally. Its cranial surface is marked by two grooves and the *scalene tubercle.* The scalene tubercle is toward the sternal extremity near the internal edge of the rib and is the site of attachment of the scalenus anterior muscle. It separates two grooves. The ventral groove is the *groove for the subclavian vein,* whereas the more dorsal groove is the *groove for the subclavian artery.* The head bears no interarticular crest; therefore, it has only a single articular facet.

Near the middle of the external surface of the *second rib* (see Fig. 5–3) is a rough *tuberosity for the serratus anterior.* Although the serratus anterior attaches along the external surface of the first eight or nine ribs, its attachment to the second rib is particularly well marked.

The 10th rib is similar to typical ribs except that there is usually no interarticular crest at the head, so that it has a single articular facet. The *11th and 12th ribs* (Figure 5–4) are the floating ribs. Each has a single, large articular facet on the head and no interarticular crest. These ribs also have no neck or tubercle. The 11th has a slight angle and a shallow costal groove, whereas the 12th demonstrates neither.

THE STERNUM

The *sternum* (Figure 5–5; see also Fig. 5–1) is composed of three parts: the manubrium, the body (or gladiolus), and the xiphoid process.

Figure 5-4 (A) The 10th rib, (B) the 11th rib, and (C) the 12th rib.

The *manubrium* is the most superior part of the sternum. At the center of its superior border is the *jugular (suprasternal) notch.* On either side of the jugular notch are the *clavicular notches,* which bear facets for articulations with the sternal ends of the clavicles.

The *body* is the largest portion of the sternum and is composed of four *sternebrae,* or segments, that become fused in adulthood. The manubrium joins the body of the sternum at the *sternal angle* (angle of Louis), an important anatomical landmark. At the sternal angle, the second costal cartilages articulate with both the manubrium and the body. The costal cartilages are composed of hyaline cartilage and run between the sternum and the ventral extremities of the ribs.

Because the second ribs lie at the level of the easily palpable sternal angle, the ribs can be counted with accuracy in the living subject. On either side of the sternum are seven *costal notches* for articulations with the costal cartilages. There is one complete costal notch and one half notch on either side of the manubrium. There are four complete notches and two half notches on each side of the body. The xiphoid process also possesses a half notch for the costal cartilage of the seventh rib on each side.

The most inferior and smallest segment of the sternum is the *xiphoid process.* It is thin and elongated. It is cartilaginous throughout youth and progressively ossifies with age. It may remain partly cartilaginous, however, throughout life. It articulates with the body of the sternum at the *xiphisternal junction.* The costal cartilages of the seventh ribs articulate with the xiphoid process.

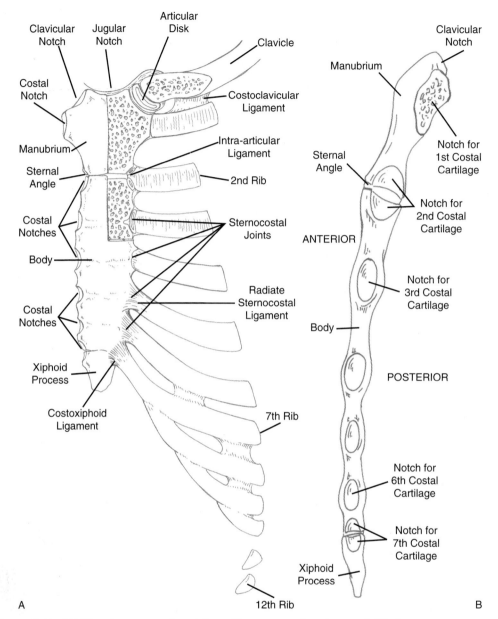

Figure 5–5   (A) The sternum and costal cartilages, anterior view, and (B) the sternum, lateral view.

ARTICULATIONS OF THE RIBS
The Costovertebral Joints

The *costovertebral joints* (Figure 5–6) are usually described as plane synovial joints. They allow gliding movement. The fibrous *articular capsule* surrounds the head of the rib and the socket formed by the demifacets on the cranial and caudal vertebrae and their intervertebral disc. The *synovial cavity* is divided in two by the *intra-articular ligament* for ribs 2 to 9, which articulate with two vertebral bodies, and is single for ribs 1, 10, 11, and 12, which articulate with a single large costal facet on a single vertebral body. The intra-articular ligament consists of short fibers extending from the interarticular crest of the head of the rib to the intervertebral disc. Joints of ribs 1, 10, 11, and 12 do not have intra-articular ligaments.

The *radiate ligaments* attach the anterior parts of each costal head to the bodies of two vertebrae and their intervertebral disc. The radiate ligament always attaches to two vertebrae even if the rib articulates with only a single vertebra; for example, the first rib articulates with T1 only, but the radiate ligament of the first rib attaches to both C7 and T1.

Costotransverse Joints

The *costotransverse joints* (see Fig. 5–6) are formed by the tubercle of the rib articulating with the *transverse costal facet* of the transverse process of a thoracic vertebra. These are also plane synovial joints, which allow sliding motion. A rib articulates with the transverse process of its corresponding vertebrae; for example, the 10th rib articulates with the transverse process of the 10th thoracic vertebra. There are no costotransverse joints associated with T11 and T12.

Each costotransverse joint is surrounded by a fibrous articular capsule. The capsule surrounds the tubercle of the rib and the transverse costal facet of the vertebra. In addition to the articular capsule, these joints are strengthened by three other ligaments:

- The superior costotransverse ligament
- The costotransverse ligament
- The lateral costotransverse ligament

The *superior costotransverse ligament* runs from the neck of the rib to the transverse process above it. Each ligament is composed of an *anterior* and a *posterior layer.* The anterior layer extends from the crest of the neck of the rib to the lower border of the transverse process above it and the posterior layer extends from the dorsal aspect of the rib's neck. The first rib possesses no superior costotransverse ligament. The 12th rib possesses an additional *lumbocostal ligament* that extends from the neck of the 12th rib to the base of the transverse process of the first lumbar vertebra.

The *costotransverse ligament,* or ligament of the neck of the rib (see Fig. 5–6), extends from the dorsal aspect of the neck posteriorly to the anterior surface of the adjacent transverse process. This ligament may be absent or rudimentary on the 11th and 12th ribs.

The *lateral costotransverse ligament,* or ligament of the tubercle of the rib (see Fig. 5–6) extends from the apex of the transverse process to the tubercle of the corresponding rib. This ligament is not present for ribs 11 and 12.

Joints of the Costal Cartilages

The joints of the *costal cartilages* are as follows:

- The sternocostal joints
- The interchondral joints
- The costochondral joints

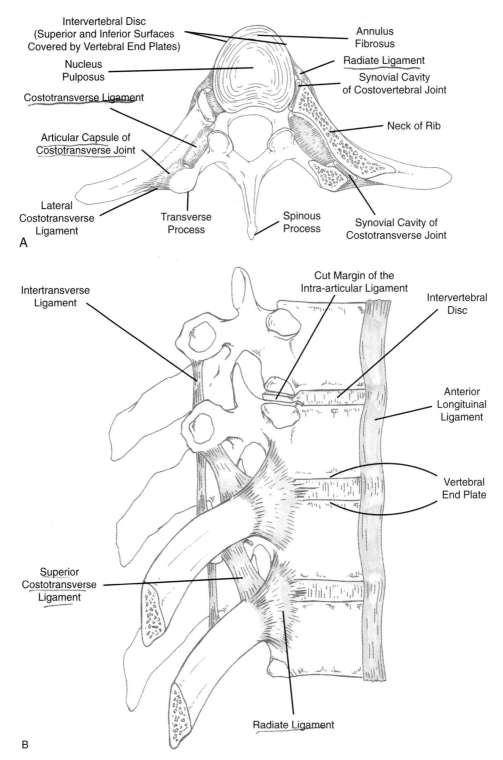

Figure 5-6   (A) Ligaments of the ribs and the intervertebral disc and (B) articulations of the ribs and thoracic vertebrae.

The *sternocostal joints* (see Figs. 5–1 and 5–5) occur between the costal notches of the sternum and the ventral ends of the costal cartilages. The first sternocostal joint is a synchondrosis, an immovable joint composed of hyaline cartilage. The second through seventh sternocostal joints are plane synovial joints. They possess a fibrous articular capsule and three ligaments:

- The radiate sternocostal ligament
- The intra-articular ligament (only at 2nd and sometimes 3rd costochondral joints)
- The costoxiphoid ligament (only at 7th costochondral joint)

The *radiate sternocostal ligament* extends from the sternal extremity of the costal cartilages to the anterior and posterior borders of the sternum. The *intra-articular ligaments* are constant only between the second costal cartilages and the sternum. The intra-articular ligaments extend from the costal cartilage to the symphysis between the manubrium and the body of the sternum. Thus it is intra-articular. Occasionally, there may be intra-articular ligaments associated with the third costal cartilages. The *costoxiphoid ligaments* connect the anterior and posterior surfaces of the seventh costal cartilage with the same surfaces of the xiphoid process. Slight movements occur at the sternocostal joints with respiration.

The *interchondral joints* (see Fig. 5–1A) are found between the 6th, 7th, 8th, 9th, and 10th costal cartilages as they articulate with each other. Those between the 6th to 9th cartilages are plane synovial joints. They are enclosed by thin fibrous articular capsules and strengthened by medial and lateral interchondral ligaments. The joint between the 9th and the 10th costal cartilages is never synovial and is sometimes absent.

The *costochondral joints* (see Fig. 5–1A) are synchondroses occurring between the ventral extremities of the ribs and their costal cartilages. The costal cartilages are persistent, unossified anterior parts of cartilaginous models preceding fully developed ribs. When separated at their junctions, the end of the costal cartilage is rounded, whereas the ventral end of the rib is depressed. The periosteum and the perichondrium are continuous across this junction. No movement occurs at these joints.

ARTICULATIONS OF THE STERNUM

The articulations of the sternum (see Figs. 5–1 and 5–5) are as follows:

- The manubriosternal joint
- The xiphisternal joint
- The sternoclavicular joints
- The sternocostal joints (discussed with joints of the costal cartilages)

The *manubriosternal joint* is a symphysis joint between the manubrium and the body of the sternum. It is located at the sternal angle. It may occasionally ossify in later life. The *xiphisternal joint* is also a symphysis, at the junction of the body of the sternum with the xiphoid process. It is usually ossified by age 40. The *sternoclavicular joints* are located between the clavicles, the clavicular notches on the superior border of the manubrium, and the costal cartilages of the first ribs. At each joint is an *articular disc* that divides the joint into two synovial cavities. These are *sellar synovial joints,* saddle-shaped joints that permit circumduction. Each joint is surrounded by a fibrous articular capsule. In addition, the joints are strengthened by several ligaments, which include the following:

- The anterior sternoclavicular ligament
- The posterior sternoclavicular ligament
- The interclavicular ligament
- The costoclavicular ligament

The *anterior sternoclavicular ligament* attaches to the anterior surface of the clavicle, the manubrium, and the first costal cartilage. The *posterior sternoclavicular ligament* covers the posterior surface of the joint. It runs from the posterior surface of the clavicle's sternal end to the posterior aspect of the upper manubrium. The *interclavicular ligament* unites the superior aspects of the sternal ends of both clavicles with one another. Some fibers attach to the superior margin of the manubrium. The *costoclavicular ligament* unites the upper part of the first rib and costal cartilage with the inferior medial surface of the clavicle.

Movement at the sternoclavicular joint occurs in conjunction with movements of the pectoral girdle and upper limbs. The joint moves anteriorly, posteriorly, and vertically and allows the lateral end of the clavicle to be raised for full elevation of the upper limb (Gray, 1995).

OSSIFICATION OF THE RIBS AND STERNUM

The Ribs

The cartilage models for the ribs are present by the 8th week in utero. At the same time, a primary center of ossification appears near the angle of the rib, usually appearing first in the 6th and 7th ribs. Three secondary centers also develop: one for the head of the rib, one for the articular portion of the tubercle of the rib, and one for the nonarticular portion of the tubercle of the rib. These secondary centers develop postnatally. They appear between 16 and 20 years of age and synostose with the rib by age 25. The 1st rib and ribs 7 to 10 have only one epiphysis for the tubercle; the 11th and 12th lack centers for the tubercle (Breathnach, 1965; Gray, 1985, 1995).

The Sternum

The sternum (Figure 5–7) is initially represented by two parallel but widely separated mesenchymal bars called the *sternal bars*. At about the 6th week in utero, the superior ends of the bars approach one another and unite; they then fuse increasingly with one another, progressing inferiorly. Ossification of the sternum begins with the manubrium in the 5th or 6th week in utero; the manubrium frequently has two centers of ossification. The body has four centers of ossification, the first appearing at 6 months in utero, the second at 7 months in utero, the third at 8 or 9 months in utero, and the fourth at birth or within the first year.

The xiphoid process has a single center of ossification that appears between ages 5 and 18. Two small *episternal centers of ossification* may appear on either side of the jugular notch and are probably vestiges of the *episternal bone* of lower vertebrates.

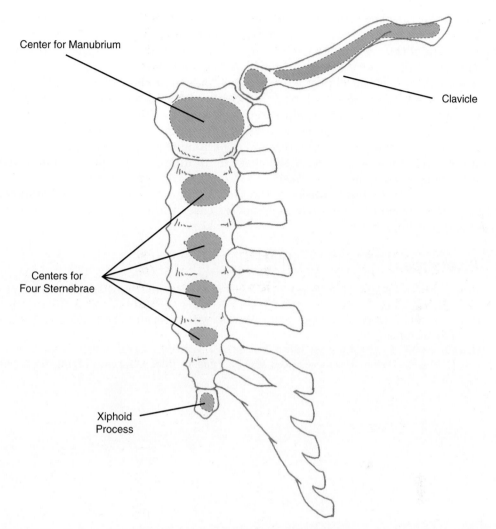

Figure 5–7   Centers of ossification of the sternum and the clavicle.

The separate ossification centers of the sternum before their synostosis with one another are known as *sternebrae*. Synostosis of the sternebrae usually begins inferiorly and works its way superiorly. By age 25 the four segments of the sternal body have synostosed. The xiphoid process synostoses with the body of the sternum most frequently after age 40, although it may occur well earlier than that. After adulthood, the manubriosternal joint may synostose in up to 10 percent of the population (Gray, 1985). Generally, the synostosis is only superficial, and remnants of the cartilaginous symphysis remain internally (Breathnach, 1965; Gray, 1985, 1995).

DISORDERS OF THE RIBS AND STERNUM

The ribs are noticeably affected by *rickets*. In rickets, the ends of the ribs adjoining the costal cartilage become enlarged. This condition is referred to as "rachitic rosary." In mild cases, the enlargement may be restricted to the internal aspect of the thorax.

Lateral to the costochondral junction, the ribs may become bowed and depressed, leaving a groove to either side of the sternum. The sternum is often forced outward by the bowing of the ribs, increasing the anteroposterior diameter of the thorax. This forward projection of the sternum is known as "pigeon breast."

"Funnel breast" is the opposite condition of "pigeon breast." It occurs in both patients with rickets and those with no evidence of rickets. In "funnel breast," the inferior end of the sternum is deeply depressed posteriorly.

Phthisical chest is sometimes associated with pulmonary tuberculosis. In this condition, the ribs show great obliquity and the scapulae are projecting. Another condition involving an enlargement of the chest in all dimensions and associated with pulmonary emphysema is *barrel chest*.

Scoliosis or other abnormalities of the thoracic spinal curvature may distort the shapes of the ribs and thoracic cavity. In severe cases these conditions may compromise heart and lung functions.

References

Breathnach, AS (Ed) (1965). *Frazer's Anatomy of the Human Skeleton* (6th ed). J and A Churchill, London.

Gray, H (1985). *Gray's Anatomy* (30th Am ed). CD Clemente (Ed). Lea and Febiger, Philadelphia.

Gray, H (1995). *Gray's Anatomy* (38th Brit ed). PL Williams, LH Bannister, MM Berry, P Collins, M Dyson, JE Dussek, and MWJ Ferguson (Eds). Churchill Livingstone, New York.

Chapter 6

Bones of the Postcranial Skeleton: The Upper Limb

The *upper limb* is attached to the trunk through the pectoral girdle (Figure 6–1). The pectoral girdle consists of the scapula and clavicle, whereas the upper limb consists of the humerus of the arm (brachium), the radius and ulna of the forearm (antebrachium), the carpal bones of the wrist (carpus), and the metacarpals and phalanges of the hand (manus).

THE PECTORAL GIRDLE

The *pectoral girdle* consists of two bones, the scapula and the clavicle. The upper limb attaches to the trunk via the glenohumeral joint between the glenoid fossa of the scapula and the head of the humerus. The upper limb is attached to the axial skeleton via the clavicle, which articulates distally with the acromion process of the scapula and proximally with the manubrium of the sternum. This sternoclavicular joint is the sole bony attachment of the upper limb to the axial skeleton.

The Clavicle

The *clavicle* (Figure 6–2; see also Fig. 6–1) forms the ventral portion of the pectoral girdle. It is a long bone, curved somewhat like the letter S, and situated almost

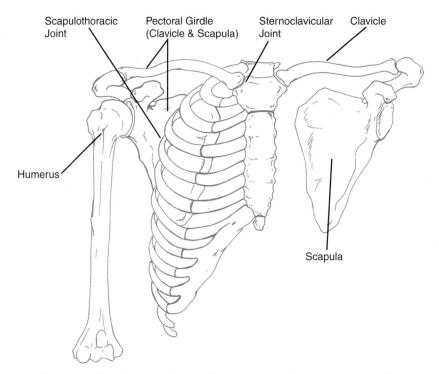

Figure 6-1 The pectoral girdle and thorax. The clavicle and scapula are visible on the right; the pectoral girdle is seen on the left in relationship to the bony thorax and the upper limb.

horizontally above the first rib. It has a sternal extremity and an acromial extremity. The double curve of the bone lies in the horizontal plane. The medial curve occupies approximately the medial two-thirds of the bone and has a posterior concavity. The lateral curve has an anterior concavity that is shorter and sharper than its medial counterpart. It occupies the lateral one-third of the bone. The medial two-thirds of the shaft of the clavicle is rounded, whereas the lateral one-third is flattened. The *sternal extremity* of the clavicle presents a small facet for articulation with the clavicular notch of the manubrium. The flattened *acromial extremity* bears a facet for articulation with the acromion process of the scapula.

The inferior aspect of the clavicle is readily identifiable by its markings for ligamentous attachments. Chief among these are the *impression for the costoclavicular ligament* on the inferior aspect of the sternal extremity, the *groove for the subclavius muscle* along the inferior surface of the midshaft, the *conoid tubercle* on the inferior surface at the dorsal border near the acromial extremity, and the *trapezoid line,* also on the inferior surface of the acromial extremity, running from the conoid tubercle ventrally and laterally. The conoid tubercle and trapezoid line provide attachment for the conoid and trapezoid ligaments, respectively. These two ligaments constitute the *coracoclavicular ligament,* which binds the clavicle to the scapula.

The Scapula

The *scapula* (refer to Figures 6–3 through 6–5 throughout the discussion of the scapula) is a flat bone lying on the posterolateral aspect of the superior part of the

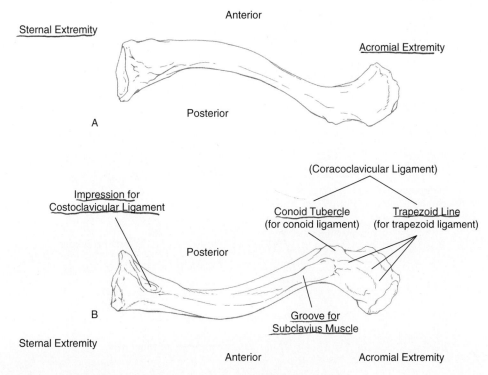

Figure 6-2   The right clavicle: (*A*) superior and (*B*) inferior views.

thorax. Superiorly, it articulates with the acromial extremity of the clavicle; laterally, it articulates with the head of the humerus. It has *three borders, three angles,* and *two surfaces.* The borders are termed *superior, vertebral* or *medial,* and *axillary* or *lateral.* The angles are *superior, inferior,* and *lateral.* The surfaces are *dorsal* and *ventral (costal).*

The *ventral surface* is concave and forms the *subscapular fossa,* the origin of the subscapularis muscle. The ventral surface has a raised rim along its vertebral border that is the origin of the serratus anterior muscle. The most prominent feature of the *dorsal surface* is the *scapular spine.* The spine divides the dorsal surface into a smaller *supraspinous fossa* for origin of the supraspinatus muscle and a much larger *infraspinous fossa* for the origin of the infraspinatus muscle. The lateral end of the spine is free as the large *acromion process,* which arises posterior to the *glenoid fossa* of the lateral angle. Deep to the acromion and posterior to the glenoid fossa is the *greater scapular notch.* The acromion process projects ventrally, cranially, and laterally. It bears a small facet for articulation with the lateral end of the clavicle.

The spine begins on the dorsal surface of the vertebral border. The *base* of the spine is located here at approximately the junction of the superior one-third and the inferior two-thirds of the vertebral border of the scapula. The levator scapulae muscle attaches along the vertebral border superior to the base of the spine. The rhomboideus minor muscle attaches to the vertebral border at the base of the spine, whereas the rhomboideus major attaches along the remaining inferior portion of the vertebral border inferior to the base of the spine.

Along the dorsal surface of the axillary border are markings for the origins of the teres major and teres minor muscles. They run from the inferior angle to the

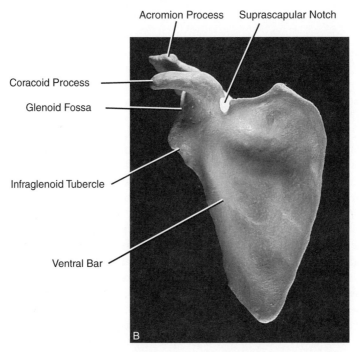

Figure 6-3   (A) Line drawing of the right scapula, ventral (costal) surface. (B) Photograph of the costal surface of the scapula.

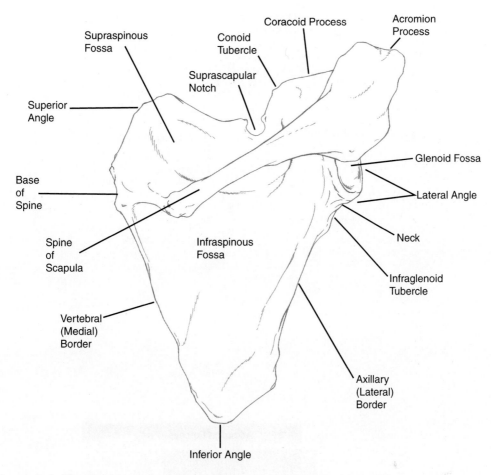

Figure 6-4   The right scapula, dorsal surface.

infraglenoid tubercle at the lateral angle. On the costal surface of the lateral border is a structural thickening, the *ventral bar* of the scapula. It runs from the glenoid fossa to the inferior angle.

The superior border is sharp in the medial portion and presents a marked *suprascapular notch* for the suprascapular nerve. This is bridged by the suprascapular ligament, which is occasionally ossified, transforming the notch into a foramen. Arising lateral to the suprascapular notch is the fingerlike *coracoid process,* which projects superiorly and then sharply bends laterally to project above the glenoid fossa. Attaching to the coracoid process are the trapezoid and conoid ligaments. On the superior surface of the bend or "knuckle" of the coracoid process is a small, roughened tubercle for attachment of the conoid ligament. This is the *conoid tubercle* of the scapula. The coracoacromial ligament runs between the coracoid process and the acromion process. The coracobrachialis, short head of the biceps brachii, and pectoralis minor all attach to the coracoid process.

The lateral angle of the scapula is not "pointed" like the superior and inferior angles and is dominated by the glenoid fossa. The glenoid fossa is oval and concave. It faces laterally and articulates with the head of the humerus. The glenoid fossa is

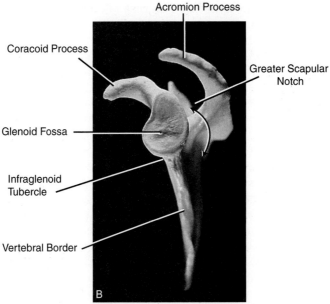

Figure 6-5   (*A*) The right scapula: axillary border demonstrating features of the lateral angle. (*B*) Photograph of the left scapula demonstrating the same features.

covered by hyaline articular cartilage and is connected with the body of the scapula by a somewhat constricted *neck.* At its apex, near the base of the coracoid process, is a slight elevation, the *supraglenoid tubercle,* to which the long head of the biceps brachii is attached.

The *infraglenoid tubercle* is located immediately inferior to the glenoid fossa. It is a rough triangular impression about an inch long that begins at the inferior border of the glenoid fossa and proceeds inferiorly along the lateral border. It is the origin of the long head of the triceps brachii.

BONES OF THE UPPER LIMB

The upper limb is divisible into the arm, the forearm, the wrist (carpus), and the hand (manus). The *arm (brachium)* is the more proximal portion of the limb, between the shoulder and the elbow. The *forearm (antebrachium)* is the portion of the upper limb from the elbow to the wrist. The humerus is the bone of the brachium, whereas the radius and ulna are the two bones of the antebrachium.

The Humerus

The *humerus* (Figure 6–6) is the large bone forming the skeleton of the upper arm, or brachium. It consists of a proximal head, a shaft (or body), and a distal extremity.

Humerus: The Proximal End

When held in anatomical position, the *head* faces medially, somewhat posteriorly and superiorly. The head is joined to the rest of the shaft by a slightly restricted *anatomical neck.* The head of the humerus articulates with the glenoid fossa of the scapula. Just distal to the head of the humerus and separated from it by the anatomical neck are two raised processes, the *greater and lesser tubercles* (sometimes referred to as *tuberosities*), which are the site of muscular attachments.

On the anterior surface of the shaft of the humerus is the *lesser tubercle.* On the lateral aspect of the proximal shaft and separated from the lesser tubercle by the *intertubercular sulcus* (or *bicipital groove)* is the *greater tubercle.* The lesser tubercle is the site of insertion of the subscapularis muscle, whereas the greater tubercle receives the supraspinatus, infraspinatus, and teres minor muscles. The intertubercular sulcus is a passageway for the tendon of the long head of the biceps brachii muscle as it passes through the capsule of the glenohumeral joint. Just distal to the greater and lesser tubercles, the shaft of the humerus narrows. This is referred to as the *surgical neck* of the humerus. The surgical neck is a common site of fractures, and fractures here can damage the anterior and posterior humeral circumflex arteries and the axillary nerve that supplies part of the shoulder region and adjacent structures.

Humerus: The Shaft

The *shaft* of the humerus runs from the surgical neck to the medial and lateral epicondyles at the distal end of the bone. On the anterior aspect of the superior portion of the shaft is the continuation of the intertubercular sulcus. It is demarcated by *medial* and *lateral lips* that are continuous with the lesser and greater tubercles,

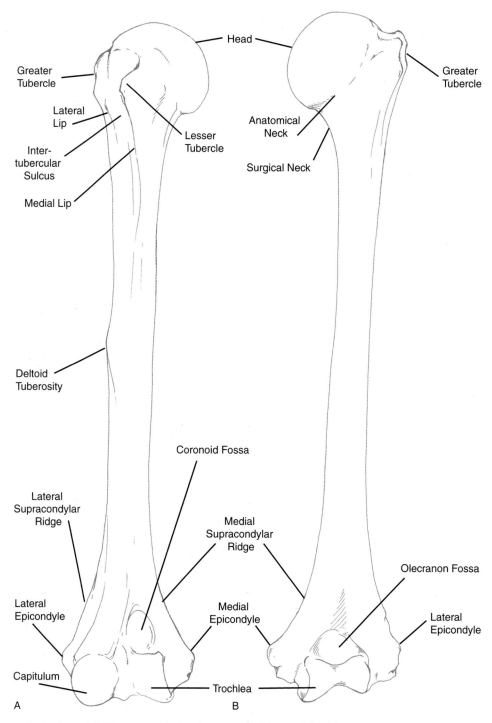

Figure 6-6   The right humerus: (*A*) anterior and (*B*) posterior views.

respectively. The medial lip of the groove has rough markings for the insertion of the teres major muscle, whereas the lateral lip is a site of attachment for the pectoralis major muscle. The latissimus dorsi muscle inserts into the floor of this shallow groove between the sites of attachment of the teres major and pectoralis major. The lateral lip of the intertubercular sulcus continues inferiorly to the anterior part of the *deltoid tuberosity,* on the lateral aspect of the shaft. The deltoid muscle inserts here.

Nearly opposite the deltoid tuberosity, on the medial aspect of the shaft, is the *impression for the insertion of the coracobrachialis muscle.* Generally, this is slightly more distal on the shaft than is the deltoid tuberosity. The *radial sulcus* is a shallow, ill-defined impression on the posterior aspect of the shaft. It passes from superomedial to inferolateral across the posterosuperior part of the humeral shaft between the sites of origin of the lateral head of the triceps superolaterally and the medial head of the triceps inferomedially. The radial nerve and the profunda brachii artery run in this groove under cover of the triceps muscle.

Humerus: The Distal End

The distal end of the humerus is broad mediolaterally and consists, more superiorly, of medial and lateral epicondyles, and inferiorly, of articular surfaces for the ulna and the radius: the trochlea and the capitulum.

The *medial* and *lateral epicondyles* are raised protuberances located at either side of the distal end of the humerus superior to the distal articular surfaces. Proceeding superiorly from the medial and lateral epicondyles are *medial* and *lateral supracondylar (epicondylar) ridges,* at the medial and lateral borders of the distal shaft, respectively. The medial epicondyle and medial epicondylar ridge serve as a common origin for the superficial flexor muscles in the forearm, whereas the lateral epicondyle and epicondylar ridge serve a similar function for the superficial extensor muscles in the forearm. The posterior surface of the medial epicondyle is marked by a groove for the ulnar nerve.

The distal articular surface of the humerus is divided into two portions, the trochlea and the capitulum. The *trochlea* is larger and is located more medially. As its name implies, it is somewhat spool shaped and consists of a deep groove defined by two well-marked borders. It receives the trochlear notch of the ulna; together, they form a hinge joint. The trochlea protrudes somewhat anteriorly, and most of its articular surface is located anteriorly and inferiorly.

Superior to the trochlea on the anterior humeral surface is the *coronoid fossa,* which receives the coronoid process of the ulna during flexion. Posterior to the trochlea is the much larger *olecranon fossa,* which receives the end of the olecranon process of the ulna during extension. The bone in the olecranon fossa is very thin and is sometimes perforated by a supratrochlear foramen. The *capitulum* is the smaller of the two distal articular surfaces and is located laterally. It is smooth and rounded and is only about half the width of the trochlea. It articulates distally with the central fossa of the head of the radius. The elbow joint is formed by articulations between the trochlea and ulna, capitulum and radius, and radial head and ulna.

The Radius

The *radius* (Figure 6–7) consists of a proximal head, shaft, and distal extremity ending in a *styloid process,* or pointed projection. It has four articular surfaces. Its proximal extremity has a surface for articulation with the capitulum of the humerus and a surface for its proximal articulation with the ulna. Distally, the radius has one articular surface for articulation with the carpus, or wrist bones, and one for its distal articulation with the ulna.

Radius: The Proximal End

The proximal end of the radius can be divided into a head, radial neck, radial tuberosity, and articular circumference. The *radial head* is an expanded disc with a central fossa for articulation with the capitulum of the humerus. Surrounding the head of the radius is a ring of subchondral bone that rests in the radial notch of the ulna, forming the *proximal radioulnar joint.* Distal to the head is a short, constricted region of the proximal shaft termed the *radial neck.* Distal to the neck, on the anteromedial part of the shaft, is the *radial (bicipital) tuberosity,* the site of the insertion of the tendon of the biceps brachii muscle. The bicipital tuberosity has a rough portion for the actual muscle insertion and a smooth portion for a bursa underlying the biceps tendon.

Radius: The Shaft

The proximal end of the radius attaches by its neck to the *radial shaft.* The shaft is more cylindrical superiorly but becomes broadened and flattened distally. The shaft has a smooth, rounded *lateral border* and a sharp, medial *interosseous crest.* To this interosseous crest attaches an interosseous membrane, which also attaches to a similar interosseous crest on the lateral aspect of the ulna. The interosseous crest continues for most of the length of the bone and ends in a small triangular area just superior to the *ulnar notch.* The ulnar notch is just superior to the distal articular surface of the radius. The ulnar notch articulates with the head of the ulna; together, they form the *distal radioulnar joint.*

Approximately one-third of the way from the proximal end of the bone on its anterior surface is the *nutrient foramen,* which is directed proximally. Running inferolaterally from the bicipital tuberosity across the anterior aspect of the shaft is the *anterior oblique line.* In a similar position on the posterior aspect of the shaft is the *posterior oblique line.* The flexor digitorum superficialis muscle arises from the anterior oblique line. Distal to the anterior oblique line is a hollow for the origin of the flexor pollicis longus muscle. The posterior oblique line divides the area of attachment of the supinator muscle superiorly from the area of attachment of the abductor pollicis longus muscle inferiorly.

Radius: The Distal End

At the *distal end* of the radius is a large articular surface for the *carpus* (wrist bones); a lateral, distally projecting *styloid process;* and a series of ridges and grooves on its posterior surface for the passage of tendons of the extensor muscles of the hand from the posterior compartment of the forearm to their distal sites of attachment.

The *carpal articular surface* of the radius is located at the distal end of the bone. It may be divided into two portions by a slight ridge or other surface irregularities. The medial portion is for articulation with the *lunate bone,* whereas the lateral portion is for the *scaphoid bone.* The articular surface of the ulnar notch is continuous with the carpal articular surface, the two surfaces meeting at an angle of

Figure 6-7   The right radius and ulna: (*A*) anterior and (*B*) posterior views.

approximately 90 degrees. The lateral aspect of the distal end comes to a projecting distal point, the *styloid process*. The radial collateral ligament of the wrist joint attaches to this process. The styloid process is also the distal attachment site of the brachioradialis muscle. The posterior aspect of the styloid process is marked by two slight grooves; the more lateral is the *groove for the extensor carpi radialis longus,* whereas the more medial is the *groove for the extensor carpi radialis brevis.*

The central region of the posterior aspect of the distal end of the radius is characterized by a raised area, known as the *extensor retinaculum tubercle* or *Lister's tubercle.* Medial to this is the prominent *groove for the extensor pollicis longus.* Medial to this groove is a second broad groove, the *groove for the tendons of the extensor digitorum* and the *extensor indicis.* Most medial is a third groove, the *groove for the tendon of the extensor digiti minimi.* This groove is completed by articulation with the head of the ulna. Lateral to Lister's tubercle are the posterior surface of the styloid process and the *grooves for the extensor carpi radialis longus* and *brevis tendons.*

The Ulna

The principal parts of the *ulna* (see Fig. 6–7) are the proximal olecranon process and the coronoid process, which contain the trochlear notch for articulation with the humerus, the shaft, and the distal ulnar head and ulnar styloid process.

Ulna: The Proximal End

The proximal end of the ulna is composed of two prominent projections, the olecranon process and the coronoid process, and two concave articular facets, the trochlear notch and the radial notch. The *olecranon process* is the proximal extension of the shaft of the ulna, and it forms the point of the elbow. Its posterior surface receives the large triceps tendon. It has a rough, more posterior portion for the actual tendon insertion and a smoother, more anterior portion for a subtendinous bursa. The *coronoid process* projects from the proximal and anterior surface of the shaft of the ulna. Its proximal surface is smooth and concave and forms the distal part of the trochlear notch of the ulna.

At the junction of the coronoid process and the shaft of the ulna is the *ulnar tuberosity,* to which attaches the tendon of the brachialis muscle. On the lateral surface of the coronoid process is the *radial notch* of the ulna. This notch receives the circumferential articular surface of the radial head; together they form the *proximal radioulnar joint.* The *trochlear notch (semilunar notch)* is a large depression formed by the coronoid and olecranon processes. It articulates with the trochlea of the humerus.

Ulna: The Shaft

The *shaft,* or body, of the ulna is three sided. Its most prominent feature is the *interosseous crest* along its lateral margin. An interosseous membrane attaches here and to the interosseous crest of the radius. The nutrient foramen of the ulna is usually located on the anterior surface of the proximal portion of the shaft. The *oblique line* separates the origin of the flexor digitorum profundus muscle from the origin of the pronator quadratus muscle. It is usually located in the distal one-fifth of the anterior surface of the shaft and runs distomedially.

The posterior surface of the ulna is divided along most of its length by a low ridge. The more medial area is occupied by the origin of the extensor carpi ulnaris. From proximal to distal, the more lateral area is occupied by the origins of three muscles: the abductor pollicis longus, the extensor pollicis longus, and the extensor indicis. Each occupies about one-third of this area, and slight separations of their origins may be detectable.

Ulna: The Distal End

The distal end of the ulna is its *head* (just the opposite of the radius). The head is composed of subchondral bone and is separated from the *ulnar styloid process* by a deep groove. To this groove attaches an intra-articular disc that separates the ulnar head from the carpal bones. The distal surface of the ulnar head is in contact with the intra-articular disc, whereas its *articular circumference* articulates with the ulnar notch of the radius at the *distal radioulnar joint.* On the posterior surface of the distal end of the ulna is a groove that becomes continuous with the groove between the head and the ulnar styloid process. This is the *groove for the tendon of the extensor carpi ulnaris muscle.*

The Hand

The skeleton of the *hand (manus)* (Figure 6–8) is composed of 27 bones consisting of three groups: the carpal bones, the metacarpal bones, and the phalanges. The *carpal bones* are most proximal; they form the wrist and articulate proximally with the radius. The *metacarpals* are a set of five small, long bones. They are numbered I through V from the radial side. Their bases articulate with the distal row of carpal bones, and their heads articulate with the proximal phalanges of each digit. Each digit has three *phalanges*—a proximal, a middle, and a distal—with the exception of the thumb, or *pollex.* The thumb has only two phalanges: the proximal and the distal.

Hand: The Carpus

The *carpus (wrist)* consists of eight small, irregularly shaped bones (Figure 6–9; refer also to Fig. 6–8 throughout the discussion of the carpal bones) arranged in two rows: a proximal and a distal. They are closely applied to one another and are held firmly in their rows by strong ligaments. As a whole, they form a strong fibrous and bony mass that is concave on the palmar side and convex dorsally. Each row consists of four bones. The *proximal row* consists, laterally to medially, of (1) the scaphoid, (2) the lunate, (3) the triquetrum (triangle), and (4) the pisiform. The *distal row* consists, laterally to medially, of (5) the trapezium, (6) the trapezoid, (7) the capitate, and (8) the hamate.

The *scaphoid* articulates medially with the lunate; proximally with the radius; and distally with the trapezium, trapezoid, and capitate. It is the largest bone of the proximal row. On the lateral part of the palmar surface of the scaphoid is its *tubercle,* to which attaches the flexor retinaculum. Some older texts may refer to the scaphoid as the *navicular.*

The *lunate* articulates laterally with the scaphoid, medially with the triquetrum, superiorly with the radius and the intra-articular disc, and inferiorly with the capitate and a small area of the hamate. The lunate may be distinguished by its deep concavity and crescentic outline. Its proximal surface is convex and smooth; it

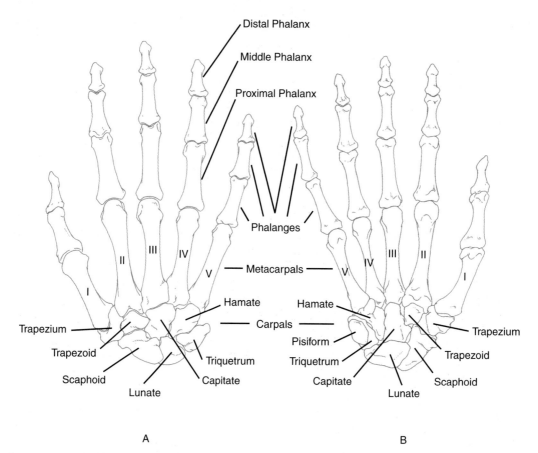

A   B

Figure 6-8 The skeleton of the right hand: (*A*) posterior or dorsal and (*B*) anterior or palmar views.

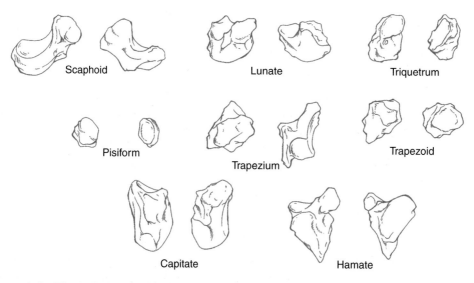

Figure 6-9 The individual carpal bones of the right hand.

articulates with the radius. Its distal surface is deeply concave; it articulates with the head of the capitate.

The *triquetrum* articulates laterally with the lunate and anteriorly with the pisiform. Inferiorly it articulates with the hamate and superiorly with the intra-articular disc at the distal ulna. It is pyramid-shaped and may be distinguished by an isolated oval facet for articulation with the pisiform bone.

The *pisiform* is a very small, more or less pea-shaped bone; it articulates posteriorly with the triquetrum. It "sits" on the palmar surface of the triquetrum. It is easily distinguished by its small size, oval shape, and single articular facet. The flexor carpi ulnaris, abductor digiti minimi, and flexor retinaculum all attach to this small bone.

The *trapezium* articulates medially with the trapezoid, superiorly with the scaphoid, inferiorly with the first metacarpal, and with a small area of the base of the second metacarpal. It may be distinguished by a deep groove on its palmar surface, which transmits the tendon of the flexor carpi radialis muscle, and its saddle-shaped articular surface for the base of the first metacarpal.

The *trapezoid* articulates laterally with the trapezium and medially with the capitate. Superiorly it articulates with the scaphoid and inferiorly with the second metacarpal. The trapezoid is the smallest bone in the distal row. It can be identified by its wedge shape; the broad end of the wedge is its dorsal surface, whereas the narrow end is its palmar surface.

The *capitate* articulates laterally with the trapezoid and medially with the hamate. Superiorly it articulates with the scaphoid and lunate. Inferiorly it articulates primarily with the third metacarpal but also with the second and fourth. It occupies the center of the wrist and is easily identified as the largest of the carpal bones. It has a rounded portion or *head* that is received into the concavity formed by the scaphoid and lunate bones. Distal to the head is a constricted *neck* that connects the head to the capitate *body*.

The *hamate* articulates laterally with the capitate, superiorly with the triquetrum and lunate, and inferiorly with the fourth and fifth metacarpals. It is readily identified by the hooklike process that projects from its palmar surface, the *hamulus*. To the apex of the hamulus attach the flexor retinaculum and the flexor carpi ulnaris. It is one of four eminences on the palmar aspect of the carpus to which the flexor retinaculum attaches. The other three attachments of the flexor retinaculum are the pisiform medially and the oblique ridge of the trapezium and the tubercle of the scaphoid laterally.

Hand: The Metacarpus

The *metacarpus* is formed by the five *metacarpal bones* (see Fig. 6–8). Each of the five metacarpal bones has a *shaft,* a proximal *base,* and a distal *head.* With the exception of the first metacarpal (for the thumb), each base has articular facets on its sides for articulation with the bases of adjacent metacarpals. On the proximal surface of the base of each is an articular facet for the particular carpal bone(s) with which that metacarpal articulates.

Hand: The Phalanges

Each *proximal phalanx* of the phalanges (see Fig. 6–8) possesses an oval, concave facet for articulation with the rounded articular surface of the head of the metacarpals. *Middle phalanges* all possess double facets for articulation with the double condyles at the distal ends of the proximal phalanges. The distal ends of the middle phalanges similarly possess these double condyles and articulate with the bases of the distal phalanges. The medial and lateral sides of the palmar (volar) surface of each proximal and middle phalanx are marked by longitudinal ridges to which the flexor retinacula attach.

The *distal phalanges* possess double concave facets at their proximal ends for articulation with the condyles of the middle phalanges. The distal tips of the distal phalanges possess flattened expansions, termed the *ungual tuberosities,* that support the fibro-fatty pulp of the fingertip. The pollex (thumb) does not possess a middle phalanx, but its distal and proximal phalanges resemble those of the other four digits. The palmar surfaces of the shafts of the phalanges of the hand are flattened. The palmar (volar) surface of the terminal phalanx of the thumb is normally marked by a deep pit for insertion of the flexor pollicis longus.

ARTICULATIONS OF THE UPPER LIMB
The Sternoclavicular Joint

The *sternoclavicular joints* (see Fig. 6–1) are located between the clavicles, the clavicular notches on the superior border of the manubrium, and the costal cartilages of the first ribs. At each joint is an *articular disc* dividing it into two synovial cavities. These are *sellar synovial joints.* Each joint is surrounded by a fibrous articular capsule. In addition, the joints are strengthened by several ligaments, which include the following:

- The anterior sternoclavicular ligament
- The posterior sternoclavicular ligament
- The interclavicular ligament
- The costoclavicular ligament

The *anterior sternoclavicular ligament* attaches to the anterior surface of the clavicle, manubrium, and first costal cartilage. The *posterior sternoclavicular ligament* covers the posterior surface of the joint. It runs from the posterior surface of the clavicle's sternal end to the posterior aspect of the upper manubrium. The *interclavicular ligament* unites the superior aspects of the sternal ends of both clavicles with one another. Some fibers attach to the superior margin of the manubrium. The *costoclavicular ligament* unites the upper part of the first rib and costal cartilage with the inferior medial surface of the clavicle.

Movement at the sternoclavicular joint occurs in conjunction with movements of the pectoral girdle and upper limbs. The joint permits motion anteriorly, posteriorly, and vertically and allows the lateral end of the clavicle to be raised for full elevation of the upper limb (Gray, 1995).

The Acromioclavicular Joint

The *acromioclavicular joint* (Figure 6–10) is a plane synovial joint. There may, however, be a slightly concave curvature on either surface, with a matching slightly convex curvature on the opposite surface. The clavicle has a narrow, oval facet that faces inferolaterally and articulates with the corresponding facet on the medial border of the acromion process. The joint is reinforced by the fibrous joint capsule as well as two ligaments: the acromioclavicular ligament and the coracoclavicular ligament. The coracoclavicular ligament is composed of the conoid ligament and the trapezoid ligament.

The fibrous joint capsule completely surrounds the joint and is reinforced superiorly by the quadrilaterally shaped *acromioclavicular ligament,* which runs from the lateral end of the superior aspect of the clavicle to the adjoining surface of the acromion process. Its fibers blend with the aponeuroses of the trapezius and deltoid muscles. The inferior aspect of the clavicle is marked by the sites of attachment for the *coracoclavicular ligament,* which include the conoid tubercle and the trapezoid line.

The conoid tubercle and trapezoid line provide attachment for the *conoid* and *trapezoid ligaments,* respectively. These two ligaments constitute the *coracoclavicular ligament,* which binds the clavicle to the scapula. It is separate from the acromioclavicular joint but is an important extrinsic ligament of the joint. There is frequently an incomplete articular disc in the superior part of the acromioclavicular joint cavity separating the two articular surfaces from one another. On rare occasions the disc is extensive enough to completely separate the joint cavity into two distinct parts.

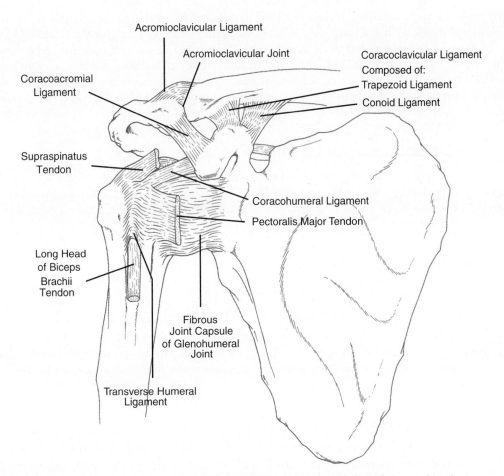

Figure 6-10   The acromioclavicular and glenohumeral joints, right side, anterior view.

Movements of the acromioclavicular joint are similar to those of the sternoclavicular joint. Each allows approximately 30 degrees of axial rotation of the clavicle; between them, rotation of approximately 60 degrees is permitted. Angulation between the scapula and clavicle can occur in any direction.

The Glenohumeral Joint

The *glenohumeral joint* (see Fig. 6–10) is a spheroidal or ball-and-socket joint between the oval-shaped humeral head and the glenoid fossa of the scapula. The humeral head has a much larger articular surface than the glenoid fossa of the scapula. Because of the relatively small bony contact between the head of the humerus and the glenoid fossa, the head of the humerus is held in contact with the glenoid fossa largely by the activities of the muscles surrounding the joint.

The fibrous joint capsule that surrounds the glenohumeral joint is very loose. It is weakest inferiorly, allowing considerable displacement of the head of the humerus from the glenoid in the absence of the surrounding muscles and ligaments. The advantage of this arrangement is the tremendous range of motion permitted by the glenohumeral joint. A disadvantage is that the head of the humerus is dislocated with relative ease (Matsen, 1980).

The articular surfaces of the glenoid and humeral head, as in all synovial joints, are covered with hyaline articular cartilage. The humeral articular surface is an oblate spheroid with its long axis located superoinferiorly. The glenoid fossa of the scapula is likewise covered with hyaline cartilage and is oval and concave to receive the head of the humerus. The area of contact between the two is made somewhat greater by the *glenoid labrum,* a fibrocartilaginous rim surrounding the margins of the glenoid fossa. In addition to the head of the humerus and glenoid fossa, the glenohumeral joint includes a number of other structures.

The Coracoacromial Ligament

The *coracoacromial ligament* extends superiorly over the top of the humeral head and reinforces the joint superiorly. The coracoacromial ligament attaches to the coracoid process more anteriorly and medially and to the acromion process more posteriorly and laterally.

The Coracoacromial Arch

The *coracoacromial arch* is an osteoligamentous arch formed by the acromion process, the coracoacromial ligament, and the coracoid process. Beneath the arch passes the tendon of the supraspinatus muscle, which arises from the supraspinous fossa of the scapula and inserts into the greater tubercle of the humerus. A bursa lies between the coracoacromial ligament and this tendon. The coracoacromial arch protects the glenohumeral joint from superior displacement, and the muscle adds stability to the joint.

The Joint Capsule

The *joint capsule* of the glenohumeral joint completely surrounds the joint. It attaches to the circumference of the glenoid fossa and to the margins of, the *glenoid labrum* at the neck of the scapula. Laterally it attaches to the margins of the humeral head along the course of the anatomical neck of the humerus, and inferiorly it encroaches on the surgical neck. In the absence of surrounding musculature, the head of the humerus can be separated from the glenoid fossa by up to 2.5 cm. The looseness of the articular capsule allows great freedom of motion of the humeral head upon the glenoid fossa. The surrounding musculature reinforces the joint and keeps the humeral head in contact with the glenoid fossa.

THE GLENOHUMERAL LIGAMENTS

In places, the fibrous joint capsule thickens to form intrinsic ligaments of the joint. These are the *glenohumeral ligaments*. These ligaments are three thickenings of the anterior aspect of the joint capsule and are termed the superior, middle, and inferior glenohumeral ligaments. They are visible only from the interior of the joint cavity. They are best seen when the joint capsule is opened posteriorly and the head of the humerus is removed with a saw or chisel.

The *superior glenohumeral ligament* runs from the top of the glenoid cavity to the greater tubercle of the humerus. The *middle glenohumeral ligament* goes from the anterior margin of the glenoid fossa to the middle of the lesser tubercle of the humerus. The *inferior glenohumeral ligament* runs from the inferior margin of the glenoid cavity to the anatomical neck of the humerus. Often, it is difficult to separate the three individual ligaments.

THE CORACOHUMERAL LIGAMENT

The *coracohumeral ligament* is a broad band of tissue strengthening the upper part of the joint capsule. It runs from the root of the coracoid process to the anterior margin of the greater tubercle of the humerus. The tendon of the long head of the biceps brachii separates this ligament from the superior glenohumeral ligament.

THE GLENOID LABRUM

The *glenoid labrum* is a fibrocartilaginous rim that surrounds the margins of the glenoid fossa to enlarge and deepen the articular surface to receive the head of the humerus. It is triangular in cross-section with a thin, sharp, free border. The fibers of the tendon of the long head of the biceps blend into the labrum as that tendon inserts into the supraglenoid tubercle above the glenoid fossa.

THE TRANSVERSE HUMERAL LIGAMENT

The *transverse humeral ligament* is a bundle of short fibers running from the greater to the lesser tubercles of the humerus from the lateral to the medial border of the bicipital groove. The fibers close the bicipital groove and help form a tunnel for the passage of the tendon of the long head of the biceps brachii as it enters the glenohumeral joint to attach to the supraglenoid tubercle.

TENDON OF THE LONG HEAD OF THE BICEPS BRACHII MUSCLE

The *tendon of the long head of the biceps brachii* is structurally important to the glenohumeral joint. This tendon is unusual in that it passes *through* the joint capsule of the glenohumeral joint; tendons are usually located outside joint capsules rather than within them. This tendon originates from the supraglenoid tubercle of the scapula, passes through the top of the glenohumeral joint, over the head of the humerus, and passes out of the joint capsule by passing under the transverse humeral ligament and into the bicipital groove. In addition to providing attachment to the muscle, this tendon helps maintain the humeral head in the glenoid fossa and limits the upward displacement of the humeral head.

The Scapulothoracic Joint

The *scapulothoracic joint* (see Fig. 6–1) is unusual in that it is neither a synarthrosis (solid connective tissue joint) nor a diarthrosis (cavitated, or synovial, joint) but rather a joint between the muscle-covered scapula and the muscle-covered thoracic wall. It is therefore sometimes referred to as a *synsarcosis.* The only bony articulations between the scapula and the rest of the skeleton are at the acromioclavicular and sternoclavicular joints. Between the subscapularis muscle, which covers the ventral or costal surface of the scapula, and the ribs and intercostal muscles lies the serratus anterior muscle, which attaches the vertebral border of the scapula to the first eight or nine ribs.

Ranges of Motion of the Shoulder Joint

As with the hip joint (the other spheroidal, or ball-and-socket, joint in the human body), the shoulder joint has a wide range of motion. This is possible because it has very little bony constraint. Abduction and adduction of the upper limb through the full range of 180 degrees of motion are caused by movement at both the glenohumeral joint and the scapulothoracic joint, with approximately 120 degrees caused by motion at the glenohumeral joint and the remaining 60 degrees caused by motion at the scapulothoracic joint. However, the great freedom of flexion, extension, abduction, and adduction permits the upper limb to be fully circumducted.

The scapula is acted on by a number of muscles that direct it along the thoracic wall. The scapula may be pulled forward *(protraction)* or backward *(retraction).* It can also be rotated upward so that the glenoid fossa faces more superiorly, or it can be rotated downward so that the glenoid fossa faces more inferiorly. In movements of the upper limb, motion at the scapulothoracic joint is almost always involved in addition to motion at the glenohumeral joint. As noted, approximately one-third of abduction and adduction of the upper limb occurs at the scapulothoracic joint. As the scapula moves, there is also motion at the sternoclavicular and acromioclavicular joints.

Disorders of the Shoulder Joint

Because the shoulder joint is relatively unconstrained, it is easily subject to dislocation. The shoulder joint capsule is weakest inferiorly, making the most frequent pattern of dislocation the *subglenoid position,* in which the head of the humerus is displaced inferiorly below the glenoid fossa. This is the region in which the joint capsule has the least reinforcement.

The long head of the triceps brachii muscle attaches to the infraglenoid tubercle and usually prevents the head of the humerus from being pushed posteriorly. As a consequence, the head of the humerus is frequently pushed secondarily into a *subco-*

racoid or *subclavicular position.* (For further discussion of clinical problems in the shoulder joint, see Edwardson, 1995; for a fuller discussion of joint mechanics, see Frankel and Nordin, 1980.)

In *ankylosis,* the bony union of the glenohumeral joint or the acromioclavicular joint, some motion of the upper limb is still possible because of motion at the scapulothoracic joint.

The Elbow Joint

The elbow is composed of a complex of joints (Figure 6–11), including the humeroulnar, humeroradial, and proximal radioulnar joints.

The Humeroulnar Joint

The *humeroulnar joint* is a ginglymus, or hinge, joint. It is located between the trochlea of the humerus and the trochlear notch, olecranon process, and coronoid process of the ulna. The trochlear notch of the ulna receives the trochlea of the humerus. The form of these joint surfaces and their investing musculature essentially permit only flexion and extension. Hyperextension is prevented by the biceps brachii and brachialis muscles and is limited by the olecranon process.

The Humeroradial Joint

The *humeroradial joint* is located between the radial head and the capitulum of the distal end of the humerus. It combines elements of a ginglymus, a trochoid or pivot joint, and a gliding joint. In fact, the humeroradial articulation resembles a ball-and-socket joint, but other associated structures—specifically the humeroulnar joint, annular ligament, and associated ligaments—effectively restrict its motion in abduction and adduction. However, the architecture of the joint permits a broad range of flexion/extension and rotation.

The capitulum of the humerus is rounded and convex, whereas the superior surface of the radial head is round and concave. As the elbow flexes and extends, the radial head slides alternately anteriorly and posteriorly over the capitulum. In pronation and supination of the forearm, the shaft and head of the radius rotate. Thus the radial head is rotating about its center relative to the surface of the capitulum.

The Proximal Radioulnar Joint

The *proximal radioulnar joint* is a trochoid (pivot) synovial joint. Around the head of the radius is a flat, circular surface that articulates with the radial notch of the lateral aspect of the proximal ulna. The *annular ligament* holds the head of the radius in contact with the radial notch of the ulna and guides its motion. This ligament attaches to the anterior and posterior borders of the radial notch; with the notch, it completes a circular collar in which the head of the radius can rotate.

THE ULNAR COLLATERAL LIGAMENT

The *ulnar (medial) collateral ligament* is triangular with thickened anterior, posterior, and inferior borders. The anterior part arises from the medial epicondyle of the humerus and attaches to the coronoid process of the ulna. The posterior part

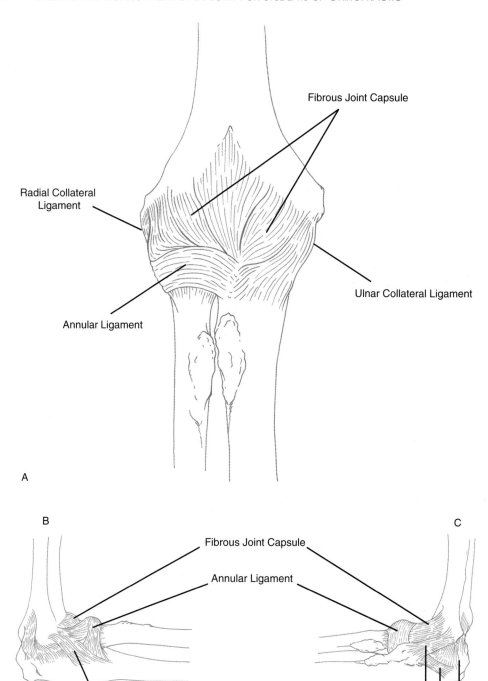

Figure 6–11   The right elbow joint: (A) anterior, (B) lateral, and (C) medial views.

runs from the back of the medial epicondyle to the medial border of the olecranon process. The inferior part, which is much more weakly developed than the anterior and posterior parts, attaches the distal portions of the anterior and posterior parts. This ligament reinforces the medial aspect of the elbow joint. A large portion of it becomes taut in flexion.

THE RADIAL COLLATERAL LIGAMENT

The *radial (lateral) collateral ligament* arises low on the lateral epicondyle of the humerus and attaches inferiorly to the annular ligament and to the supinator crest of the ulna. It blends with the attachments of the supinator muscle and the extensor carpi radialis brevis muscle. It reinforces the lateral aspect of the elbow joint and tightens in flexion.

THE JOINT CAPSULE

The *fibrous joint capsule* attaches on the humerus anteriorly above the coronoid fossa and blends with the radial and ulnar collateral ligaments. Anteriorly it shares some fibers with the brachialis muscle. Posteriorly it attaches behind the trochlea and capitulum and extends down to attach to the medial and lateral margins of the olecranon process. The synovial membrane lines the fibrous capsule and is thrown into a fold that projects from the posterior part of the capsule to partly separate the humeroradial from the humeroulnar joint.

Ranges of Motion of the Elbow Joint

Because of the shapes of the olecranon fossa and the humeral trochlea, flexion and extension of the humeroulnar joint are accompanied by a small degree of torsion or rotation of the ulna. The ulna is *very slightly* pronated in extension and *very slightly* supinated in flexion. In the anatomical position, when the forearm is extended and supinated, the long axis of the ulnar shaft and the long axis of the humeral shaft meet at an obtuse angle because of the obliquity of the trochlea in relation to the humeral shaft. This is called the *carrying angle*. This angle deflects the hand and distal ends of the radius and ulna laterally away from the body. From extreme flexion (hyperflexion) to maximum extension (hyperextension), the elbow joint is capable of motion through approximately 140 degrees.

Disorders of the Elbow Joint

Lateral epicondylitis ("tennis elbow") and medial epicondylitis ("golfer's elbow") are two of the most common problems encountered at the elbow joint. *Lateral epicondylitis* is an inflammation of the common extensor tendon, which attaches to the lateral epicondyle. This is caused by repetitive motion injuries of the wrist extensors that attach here, particularly the extensor carpi radialis brevis muscle. *Medial epicondylitis* is an inflammatory response to repetitive motion injuries of the wrist flexors.

The elbow may be displaced posteriorly by a dislocation of the ulna and is complicated by fractures of the coronoid process of the ulna. The medial epicondyle of the humerus is frequently separated from the remainder of the bone in lateral dislocations because of the very strong ulnar collateral ligament.

The radial head is frequently dislocated anteriorly with rupture of the annular ligament, particularly in falls when the hand is used to break a fall with the forearm extended; it occurs most commonly in children. In children, the head of the radius may be displaced inferiorly through the annular ligament. In this situation, the annular ligament becomes entrapped between the capitulum and the radial head, and the forearm becomes fixed in semiflexion, midway between supination and pronation. The small radial head predisposes children to this disorder.

Tears and dislocations of bony articulations in children are also attributable to inherent weakness of the epiphyses, particularly at the medial epicondyle of the humerus and the head of the radius. (For further discussion of clinical problems in the elbow joint, see Edwardson, 1995; for a fuller discussion of joint mechanics, see Frankel and Nordin, 1980.)

The Radioulnar Articulations

There are three joints between the radius and ulna: the proximal radioulnar joint, the middle radioulnar joint (radioulnar syndesmosis), and the distal radioulnar joint (Figure 6–12). The proximal radioulnar joint has been discussed with the elbow joint.

The Radioulnar Syndesmosis

The shafts of the radius and ulna are joined to one another throughout their lengths by two interosseous ligaments: the interosseous membrane and the oblique cord, creating the *radioulnar syndesmosis,* or *middle radioulnar joint.*

THE INTEROSSEUS MEMBRANE

The *interosseous membrane* is a broad, flat membrane composed primarily of dense connective tissue with fibers running inferiorly and medially to attach the interosseous crest of the radius to the interosseous crest of the ulna. The membrane helps bind the two bones together and creates a large surface for origins of the flexor and extensor muscles in the forearm. In fractures of the upper limb that require immobilization of this membrane, the forearm is always casted (or immobilized) in the supine position. This keeps the membrane taut, preventing atrophy.

THE OBLIQUE CORD

The *oblique cord* is a ligament running from the coronoid process of the ulna to the shaft of the radius slightly distal to the radial tuberosity. Its fibers run inferiorly and laterally; sometimes it is absent.

The Distal Radioulnar Joint

The *distal radioulnar joint* is nearly the inverse of the proximal joint. The head of the ulna is located distally and presents a circular margin that articulates with the ulnar notch on the distal radius. This trochoid joint is surrounded by a loose articular capsule lined with a synovial membrane. The joint is reinforced by the presence of an articular disc. The fibrous joint capsule is thickened posteriorly and anteriorly. The synovial lining of the joint extends a short distance proximally between the radius and ulna to form a *sacciform recess.*

Figure 6-12   Pronation and supination of the forearm skeleton, right side.

The *articular disc* is triangular and extends transversely across the distal end of the ulnar head. Its apex attaches to the depression between the head and styloid process of the ulna, and its base attaches to the medial edge of the distal articular surface of the radius. Its center is thinner than its periphery and may occasionally be perforated. It helps bind the distal ends of the radius and ulna together and separates the ulnar head from articulation with the carpals. It also separates the ulnar notch from the wrist joint. The disc's inferior surface is concave to receive the medial part of the lunate bone. Proximally the disc itself rotates relative to the head of the ulna, whereas distally the carpal bones move relative to the disc in flexion/extension or abduction/adduction of the wrist.

The Wrist

The *wrist* (Figure 6–13; refer also to Fig. 6–12 throughout the discussion of the wrist) can be loosely defined as the region between the hand and the forearm. Two separate

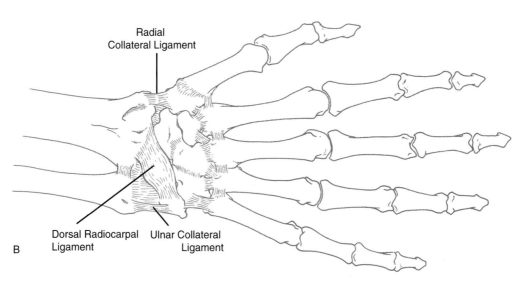

Figure 6-13   Ligaments of the wrist: (*A*) anterior or palmar and (*B*) posterior or dorsal views, right side.

joints lie within the wrist: the *distal radioulnar joint* and the *radiocarpal joint*. The distal radioulnar joint is described in the preceding section.

The Radiocarpal Joint

The *radiocarpal joint* (wrist joint proper) is an ellipsoid synovial joint. It is formed by the articulation of the distal end of the radius and the articular disc superiorly with the scaphoid, lunate, and triquetrum of the proximal row of carpal bones inferiorly.

THE LIGAMENTS

A fibrous articular capsule surrounds the joint. The joint is reinforced by a number of ligaments, including the following:

PALMAR RADIOCARPAL LIGAMENT: The palmar radiocarpal ligament runs from the anterior distal radius and ulna to the palmar surfaces of the scaphoid, lunate, and triquetrum bones. A few fibers may attach to the capitate. It is essentially a reinforcement of the anterior portion of the joint capsule.

DORSAL RADIOCARPAL LIGAMENT: The dorsal radiocarpal ligament is weaker and less well developed than the palmar ligament. It attaches to the posterior distal radius and runs inferiorly to attach to the dorsal aspects of the scaphoid, lunate, and triquetrum. Like its palmar counterpart, it is again a strong posterior reinforcement of the radiocarpal joint capsule.

ULNAR COLLATERAL LIGAMENT: The ulnar collateral ligament attaches superiorly to the styloid process of the ulna and runs inferiorly along the medial aspect of the wrist to attach below to the triquetrum and pisiform as well as to the transverse carpal ligament. The ulnar collateral ligament, along with the radial styloid process, guides abduction or radial deviation of the hand at the wrist joint.

RADIAL COLLATERAL LIGAMENT: The radial collateral ligament runs from the styloid process of the radius to the lateral aspect of the scaphoid with a few additional fibers running to the trapezium and flexor retinaculum. The radial collateral ligament, along with the ulnar styloid process, guides adduction or ulnar deviation of the hand at the wrist joint. The aforementioned four ligaments reinforce the fibrous joint capsule and essentially surround its entire external aspect.

FLEXOR RETINACULUM (TRANSVERSE CARPAL LIGAMENT): The flexor retinaculum is a strong ligamentous band that runs from the pisiform and the hook of the hamate laterally to the scaphoid tuberosity and the palmar side of the trapezium. The space beneath the retinaculum and anterior to the carpal bones is the *carpal tunnel*. The carpal tunnel is completely lined with synovial membranes that provide lubrication for the tendons of the long flexors of the hand. The tunnel provides a passage for these tendons to reach their distal attachments in the hand. Accompanying these tendons is the median nerve.

Ranges of Motion of the Wrist Joint

As noted, the wrist joint is an ellipsoid synovial joint. Motions permitted include abduction, adduction, flexion, and extension. The long axis of the articular surfaces is oriented in a coronal plane, whereas the short axis is along a parasagittal plane. As a result of the different lengths of these axes, abduction and adduction along the coronal plane are permitted, and flexion and extension along a parasagittal plane are permitted, but rotation is much more limited. Movement also occurs between the carpal bones. *Circumduction* of the hand at the wrist is carried out by sequential movement of flexion, abduction, extension, and abduction, because little rotation can occur. The degree of abduction of the hand is considerably less than the degree of adduction, perhaps because of a more distal styloid process on the radius relative to that on the ulna.

Disorders of the Wrist Joint

Of the bones of the wrist, the scaphoid is the most frequently fractured, usually fracturing transversely across its long axis. These fractures occasionally fail to unite, generally because the proximal fragment frequently has no nutrient artery and so loses its blood supply. As a result, avascular necrosis is a common complication in fractures of the scaphoid. *Palmar dislocation of the lunate* is also a frequent complication of fractures of the scaphoid. When this occurs, the displaced lunate may compress the median nerve against the flexor retinaculum.

Carpal tunnel syndrome can be considered a wrist disorder. It is caused by inflammation of the synovium surrounding the tendons as a result of repetitive motion injuries, fractures, arthritis, or other conditions. The inflammation results in compression or impingement of the median nerve, causing weakness, numbness, and pain of the hand. (For more details, see Edwardson, 1995.)

Joints of the Hand

The hand is composed of a number of small bones separated by a multitude of synovial joints. We touch on the basics of their anatomy here.

The Intercarpal Joints

The joints between the carpal bones may be defined as plane synovial joints. The basic type of motion between carpal bones is gliding, or translatory, motion. The *midcarpal joint* is the joint between the *proximal* (scaphoid, lunate, and triquetrum) and *distal* (trapezium, trapezoid, capitate, and hamate) rows of carpal bones. Motion at the midcarpal joint is largely analogous to that in a ball-and-socket joint, with the proximal row approximating the sides of the "socket" and the distal row forming a proximally projecting "ball" centered around the head of the capitate. This is only a partial analogy, however, because motion among these elements is complex. Bones in the individual rows are bound to one another by *dorsal* and *palmar ligaments* and by *interosseous ligaments.*

Ranges of Motion of the Joints of the Hand

Flexion/extension and abduction/adduction occur at the *midcarpal joint* as well as at the *radiocarpal joint.* Movements of the hand and wrist involve movements at both these joints. The combined range of typical motion is *flexion:* 85 degrees, *extension:* 85 degrees, *adduction (ulnar deviation):* 45 degrees, and *abduction (radial deviation):* 15 degrees. Thus these joints can be circumducted.

The Carpometacarpal Joints

The *first carpometacarpal joint* is between the base of the proximal phalanx of the thumb (pollex) and the trapezium. It is a *sellar synovial joint,* capable of flexion/extension and abduction/adduction as well as circumduction. This is also true of the other four carpometacarpal joints, but motion is much more limited in them.

The first carpometacarpal joint has unique features that greatly enhance its motion. First, as noted, it is a sellar synovial joint. Second, the thumb (pollex) is rotated 90 degrees relative to the other fingers. For the pollex, the plane of flexion/extension is parallel to the plane of the palm of the hand, rather than perpendicular to it as for the other fingers. The plane of abduction/adduction for the pollex is perpendicular to the plane of the palm, whereas for the other fingers it is parallel to the palm. Also, the pollex may be *opposed* to the other fingers (bringing the pad of the tip of the thumb into contact with the pad, or palmar surfaces, of the other fingers). *Opposition* of the pollex is carried out by simultaneously flexing and medially rotating the abducted thumb. The sellar-shaped joint surfaces of the trapezium and the base of the first metacarpal allow this action to be brought about easily.

Opposition of the pollex is a hallmark of primates in general and of humans in particular. In humans, opposition is particularly strong because of the relative shortness of the other digits, permitting "pulp-to-pulp" contact of their tips with that of the thumb. Opposition allows the manipulation of objects and the environment and enables humans to carry out complex tasks, such as writing, with great ease.

The Second through Fifth Carpometacarpal Joints

The remaining carpometacarpal joints do not permit the freedom of motion of the first. Their joint surfaces are usually described as plane, although they possess some curvature and are somewhat more complex than the term *plane* implies. The carpals and metacarpals are joined together by synovial articular capsules, by dorsal and palmar ligaments, and by interosseous ligaments. These joints allow flexion/extension and abduction/adduction. They also permit a very limited amount of rotation. This can be demonstrated by grasping a small round object, such as a tennis ball or an apple. When the hand cups the object, the metacarpals rotate somewhat, resulting in a cupping of the palm.

The fifth metacarpal rotates more do the second through fourth. Thus the fifth metacarpophalangeal joint may be easily circumducted. During opposition, the second through fifth metacarpals rotate sufficiently to allow the second through fifth digits to come into contact with the first, although most of the movement takes place in the pollex.

The Metacarpophalangeal Joints

The *metacarpophalangeal joints* are usually considered *ellipsoid joints,* but the metacarpal heads are divided on their palmar aspects, making these joints almost bicondylar. The joints are surrounded by a fibrous joint capsule. Each also has a *palmar ligament* reinforcing the capsule anteriorly and two *collateral ligaments,* one on each side of the joint.

The second through the fifth metacarpophalangeal joints are joined to one another on their palmar surfaces by the *deep transverse metacarpal ligaments*. These joints permit flexion/extension, abduction/adduction, and a limited amount of rotation that may accompany flexion/extension. They may be flexed nearly 90 degrees, but extension is limited to just a few degrees.

The Interphalangeal Joints

Because each digit except the thumb has three phalanges, the second through fifth digits have both a proximal and a distal *interphalangeal joint*. The interphalangeal joints are *ginglymi*, or uniaxial hinge joints. Each has a medial and lateral collateral ligament and a palmar ligament to reinforce the fibrous joint capsule. These joints allow a great deal of flexion, but extension is considerably limited by the tension of the tendons of the flexor muscles. A *slight* amount of rotation occurs during flexion and extension. In flexion, the phalanges rotate slightly laterally such that the pads of the fingers meet the pad of the terminal pollex. In extension, slight medial rotation occurs.

OSSIFICATION OF THE UPPER LIMB BONES
The Scapula

There are normally at least seven centers of ossification for the scapula (Figure 6–14). The primary center of ossification is for the scapular body, which appears about the second month in utero. Ossification begins near the glenoid fossa and spreads throughout the body. The spine of the scapula arises from the dorsal aspect

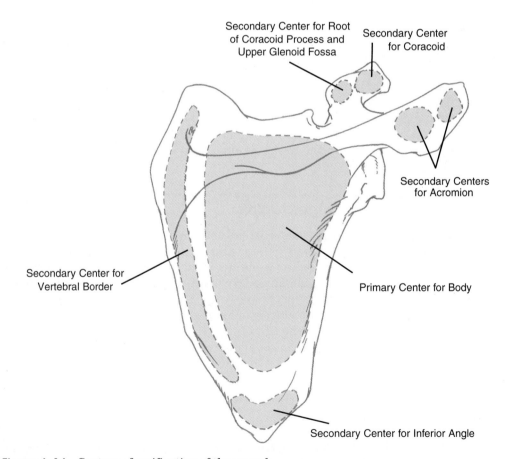

Figure 6–14   Centers of ossification of the scapula.

of the body around the third fetal months as an extension of the center for the body. At birth, the glenoid, vertebral border, inferior angle, coracoid process, and acromion process are still cartilaginous.

The secondary center of ossification in the middle of the coracoid appears at about 1 year and unites with the rest of the bone at about 15 years. The upper third of the glenoid ossifies from a subcoracoid center of ossification. It appears between ages 10 and 11 and fuses with the remainder of the bone between ages 16 and 18. Between the 14th and 20th years, ossification of the remainder of the scapula takes place rapidly. In order, the secondary centers for the root of the coracoid process, the base of the acromion, the inferior angle, the tip of the acromion, and the remainder of the vertebral border all ossify between 14 and 20 (Breathnach, 1965; Gray, 1985; Krogman, 1962).

The Clavicle

The clavicle (Figure 6–15) ossifies from three centers: a medial and a lateral center for the shaft (both primary centers) and a secondary center for the sternal end. The clavicle demonstrates both intramembranous and endochondral ossification. The shaft forms by intramembranous ossification, whereas the sternal end forms by endochondral ossification. The primary centers for the shaft appear between 5 and 6 weeks in utero. As a consequence, the clavicle is the first bone in the body to ossify. The secondary center at the sternal end appears at about age 18 to 20 and unites with the shaft of the bone at about age 25. As a result, it is one of the last epiphyses in the body to undergo synostosis (Breathnach, 1965; Gray, 1985; Krogman, 1962).

The Humerus

The humerus (Figure 6–16) normally has eight centers of ossification: one primary center for the diaphysis and seven secondary centers. The proximal end of the humerus forms from a compound epiphysis formed by the union of three secondary centers of ossification. The distal epiphysis is also a compound epiphysis formed from the union of three secondary centers of ossification. The medial epicondyle has a single center of ossification and is isolated from the others. The primary center for the shaft of the humerus appears at about 7 to 8 weeks in utero.

PROXIMAL END: The center for the head of the humerus appears either at birth or in the first few months of life; for the greater tubercle, at 3 years; and for the lesser tubercle, at 5 years. The three unite between ages 5 and 6. This compound epiphysis finally synostoses with the shaft at about 18 to 20 years. As with most other epiphyses, this occurs at a younger chronological age in girls than in boys.

DISTAL END: The ossification center for the capitulum appears at approximately 2 years; for the trochlea, at 9 to 10 years; and for the lateral epicondyle, at 11 to 13 years. These three fuse at about puberty; the resulting compound epiphysis fuses with the distal end of the diaphysis at 14 to 17 years.

MEDIAL EPICONDYLE: The secondary center of ossification for the medial epicondyle appears at 5 to 7 years and fuses with the rest of the bone at about 15 to 18 years (Breathnach, 1965; Gray, 1985; Krogman, 1962).

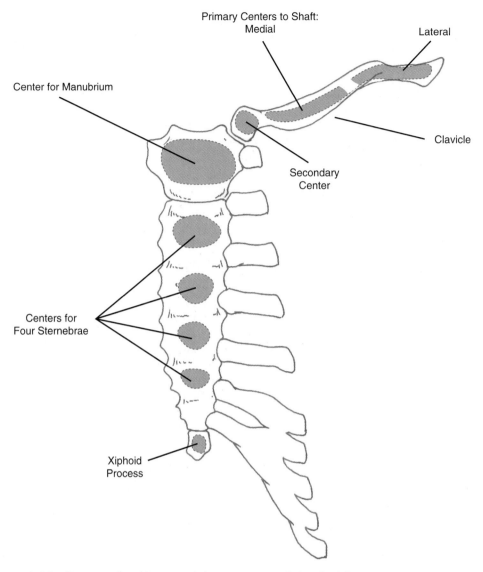

Figure 6-15   Centers of ossification of the sternum and the clavicle.

The Radius

The radius (see Fig. 6–16) ossifies from three centers: one for the head, one for the shaft, and one for the distal end. The primary center of ossification is in the diaphysis, which begins ossification at about 8 weeks in utero. The secondary center of ossification in the radial head appears at 5 years and fuses with the shaft between 15 and 18 years. The secondary center for the distal end appears at 2 years of age and fuses with the shaft between 17 and 20 years of age. As with other epiphyses, ossification and fusion occur somewhat earlier in girls than in boys (Breathnach, 1965; Gray, 1985; Krogman, 1962).

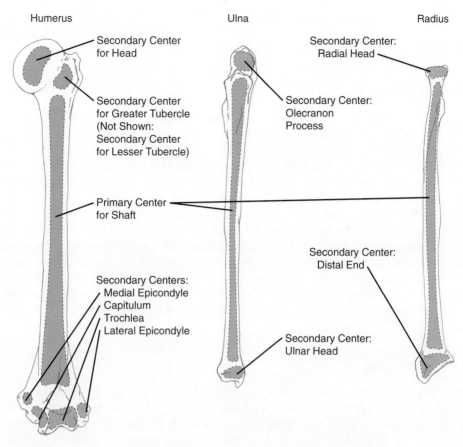

Figure 6-16   Centers of ossification of the humerus, the ulna, and the radius.

The Ulna

Like the radius, the ulna (see Fig. 6–16) ossifies from three centers: one for the proximal end of the olecranon process, one for the shaft, and one for the distal end (ulnar head). The center of ossification for the shaft appears at about 8 weeks in utero. The proximal epiphysis appears at about 10 years and fuses with the rest of the olecranon at about age 16. Most of the olecranon ossifies by a continuation of the ossification of the shaft. The center for the ulnar head appears at about 5 to 6 years and fuses with the shaft by age 20. As with all the long bones, union of epiphyses occurs earlier in girls than in boys (Breathnach, 1965; Gray, 1985; Krogman, 1962).

The Carpals

Each carpal has only a single center of ossification. The capitate and hamate ossify at 1 year; the triquetrum, at 3 years; the lunate, at 4 years in girls and at 5 years in boys; the trapezium, trapezoid, and scaphoid, at 5 years in girls and at 6 or 7 years in boys; and the pisiform, at 9 years in girls and at 11 years in boys. Occasionally, a small bone, the *os centrale*, may appear in the wrist. When present, it is found on the dorsum of the wrist between the scaphoid, trapezoid, and capitate. This bone is constant in some other primates, but not in humans. Ordinarily, the cartilage anlage for the os centrale fuses with the anlage of the scaphoid at about 2 months in utero (Breathnach, 1965; Gray, 1985; Krogman, 1962).

The Metacarpals

Metacarpals II through V all ossify from two centers: one for the shaft and one for the head (distal end). Metacarpal I (for the pollex) ossifies from two centers as well, but its epiphysis is at its proximal rather than its distal end. In this regard it follows the pattern of the phalanges. It has been suggested that the first metacarpal is phylogenetically the proximal phalanx of the first digit, with the bone homologous to the other four metacarpals lost in the course of evolution (Gray, 1985).

The shafts of the metacarpals begin ossification at the eighth or ninth week in utero. The centers for the second and third metacarpals appear first; the center for the first metacarpal appears last. At about age 3 the epiphyses of all five metacarpals begin to ossify, and they unite with the shafts of the metacarpals between ages 18 and 20. There can be a secondary center at the base of the third metacarpal, forming its "styloid process." It is occasionally present and, by failing to fuse with the rest of the bone, may form a separate bone (Breathnach, 1965; Gray, 1985; Krogman, 1962).

The Phalanges

The phalanges, like the first metacarpal, all ossify from two centers: one for a proximal epiphysis and one for the shaft. Like the metacarpals, the centers for the shafts of the phalanges appear at the eighth or ninth week in utero. The distal phalanges ossify from their distal ends first, instead of from the centers of the shafts as with the proximal and middle phalanges. Along with the clavicle, the distal phalanges are among the first bones in the body to ossify. The proximal epiphysis, or phalangeal base, begins to ossify at age 2 in the proximal phalanges and at age 3 in the middle and distal phalanges. The epiphyses of all three phalanges of each digit fuse with the shaft by age 20 (Breathnach, 1965; Gray, 1985; Krogman, 1962).

References

Breathnach, AS (Ed) (1965). *Frazer's Anatomy of the Human Skeleton* (6th ed). J and A Churchill, London.

Edwardson, BM (1995). *Musculoskeletal Disorders: Common Problems.* Singular Publishing Group, San Diego.

Frankel, VH, and Nordin, M (Eds) (1980). *Basic Biomechanics of the Skeletal System.* Lea and Febiger, Philadelphia.

Gray, H (1985). *Gray's Anatomy* (30th Am ed). CD Clemente (Ed). Lea and Febiger, Philadelphia.

Gray, H (1995). *Gray's Anatomy* (38th Brit ed). PL Williams, LH Bannister, MM Berry, P Collins, M Dyson, JE Dussek, and MWJ Ferguson (Eds). Churchill Livingstone, New York.

Krogman, WM (1962). *The Human Skeleton in Forensic Medicine.* Charles C Thomas, Springfield, IL.

Matsen, FA (1980). Biomechanics of the shoulder. In VH Frankel and M Nordin (Eds), *Biomechanics of the Skeletal System* (pp 221–242). Lea and Febiger, Philadelphia.

Chapter 7

Bones of the Postcranial Skeleton: The Lower Limb

THE PELVIC GIRDLE: THE OS COXAE

The *pelvic girdle* attaches the lower limb to the axial skeleton. The pelvic girdle consists of the two *ossa* (singular: *os*) *coxae*, better known as the *hip bones* or *innominate bones* (refer to Figures 7–1 through 7–3 throughout the discussion of the innominate or hip bone). The innominates articulate with the sacrum at the sacroiliac joint; together they form the bony *pelvis*. Each innominate articulates with the lower limb at the hip joint.

In the adult, the innominate is present as a single, irregularly shaped bone. In the child, however, it consists of three separate bones—the ilium, the ischium, and the pubis—which are united by a Y-shaped hyaline growth cartilage in a central depression called the acetabulum (the hemispherical socket for the femur). At adolescence these three bones fuse. The upper bladelike bone is the *ilium*. At the *acetabulum* (Latin meaning "vinegar cup") it is fused to the *pubis* anteriorly and the *ischium* inferiorly. The two innominates are joined to the sacrum at the bilateral *sacroiliac joints* and to each other at the anterior *pubic symphysis*.

Much of the internal surface of the ilium is taken up by the *iliac fossa*, from which the iliacus muscle originates. The blade itself is surmounted by the *iliac crest*, which is formed by a separate apophysis during development. As noted in Chapter 2, an *apophysis*, or *traction epiphysis*, is a secondary center of ossification forming

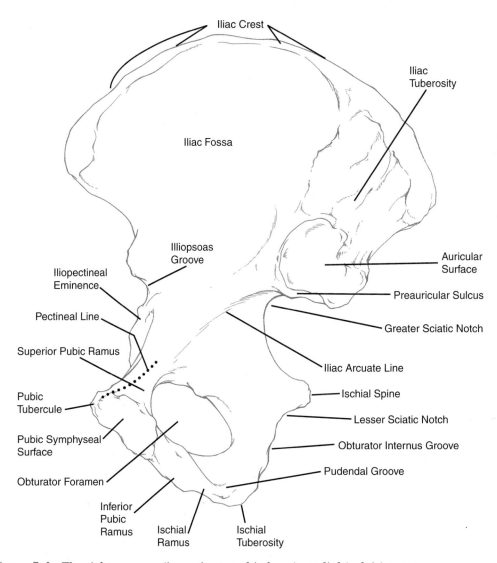

Figure 7-1   The right os coxae (innominate or hip bone), medial (pelvic) aspect.

under a muscle attachment. The iliac crest serves as an attachment for the internal and external oblique and transversus abdominus muscles of the abdominal wall. Its anteriormost projection is the *anterior superior iliac spine*, which provides attachment for the sartorius muscle. Inferior to this is the *anterior inferior iliac spine*, which is also formed from a separate apophysis. The upper portion of the anterior inferior iliac spine gives origin to the straight head of the rectus femoris muscle. A teardrop-shaped lower portion, with the teardrop pointed posteriorly, gives origin to the iliofemoral ligament and directly abuts the rim of the acetabulum.

The second head of the rectus femoris muscle arises from a small depression a few millimeters above the acetabular rim more posteriorly. Just anteromedial and inferior to the anterior inferior iliac spine is the *iliopsoas groove*, which provides passage for the iliopsoas muscle as it passes over the femoral head to its insertion on the

Figure 7–2   The right os coxae (innominate or hip bone), lateral aspect.

lesser trochanter of the femur. The medial wall of this groove is sometimes formed by
the bossing (swelling) that results from the fusion point of the ilium and the pubis.
This is called the *iliopectineal (iliopubic) eminence.*

A sharp border between the iliac blade bearing the origin of the iliacus and its
more inferior portion forms the true pelvis. This border is called the *iliac arcuate
line.* It junctures the *auricular surface* at its apex. Just inferior to the auricular surface is the *preauricular sulcus,* also known as the *paraglenoid sulcus.* This groove is
more common and better developed in females than in males. Its origin and function
are controversial but may be related to changes in adjacent ligaments induced by
hormones associated with pregnancy and childbirth.

Between the auricular surface and the iliac crest is a very rugose (roughened)
region called the *iliac tuberosity.* This tuberosity is for the attachment of the *interosseous sacroiliac ligament.*

The *exterior surface of the ilium* (Figure 7–4; refer also to Figs. 7–2 and 7–3
throughout the remainder of the discussion of the ilium) gives rise to two important
muscles of gait, the gluteus medius and gluteus minimus. The minimus occupies the

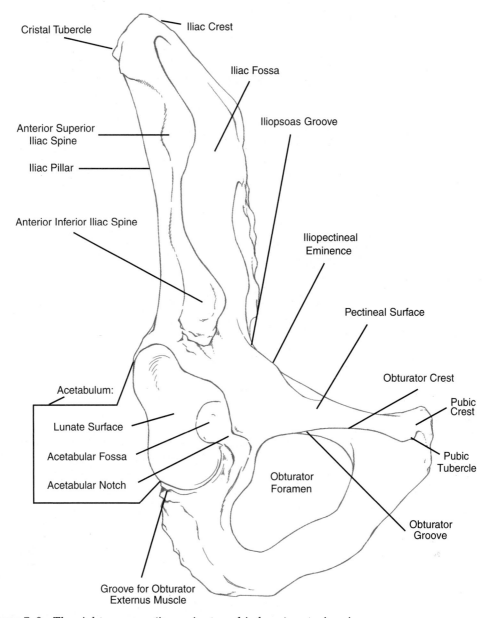

Figure 7–3   The right os coxae (innominate or hip bone), anterior view.

anterior portion, with its attachment outlined by the anteriormost extent of the ilium, the anterior iliac crest, and a line originating from the iliac crest and passing posteroinferiorly toward the *greater sciatic notch*. This is the *anterior gluteal line*.

The medius is attached posterior to the anterior gluteal line from an almost circular area outlined by the iliac crest and a second line, the *posterior gluteal line*. The posterior gluteal line is a short continuation of the iliac crest toward the greater sciatic notch. The posterior terminus of the iliac crest is the *posterior superior iliac spine*.

Anterior Gluteal Line

Posterior Gluteal Line

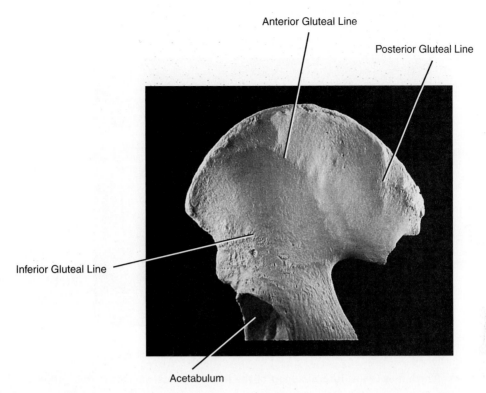

Inferior Gluteal Line

Acetabulum

Figure 7-4   The left os coxae, lateral aspect of the ilium demonstrating the gluteal lines.

Note that the posterior gluteal line and the posterior part of the iliac crest (anterior from the posterior superior spine for a distance of approximately 1 to 2 inches) form a rugose triangular area. To this area is attached a portion of the gluteus maximus muscle, originating predominantly from the sacrum. A vague line may run from the anterior inferior iliac spine to the greater sciatic notch, delineating the inferior extent of the gluteus minimus origin. This is the *inferior gluteal line.*

Also note that the iliac blade is bent back relative to the massive portion of the innominate that houses the acetabulum. The ilium's inferior surface thus forms the greater sciatic notch, which is shaped in males very much like an inverted fishhook and in females very much like a boomerang; that is, the walls of the notch are much more divergent from one another in females than in males. The posterior terminus of this notch is the *posterior inferior iliac spine.* The anterior terminus of the notch is actually located on the ischium and is called the *ischial spine.*

In external view the ilium displays a distinct thickening of its body about one-third of the distance from the anterior superior iliac spine to the posterior superior iliac spine. This thickened region runs from the iliac crest to the acetabular lip. It is called the *iliac pillar* (Figure 7–5). At the juncture of the pillar with the crest is a thickening of the crest called the *cristal tubercle.* The pillar is crossed by the anterior gluteal line.

The lower portion of the acetabulum is formed by the *corpus* or *body* of the *ischium* (see Figs. 7–1 through 7–3 throughout the discussion of the ischium). From this corpus a large *ischial ramus* projects anteriorly and joins the inferior ramus of the pubis. The inferior portion of the corpus is surmounted by a large rugose region

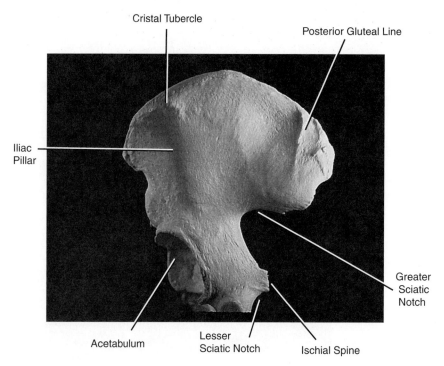

Figure 7-5   The left os coxae, lateral aspect of the ilium demonstrating the iliac pillar.

called the *ischial tuberosity*. The tuberosity is formed by the posterior terminus of a separate apophysis that surmounts the length of the ischiopubic ramus. The ischial tuberosity's surface is highly rugose and faceted. These facets are for the origin of the so-called hamstring muscles. The superiormost facet gives origin to the semimembranosus muscle. The next facet is for the biceps femoris muscle, with the most inferior facet for the origin of the semitendinosus muscle. These three muscles arise from the more vertical portion of the tuberosity before it becomes sharply angled to provide a horizontal surface for the attachment of the adductor magnus muscle.

A distinct groove lies between the ischial tuberosity and the remaining surface of the ischium on its internal surface. This is the *pudendal groove* for the pudendal nerve and the internal pudendal vessels. Between the ischial tuberosity and the ischial spine is a second involution of the lesser pelvis, called the *lesser sciatic notch*. A groove called the *obturator internus groove* may occasionally be palpated just inferior to the ischial spine for the obturator internus muscle. A second groove is formed by the anterosuperior edge of the ischial tuberosity and the lower lip of the acetabulum. This is the *obturator externus groove*. The pubis and ischium together surround a large opening called the *obturator foramen*. It is closed by a membrane during life. Its outer surface gives attachment to the obturator externus muscle, whereas its internal surface gives attachment to the obturator internus muscle.

The pubis (see Figs. 7–1 through 7–3 throughout the discussion of the pubis) is formed by two separate portions called *rami* (the *superior* and *inferior rami*) and a central portion called the *corpus* or *body* that provides attachment to the two rami and to the pubic symphysis. The arcuate line of the ilium is continuous onto the superior ramus of the pubis and may be followed anteriorly to a large anterior projection called the *pubic tubercle.* The continuation of the iliac arcuate line on the pubis is called the *pectineal line* or *pecten* (Figure 7–1).

The iliac arcuate line and the pectineal line together form the *linea terminalis.* The pectineal line, the iliac arcuate line, and the *sacral promontory* form the brim of the lesser, or "true," pelvis, the area inferior to this brim. Medial to the pubic tubercle is the *pubic crest.* The surface of the superior ramus just anterior to the pectineal line is called the *pectineal surface.* A second ridge or line runs from the pubic tubercle to the acetabular rim. This is the *obturator crest.* It gives attachment to the pubofemoral ligament.

The inferior ramus of the pubis joins the ramus of the ischium. It gives origin to the three adductor muscles of the thigh. At the apex of the obturator foramen on the inferior and posterior aspect of the superior ramus of the pubis is the *obturator groove* for the passage of the obturator nerve and vessels. In life this is converted to the obturator canal by the obturator membrane.

The acetabulum bears a *lunate (articular) surface,* an *acetabular notch,* a *rim,* and a central nonarticular portion, the *acetabular fossa.* The acetabulum is traditionally described as being composed of two-fifths ilium, two-fifths ischium, and one-fifth pubis. In life, a fibrocartilaginous labrum attaches to and deepens the acetabular rim. The acetabular notch is a gap in the acetabular rim and is actually closed in life by the *transverse acetabular ligament.* Additionally, a small ligament of the femoral head runs from this transverse acetabular ligament to the fovea capitis, a small depression in the center of the femoral head.

The innominate bone and pelvis are very important in the identification of both gender and age in unidentified skeletal remains and in radiographs. There are a

Figure 7–6   Gender-related differences in the male and female pelvis: (*A*) superior views, (*B*) anterior views. Note the much greater relative mediolateral diameter of the pelvic inlet and outlet in the female and the absolutely greater subpubic angle of the female.

number of sexual differences in the morphology of the innominates (see Fig. 7–6). As noted previously, in females the greater sciatic notch is broad and shallow, whereas it is deep and narrow in males. Among females, the *superior pubic ramus* is relatively long and the *subpubic angle,* formed by the meeting of the two inferior pubic rami at the pubic symphysis, is obtuse, whereas in males it is acute.

Important age-related changes also occur at the pubic symphysis and the auricular surface of the ilium. In young adulthood both of these surfaces are covered with ridges and furrows that progressively fill and become smoother with age. Other degenerative changes occur with age as well. These changes occur with some regularity and can be used by trained observers to estimate an age at death with reasonable certainty.

Additionally, throughout the skeleton, the appearance and fusion of ossification centers occur with a high degree of regularity. Therefore, the appearance and fusion of apophyses and epiphyses are an excellent means of determining skeletal age in subadults, either in x rays or in unidentified skeletal remains. Likewise, the appearance of tooth buds and the eruption sequence of teeth can be used to determine age in subadult skeletons. Anyone interested in the subject of diagnosis of age and gender in human skeletal remains would do well to consult as a starting point *The Human Skeleton in Forensic Medicine* (1st ed., Krogman, 1962; 2nd ed., Krogman and Iscan, 1986). See the References and Further Readings and Resources at the end of the text for additional information.

BONES OF THE LOWER LIMB

The *lower limb* is divisible into a more superior thigh (femur), running from the hip to the knee, and a more inferior leg (crus), running from the knee to the ankle. The femur (os femoris) is the bone of the thigh (Figure 7–7), whereas the tibia and fibula are the two bones of the leg (Figure 7–8). Strictly speaking, the term *femur* refers to the thigh, whereas *os femoris* refers to the bone of the thigh. Convention uses *thigh* to refer to bone and soft tissue, whereas *femur* is generally used to mean the bone alone.

The Femur

The *femur* is the largest bone of the body and the skeleton of the thigh. It consists of a proximal head; a neck; two large proximal protuberances, the greater and lesser trochanters; a shaft, or body; and a distal extremity composed of medial and lateral articular condyles.

Femur: The Proximal End

The *head* of the femur approximates a sphere. It is covered with hyaline articular cartilage and articulates with the acetabulum of the os coxae (innominate bone). The *fovea capitis* is a superomedial depression in the head, lacking articular cartilage. The fovea capitis receives the ligament of the head of the femur. The head is joined to the shaft by the *femoral neck.* There are two trochanters, or projections, on the proximal femur; they are formed by means of separate apophyses. The larger and more lateral projection is the greater trochanter, whereas the smaller, more medial projection is the lesser trochanter.

Viewed laterally, the *greater trochanter* approximates a square. The square is divided into two triangular areas by a transverse ridge beginning at its superoposterior corner and running to its anteroinferior corner. The ridge is the insertion of the gluteus medius. The upper of the two triangles is also covered by the gluteus medius. The area may underlie a bursa. The lower of the two triangles also underlies a bursa

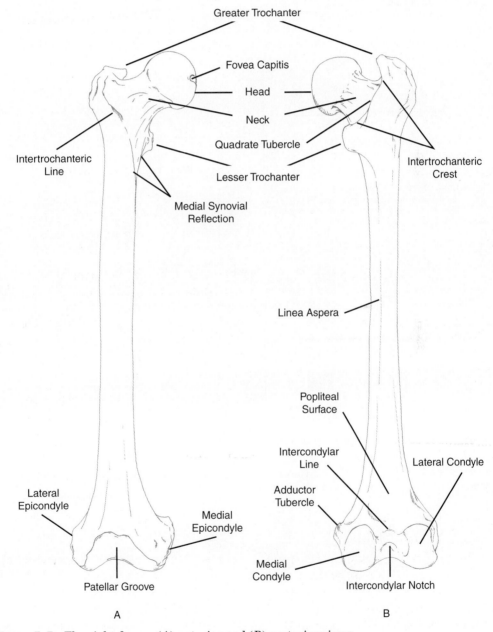

Figure 7–7   The right femur: (*A*) anterior and (*B*) posterior views.

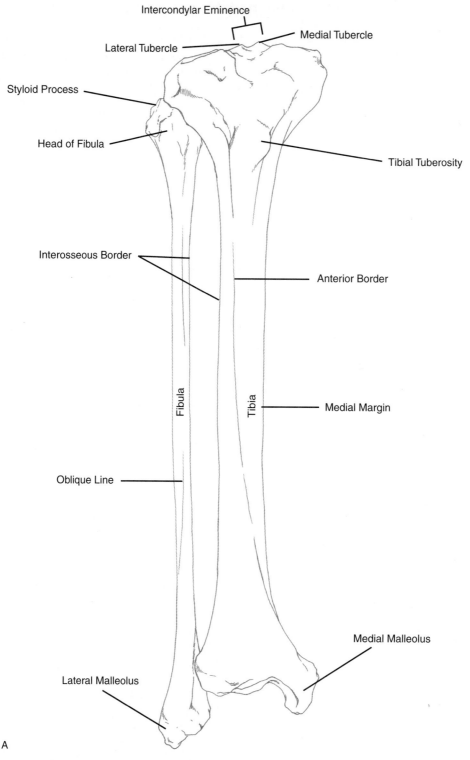

Figure 7–8 The right fibula and tibia: (A) anterior.

Intercondylar Eminence

Styloid Process

Lateral Articular Surface
(for lateral condyle of femur)

Medial Articular Surface
(for medial condyle of femur)

Head of Fibula

Soleal Line

Interosseous Border

Tibia

Fibula

Medial Margin

Malleolar Groove

Groove for Peroneal Tendons

Medial Malleolus

Lateral Malleolus

B

Figure 7–8 (*Continued*) (*B*) posterior.

that aids movement of the gluteus maximus covering this region. The greater trochanteric surface continues onto the anterior surface of the femoral shaft. There an inferior ovoid region may be distinguished, which receives the insertion of the gluteus minimus.

At the juncture of the femoral neck and shaft on the anterior surface is a linear rugosity that runs from the greater trochanter inferomedially toward the *lesser trochanter*. Before the rugose area reaches the lesser trochanter, however, it begins to ascend superomedially, forming a V. The entire line is called the *intertrochanteric line*. The V-shaped portion is referred to as the *medial synovial reflection*. The path of the line marks the insertion of a portion of the hip joint capsule called the *iliofemoral ligament*. The intertrochanteric line continues around the posterior aspect of the femur as the *spiral line* and eventually reaches the *linea aspera,* a raised ridge on the posterior aspect of the femur.

The medial surface of the greater trochanter displays a deep fossa, the *trochanteric fossa,* which receives the insertion of the obturator externus muscle. A groove may be palpated running across the posterior aspect of the neck superolaterally in the direction of the fossa. This is the *obturator externus groove.* Just anterior to the fossa, the insertions of the obturator internus and gemelli may be detected. Above them, on the superior surface of the trochanter, is an oval region to which the piriformis attaches.

On the posterior aspect of the proximal femur, the posterior surface of the greater trochanter is connected via a thick, broad elevation to the lesser trochanter. This ridge is called the *intertrochanteric crest.* Midway between the two trochanters on this crest is the *quadrate tubercle.* The quadratus femoris muscle inserts onto the quadrate tubercle and the portion of the intertrochanteric crest between the quadrate tubercle and the lesser trochanter. The lesser trochanter is the site of insertion of the combined iliopsoas muscle. The apex of the lesser trochanter receives the psoas major portion of the muscle; just distal to this is the insertion of the iliacus portion of the muscle.

Femur: The Shaft

The most prominent feature of the *shaft* of the femur is the *linea aspera* (literally, the "rough line"), the rugose line that runs two-thirds the length of the shaft on its posterior aspect. The linea aspera may be thought of as the arcs of two circles of very large diameter that intersect at approximately the center of the shaft. As the linea aspera approaches either end of the shaft, it divides into two crests or lips, a medial and a lateral. Proximally the lateral crest passes directly into a very long and thick rugosity, the *gluteal tuberosity.* The gluteal tuberosity receives the insertion of a part of the gluteus maximus.

An additional apophysis may occasionally be present at this site; it is termed the *third trochanter.* Although it is present only occasionally in *Homo sapiens,* it is a constant feature in some quadrupeds. The medial divergence of the proximal linea aspera receives the tendon of the pectineus muscle and is called the *pectineal line* (superior to the *spiral line*).

The central third of the linea aspera is densely occupied by numerous origins and insertions of thigh and hip muscles. Inserting upon it are the adductor brevis, adductor magnus, and adductor longus. Originating from it are the vastus medialis, the vastus lateralis, and the short head of the biceps femoris.

Femur: The Distal Extremity

As the distal extremity of the bone is approached, the linea aspera again divides into medial and lateral portions that descend to *medial* and *lateral condyles* of the femur. In doing so, they define a distinct triangular area on the posterior surface of the distal femur. This is called the *popliteal surface* of the femur. The less distinct medial portion of the divided linea aspera may be seen to terminate just proximal to the medial condyle at a small roughening called the *adductor tubercle.* The "hamstring" portion of the adductor magnus muscle inserts on this tubercle. At the base of the triangular popliteal surface superior to the medial and lateral condyles are two local elevated areas for the origins of the medial and lateral heads of the gastrocnemius muscle.

The dominant feature of the distal femur is its articular surface, composed of the large *medial* and *lateral femoral condyles.* The two condyles are confluent anteriorly and proximally to form the *patellar groove* or *surface,* but they are separated distally and posteriorly by the *intercondylar notch.* Each of the condyles bears a slight depression that may be easily palpated on the dry bone. These depressions represent the anterior limits of the intra-articular menisci of the knee joint.

Within the intercondylar notch may be found two distinctly smooth areas, one on each condyle. The one on the lateral condyle is more posterior and is the site of attachment of the *anterior cruciate ligament,* whereas the one on the medial condyle is more anterior and is the site of attachment of the *posterior cruciate ligament.* A slight ridge may be seen to join the two condyles at the posterior limit of the intercondylar notch; this is called the *intercondylar line.*

The medial surface of the medial condyle and the lateral surface of the lateral condyle both bear *epicondyles* above the articular surfaces. The *medial epicondyle* is the larger of the two, about the size of a quarter. The tibial (or medial) collateral ligament of the knee takes origin from it. The *lateral epicondyle* is smaller, about the size of a nickel, and gives origin to the fibular (or lateral) collateral ligament. A smooth depression may be located posteroinferior to the lateral epicondyle. This is the origin of the popliteus muscle.

Important Facts about the Femur

There are important age- and gender-related variations in the femur. Relative to femoral length, women have greater interacetabular widths than do men. As a result of this, women have a greater *bicondylar angle,* the angle formed between the shaft of the femur and a vertical parasagittal plane.

Because the proximal femur is an area particularly affected by age-related osteoporosis, x rays of the proximal femur can help to establish age in undocumented human skeletal material. Such features, together with other features of the skull and pelvis, are useful in medicolegal contexts in gender identification in unidentified or archeological human skeletal remains. The femur is also a particularly frequent site for histological and other methods of age-at-death determination from bone. (See Walker and Lovejoy, 1985; Walker et al., 1994; and other references at the end of the text for further information.)

The Patella

The *patella* (Figure 7–9) is a flat, rounded, triangular bone at the front of the knee joint. It is generally regarded as a large sesamoid bone in the tendon of the quadriceps

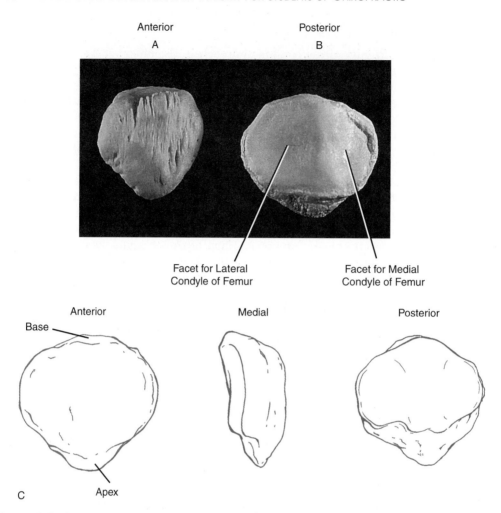

Anterior
A

Posterior
B

Facet for Lateral
Condyle of Femur

Facet for Medial
Condyle of Femur

Anterior
Base

Medial

Posterior

Apex

C

Figure 7-9   The right patella: (A) anterior surfaces and (B) articular (posterior) surfaces. (C) Diagrammatic representation from anterior, medial, and posterior aspects.

femoris muscle. It protects the front of the knee joint and increases the effectiveness of the quadriceps femoris muscle as an extender of the leg on the knee by increasing its moment arm about the knee. It has an anterior surface, a posterior surface, a base, and an apex.

The anterior surface is subcutaneous, whereas the posterior surface has a smooth oval articular area divided into two facets by a vertical ridge. The ridge contacts the patellar groove of the femur in extension, whereas the two demifacets on either side of this ridge contact the articular surfaces of the medial and lateral condyles of the femur in flexion. The base is proximal and receives the quadriceps tendon proper. The apex is distal.

Running between the apex of the patella and the tibial tuberosity on the proximal anterior tibia is the *patellar ligament* (patellar tendon). It is properly termed a *ligament* because it connects bone to bone, but functionally it is a part of the tendon of the quadriceps and possesses the histological features and receptors characteristic of a tendon.

The Tibia

The *tibia* (see Fig. 7–8) is the main weight-bearing bone of the leg. The fibula transmits only 10 percent of the force through the leg. With the exception of the femur, the tibia is the largest bone of the skeleton. It has five articulations: three (superior, middle, and inferior) for the fibula and one each for the talus (the large tarsal bone of the ankle joint) and the femur.

Tibia: The Proximal End

The femur rests upon the superior surface of the tibia. This superior surface is called the *tibial plateau.* The plateau supports two articular surfaces called the *medial* and *lateral articular facets* on its superior aspect and has a narrow nonarticular area separating them. The medial and lateral aspects of the tibial plateau that support the articular surfaces are often incorrectly referred to as *condyles.* A condyle is a convex, somewhat knuckle-shaped articular surface that articulates with a complementary concave surface on another bone. Thus the femur possesses *medial* and *lateral condyles* that articulate with medial and lateral articular surfaces on the tibial plateau. The medial articular surface of the tibial plateau is ovoid and usually concave, whereas the lateral articular surface of the tibial plateau is usually, but not always, convex.

The area between the articular surfaces is divided into anterior and posterior regions. The anterior region is triangular and is called the *anterior intercondylar area.* It typically has a deep groove where it borders the lateral articular surface. The anterior attachment of the lateral meniscus lies in this groove.

The anterior attachment of the medial meniscus is less well defined. A depression may usually be found near the anteromedial edge of the anterior intercondylar area. This is the site of attachment of the anterior cruciate ligament. (The names of the cruciate ligaments are based on their attachments to the tibia.)

In the center of the superior surface of the tibia are the *medial* and *lateral tubercles* that form the *intercondylar eminence.* This structure slopes posteriorly into the *posterior intercondylar area.* The medial and lateral menisci are attached in the depressions at the junctures of the medial and lateral tubercles of the intercondylar eminence within this area. The posterior cruciate ligament attaches in the center of this area.

The anterior portion of the proximal tibia is marked by a large triangular area. The inferior apex of this triangle is marked by the *tibial tuberosity.* It has a superior smooth portion and an inferior rough portion. The rough portion is the site of insertion of the patellar ligament, whereas the smooth portion underlies the infrapatellar bursa. Lateral and superior to the tibial tuberosity is a ridge marking the site of attachment of the iliotibial tract.

The thick, shelflike form of the two tibial "condyles" is broken posteriorly by a gap beneath the posterior interarticular area. Just medial to this gap, on the border of the medial articular surface, is a distinct groove, the site of attachment of the semimembranosus tendon. Just lateral to the gap, on the lateral aspect of the proximal tibia, is the articular facet for the fibula. Ligaments binding these two bones are attached around the circumference of this facet. Inferomedial to the tibial tuberosity is the site of the combined insertions of the sartorius, semitendinosus, and gracilis muscles. The marking for this triple tendon complex is called the *pes anserinus* (Latin meaning "goose foot").

Tibia: The Shaft

Descending from the fibular facet posteriorly and coursing medially is the *soleal line* (spiral line). It marks the origin of the soleus muscle from the fibular head to the proximal two-fifths of the tibia. Superior to this line is a broad, undefined triangular region that gives origin to the popliteus.

Almost joining the soleal line at the fibular facet is a distinct angular elevation running the length of the lateral surface of the tibia. This is the *interosseous border (interosseous margin)*, which separates the lateral surface of the shaft on its anterior side from the posterior surface of the shaft on its posterior side and gives attachment to the interosseous membrane running between the tibia and the fibula. The *anterior border* of the tibial shaft proceeds distally from the tip of the tibial tuberosity along the length of the shaft. It terminates on the anterior surface of the medial malleolus, the projection at the ankle.

The *medial margin* is ill defined. It develops from the expanded buttress of the medial side of the tibial plateau and descends to the posterior surface of the medial malleolus. It is more defined in its lower half. Much of its proximal portion is the soleal line. Just anterior to the medial margin, where the buttressing of the tibial plateau blends with the shaft, is usually a roughened, poorly defined region that is the insertion of the tibial (medial) collateral ligament of the knee.

The proximal two-thirds of the lateral surface of the tibial shaft give rise to the tibialis anterior. The posterior surface of the tibial diaphysis gives rise to the tibialis posterior laterally and the flexor digitorum longus medially (as well as the soleus and popliteus). Their origins are variable but occur along the middle third of the shaft. The tibialis posterior origin extends to the lower portion of the soleal line and bears the nutrient foramen in most cases. The tibialis posterior and anterior are separated from one another by the interosseous membrane.

Tibia: The Distal End

The prominent projection of the distal end of the tibia is the *medial malleolus*. Its inferior surface is occasionally pierced by vascular channels. Its posterior surface bears a deep groove that upon palpation is usually felt to be double. This double groove is for the tibialis posterior and flexor digitorum longus tendons. It is called the *malleolar groove*.

Another groove may also be detectable on the lateral portion of the posterior surface of the distal tibia. This is the *groove for the flexor hallucis longus tendon*. The lateral surface of the distal end bears the *fibular notch*. The inferior end of the medial malleolus, when viewed medially, usually appears notched. The deltoid ligament originates in this notch. The inferior articular surface, for the talus, frequently bears on its anterior edge articular extensions that contact the talus in extreme dorsiflexion of the foot. These are called *squatting facets*. They are not a constant feature, and their frequency varies from population to population.

Fibula

The *fibula* (see Fig. 7–8) bears approximately 10 percent of the force transmitted through the leg. It has three articular surfaces: two (proximal and distal) for the tibia and one distally for the talus. The joint between the distal fibula and the talus is synovial, whereas the distal joint between the fibula and tibia is more fibrous but at least in part synovial.

Fibula: The Proximal End

The proximal enlargement of the fibula is the *head*. It bears a flat articular facet for the corresponding facet on the lateral aspect of the tibial plateau. Surrounding it are the insertions of the tibiofibular joint capsule. The head has a distinct superiorly directed apex, the *styloid process*. The lateral surface of the head receives the tendon of the biceps femoris muscle. The posterior surface of the head receives the origin of the soleus muscle. The lateral aspect also receives the fibular (lateral) collateral ligament of the knee joint and gives origin to the fibularis (peroneus) longus muscle. The extensor digitorum longus arises from the anterior aspect of the head. *None of these origins and insertions are clearly defined osteologically.*

Fibula: The Shaft

The shaft is highly variable, and its muscular markings are usually difficult to interpret. The shaft is prismatic in cross-section. The lateral surface is usually the widest and smoothest. Note that it twists as it descends distally and begins to face more posteriorly. It terminates on the lateral surface of the distal end of the fibula, which is called the *lateral malleolus*. The fibularis (peroneus) longus muscle originates from the proximal two-thirds of the fibula. This overlaps the region of origin of the fibularis (peroneus) brevis muscle from the fibular's distal two-thirds. The tendons of these muscles pass through a groove on the posterior surface of the lateral malleolus.

Directly opposite the lateral surface of the shaft is the *interosseous crest* of the fibula, affording attachment to the interosseous membrane. It divides the remainder of the fibular surface into a medial and a posterior surface. The medial surface is usually grooved and gives rise to the extensor digitorum longus, peroneus tertius, and extensor hallucis longus. The posterior surface is frequently divided by a prominent line, the *oblique line;* it divides the posterior surface into two parts, one facing more medially and giving rise to the tibialis posterior, and the other facing more posteriorly and giving rise to the soleus and the flexor hallucis longus.

Fibula: The Distal End

The distal extremity of the fibula is the *lateral malleolus*. Its medial surface is composed of the more anterior *malleolar articular surface* and the more posterior *lateral malleolar fossa*. In the latter are the origins of the posterior tibiofibular ligament and the posterior talofibular ligament. The distal extension of the posterior face of the lateral malleolus bears a *groove for the tendon of the fibularis (peroneus) longus* and *brevis muscles*. The anterior border of the lateral malleolus gives attachment to the anterior tibiofibular ligament, the anterior talofibular ligament, and the calcaneofibular ligament. The articular surface of the lateral malleolus is for articulation with the talus. The distal tibiofibular joint is a syndesmosis and therefore has no subchondral bone.

The Foot

The skeleton of the *foot* (Figure 7–10) is composed of 26 bones consisting of three groups: *the tarsal bones, the metatarsal bones,* and *the phalanges.* The *tarsal bones* are most proximal, form the ankle and heel, and articulate proximally with the tibia and fibula. The *metatarsals* are a set of five small long bones. They are numbered I

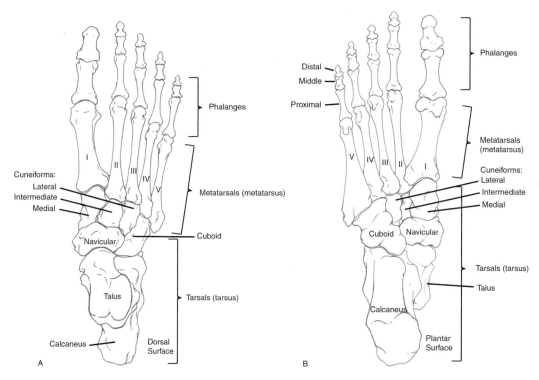

Figure 7-10 The skeleton of the right foot: (*A*) dorsal, (*B*) plantar.

through V from the medial (big toe) side. Their bases articulate with the distal row of tarsal bones; their heads articulate with the proximal phalanges of each of the digits. Each digit has three *phalanges*—a proximal, a middle, and a distal—with the exception of the big toe, or *hallux*. The hallux has only two phalanges, proximal and distal.

Foot: The Tarsus

The *tarsus* (see Fig. 7–10) consists of seven small, irregularly shaped bones, arranged in three rows: a proximal row, an intermediate row, and a distal row. They are closely applied to one another and are held firmly in their rows by strong ligaments. As a whole they form a strong fibrous and bony mass. The *proximal row* consists of the talus and the calcaneus. The talus rests on the superior surface of the calcaneus, between the latter and the medial and lateral malleoli. The *intermediate row* consists of a single bone, the navicular, situated between the head of the talus and the distal row of tarsals. Medially to laterally, the *distal row* consists of the medial cuneiform, the intermediate cuneiform, the lateral cuneiform, and the cuboid.

The *talus* (Figure 7–11A; see also Fig. 7–10) is the largest bone of the body that lacks any muscle attachments. The three major portions are the *corpus, neck,* and *head.* The *superior articular surface (trochlear surface),* on which the tibia rests, and the two *malleolar surfaces (medial malleolar surface* and *lateral malleolar surface)* constitute the *trochlea* of the talus. Immediately posterior to the medial malleolar facet is a vascularized area; behind this is a roughened area for the insertion of the deltoid ligament, which firmly binds the medial malleolus with the talus and calcaneus.

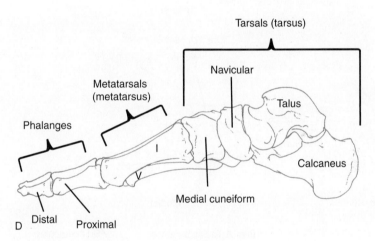

Figure 7-10 (*Continued*) (*C*) lateral and (*D*) medial views.

The posterior surface of the talus is marked by a deep groove for the tendon of the flexor hallucis longus. On either side are the lateral and medial tubercles of the talus. The *lateral tubercle* receives the posterior talofibular ligament. The *medial tubercle* receives the medial talocalcaneal ligament.

The inferior surface of the corpus is occupied by the *posterior calcaneal articular surface.* The inferior surface of the neck of the talus is occupied by the *anterior calcaneal articular surface.* Occasionally this is divided into a smaller *anterior* and larger *middle calcaneal articular surface,* to correspond with a similar division on the calcaneus. Between these two articular areas is the deep *talar groove.* This groove is occupied by the interosseous talocalcaneal ligament, a dense band filling the entire length of the groove.

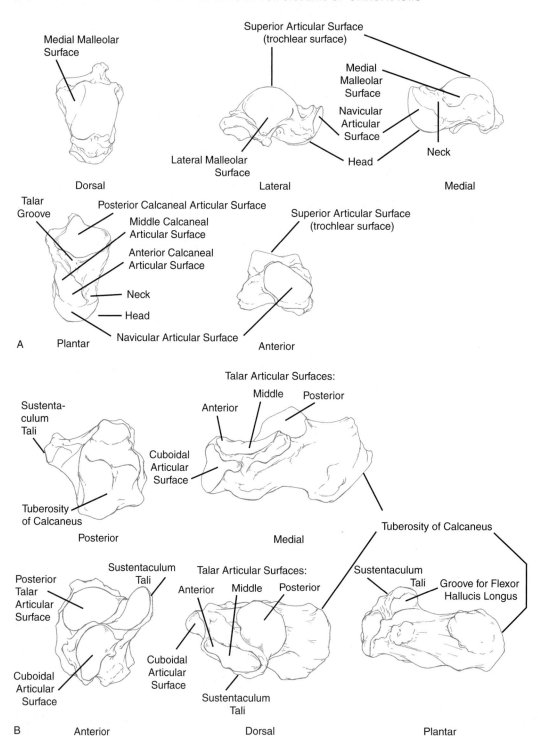

Figure 7–11   (A) Right talus and (B) right calcaneus.

Anterior to the neck of the talus is the *talar head*. Its articular surface is usually distinguishable into three planes. The most superior of these is the *navicular articular surface*. The other two planes, if present, define the anterior and middle parts of the anterior calcaneal articular surface.

The *calcaneus* (see Figs. 7–10 and 7–11*B*) is the only bone of the tarsus with an *apophysis,* which develops at the site of insertion of the gastrocnemius-soleus (calcaneal, or Achilles) tendon. It appears before the age of 10 and unites during the late teens. The large posteroinferior buttress is called the *tuberosity of the calcaneus.* The superior surface usually has three facets for articulation with the talus: the *anterior, middle,* and *posterior talar articular surfaces,* although the anterior and middle facets are often conjoined. The anterior surface of the bone is defined by the *cuboidal articular surface.*

When you articulate the talus and calcaneus, note that the talar groove has a corresponding floor on the calcaneus. This channel between the talus and calcaneus is called the *tarsal sinus.* The floor is called the *calcaneal groove.* The sinus and groove contain the *interosseous talocalcaneal ligament,* which also attaches in the talar groove.

The rough inferior surface ends posteriorly in an abrupt fashion as it develops into the *tuberosity of the calcaneus.* A well-defined anteriorly projecting spike of bone from this tuberosity is the site of origin of the long plantar ligament, which passes anteriorly to attach to the cuboid and four lateral metatarsal bases. The superior part of the calcaneal tuberosity is smooth, whereas the inferior part presents definite striations. The superior part underlies the bursa deep to the calcaneal tendon, whereas the rough inferior part receives the calcaneal tendon.

When the talus and calcaneus are articulated, the lateral malleolar surface of the talus comes to a point, which "points" inferiorly to a small but well-defined area of bone that is the *fibular (peroneal) trochlea* of the calcaneus. Posterior to this is a slight *groove for the fibular (peroneal) muscles.* Superior to the groove, at about the midpoint along the length of the bone, is a roughened area for the insertion of the calcaneofibular ligament.

The process on which the middle talar articular facet is found is called the *sustentaculum tali.* The sustentaculum tali projects medially and is easily identified in even fragmentary specimens by its presence. Note the deep groove for the flexor hallucis longus tendon on the undersurface of this structure.

The *navicular bone* (Figure 7–12) separates the talus and the three cuneiform bones. Its *posterior surface* is deeply concave for articulation with the head of the talus. Its *anterior surface* has three distinct facets for the three cuneiform bones. The largest of these is for the medial or first cuneiform. Extending out medially from the navicular is the *navicular tuberosity,* which receives the tendon of the tibialis posterior muscle. Its superior surface is convex.

The *medial (first) cuneiform* (see Fig. 7–12) is the largest of the three cuneiform bones. Its largest facet is kidney shaped and defines the anterior surface. It articulates with the first metatarsal. Opposite the medial cuneiform, on the posterior surface, is a concave facet for the navicular. The lateral surface has an L-shaped facet for articulation with the second cuneiform. On the medial surface is a smooth area that is actually a groove for the tendon of the tibialis anterior. The inferior surface of the wedge-shaped bone is narrow, whereas the superior surface is broad. The inferior surface receives the insertion of the tibialis anterior, tibialis posterior, and peroneus longus muscles.

The *intermediate (second) cuneiform* (see Fig. 7–12) is the smallest of the cuneiform bones. Two of its surfaces, the anterior and the posterior, are completely

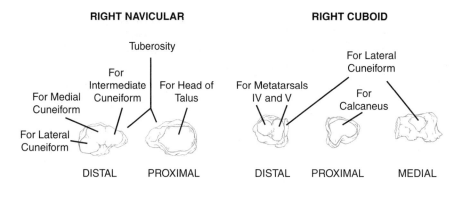

RIGHT NAVICULAR

Tuberosity

For Intermediate Cuneiform

For Medial Cuneiform

For Head of Talus

For Lateral Cuneiform

DISTAL   PROXIMAL

RIGHT CUBOID

For Lateral Cuneiform

For Metatarsals IV and V

For Calcaneus

DISTAL   PROXIMAL   MEDIAL

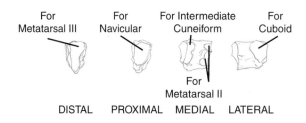

LEFT LATERAL CUNEIFORM

For Metatarsal III

For Navicular

For Intermediate Cuneiform

For Cuboid

For Metatarsal II

DISTAL   PROXIMAL   MEDIAL   LATERAL

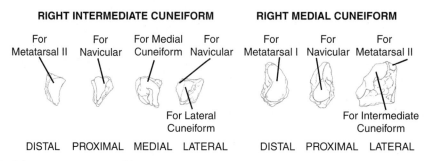

RIGHT INTERMEDIATE CUNEIFORM

For Metatarsal II

For Navicular

For Medial Cuneiform

For Navicular

For Lateral Cuneiform

DISTAL   PROXIMAL   MEDIAL   LATERAL

RIGHT MEDIAL CUNEIFORM

For Metatarsal I

For Navicular

For Metatarsal II

For Intermediate Cuneiform

DISTAL   PROXIMAL   LATERAL

Figure 7-12   The remaining tarsal bones.

covered by subchondral bone. The posterior concave surface articulates with the navicular; the anterior convex surface articulates with the second metatarsal. An L-shaped articular facet is located on its medial surface and matches the facet on the first cuneiform. The inferior surface receives an insertion of the tibialis posterior.

The *lateral (third) cuneiform* (see Fig. 7–12) also has anterior and posterior surfaces completely covered by subchondral bone. The large anterior surface articulates with the third metatarsal; the smaller posterior surface articulates with the navicular. The navicular facet continues on to the medial surface of the bone to form the articular surface for the second cuneiform.

The *cuboid* (see Fig. 7–12) is quite distinctive in shape. Note that it has only three articular facets. One of these is small and isolated. It is for the third cuneiform and matches the corresponding facet on that bone. The superior surface is broad; the inferior surface has a prominent ridge. The smaller of the two remaining articular facets is anterior and is subdivided for the fourth and fifth metatarsals. The posterior surface is saddle shaped with a prominent projection. It articulates with the calcaneus. The prominent ridge on the inferior surface is for the *attachment of the long plantar ligament.* Anterior to this is a deep *groove for the tendon of the fibularis (peroneus) longus muscle.* The notch on the very small lateral surface of the bone is an artifact of the peroneus longus groove.

Foot: The Metatarsus

The *metatarsus* (see Fig. 7–10) is formed by the five *metatarsal bones.* Each of these bones has a *shaft,* a proximal *base,* and a distal *head.* The first metatarsal is the most robust and the shortest. The peroneus longus and tibialis anterior insert at the inferior surface of its base. There is occasionally a facet for the articulation with the second metatarsal. The head is subdivided into *two grooves* by a prominent inferior ridge. These grooves are for the *two sesamoid bones* in the tendons of the flexor hallucis brevis. The nutrient foramen is usually clearly identifiable.

If all are present, the rest of the metatarsals may be easily identified as follows: The *second* is the longest; the *third, fourth,* and *fifth* successively decrease in length. The fifth is especially distinctive because of the presence of a prominent inferolateral *tuberosity* that receives the tendon of the fibularis (peroneus) brevis muscle. The bases of the second and third metatarsals have distinctive triangular articular facets for the second and third cuneiforms. The second is much longer, and its facet is more concave, well rounded, and distinctly nonangular.

Foot: The Phalanges

There are three phalanges (see Fig. 7–10) in each toe: a *proximal,* a *middle,* and a *distal,* with the exception of the hallux, which possesses only a proximal and a distal, just as does the *pollex.* The phalanges of the toes are similar to the phalanges of the hand in general morphology; they are, however, generally shorter. The phalanges of the hallux are very robust, much more so than those of the pollex.

The *distal phalanx of the hallux* is distinctive. It is very large and the bone shows considerable torsion along its long axis. The flexor digitorum brevis inserts upon the middle phalanges of the second through fifth digits.The distal phalanges receive the tendons of the flexor digitorum longus and extensor digitorum longus. Unlike the palmar surfaces of the phalanges of the hand, the plantar surfaces of the phalanges of the foot are rounded.

ARTICULATIONS OF THE LOWER LIMB

The joints of the lower limb consist of the joints of the hip, knee, ankle, and foot. The pelvic girdle is intimately associated with the hip joint; we consider it here with the lower limb joints.

Articulations and Ligaments of the Pelvis

The bony pelvis, which includes the sacrum, is joined to the lumbar vertebrae via the anterior and posterior longitudinal ligaments, the L5-S1 intervertebral disc, the ligamenta flava, the interspinous and supraspinous ligaments, and the articular capsules of the zygapophyseal joints (refer to Figures 7–13 through 7–15 throughout the

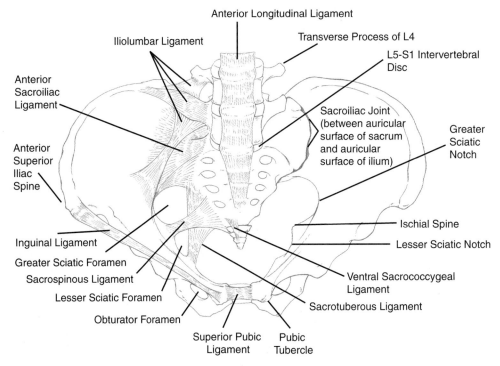

Figure 7–13   Ligaments of the pelvis, anterior view.

discussion of the articulations and ligaments of the pelvis). Additionally, the fifth lumbar vertebra (and occasionally the fourth) is joined with the pelvis via one additional ligament on each side, the *iliolumbar ligament.* Each iliolumbar ligament consists of a *superior band* and an *inferior band;* the inferior band is also known as the *lumbosacral ligament.*

Both bands attach medially to the transverse process of L5 and sometimes to L4 as well. The superior band runs from the transverse process of L5 to the crest of the ilium immediately lateral to the sacroiliac articulation. The inferior band runs from the transverse process of L5 to the base of the sacrum, where it blends with the *anterior sacroiliac ligament.* These two bands limit lateral flexion of the lumbar spine.

Other articulations of the pelvis can be divided into four groups: (1) those connecting the sacrum and ilium, (2) those passing between the sacrum and ischium, (3) those uniting the sacrum and coccyx (discussed with the vertebral articulations in Chap. 4), and (4) those between the two pubic bones.

The Sacroiliac Articulation

The *sacroiliac articulation* occurs between the *auricular surface of the ilium* and the matching *auricular surface of the sacrum.* This joint is a synchondrosis. It has a very special character because the sacral portion develops from somitic mesoderm, whereas the innominate portion develops from lateral plate mesoderm. The sacral portion presents a typical chondral surface and is also a growth center, or epiphysis. The surface of the innominate portion has a different texture and includes a significant amount of fibrocartilage. The two parts of the joint are united by patches of

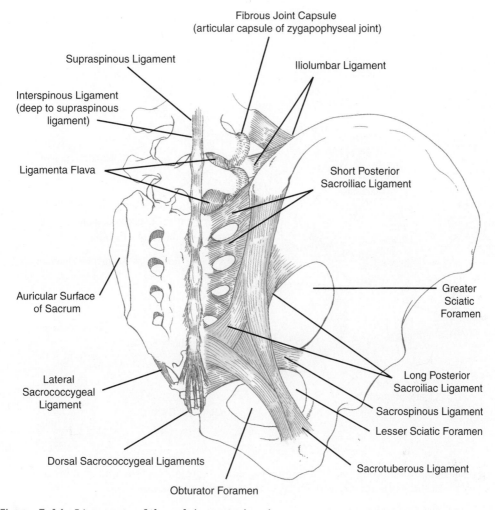

Figure 7–14   Ligaments of the pelvis, posterior view.

softer fibrocartilage. Over a considerable portion of the joint, especially in later life, there may be a synovial cavity, so that it exhibits some characteristics of a plane synovial joint. The joint has three ligaments:

1. The anterior sacroiliac ligament
2. The posterior sacroiliac ligament
3. The interosseous sacroiliac ligament

The *anterior sacroiliac ligament* extends from the base and the lateral parts of the ventral surface of the sacrum to the margins of the auricular surface of the ilium. The *posterior sacroiliac ligament* consists of both long and short fibers. The *short posterior sacroiliac ligament* runs from intermediate and lateral sacral crests to the posterior superior iliac spine and internal lip of the iliac crest at its dorsal end. The *long posterior sacroiliac ligament* runs from the lower part of the lateral sacral crest to the posterior superior iliac spine, where some of its fibers merge with the fibers of the *sacrotuberous ligament*.

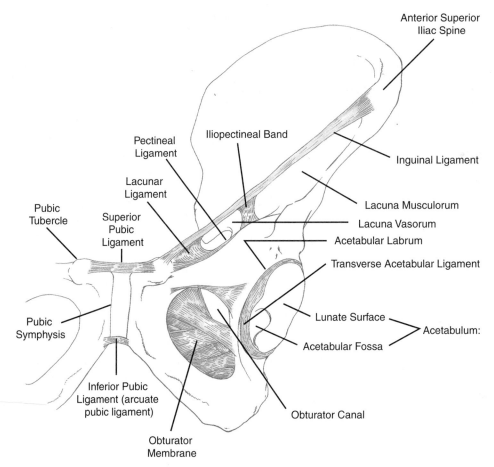

Figure 7-15   Inguinal and associated ligaments, pubic ligaments, obturator membrane, transverse acetabular ligament, and acetabular labrum, left anterior view.

The *interosseous sacroiliac ligament* is located between the sacroiliac joint and the posterior sacroiliac ligaments, uniting the tuberosities of the ilium and the sacrum. It is a large syndesmosis lying deep to the posterior sacroiliac ligament.

During flexion and extension of the trunk, some rotation may occur at the sacroiliac articulation (Soames and Atha, 1981). The axis of rotation is located 5 to 10 cm inferior to the sacral promontory. The greatest amount of motion of the sacrum relative to the innominate bones occurs in rising from a sitting position. The sacral promontory moves forward, a movement called *nutation*, as much as 5 or 6 mm as body weight pushes down on the top of the sacrum. Less posterior motion occurs at the sacral apex.

The range of motion is the same in males and nonpregnant females, but *nutation* and *counternutation* increase in pregnancy. The sacroiliac joint may be injured by falls, automobile accidents, childbirth, and other causes, with resultant pain in walking, climbing stairs, and moving from a sitting to a standing position and vice versa. The patient may walk with a limp. (For more details, see Edwardson, 1995.)

Ligaments Connecting the Sacrum and Ischium

The two ligaments connecting the sacrum and the ischium are the sacrotuberous ligament and the sacrospinous ligament.

The *sacrotuberous ligament* extends from the posterior inferior iliac spine, the fourth and fifth transverse tubercles, and the caudal part of the lateral margin of the sacrum and coccyx to the inner margin of the tuberosity of the ischium. Its more proximal fibers fuse with the long posterior sacroiliac ligament.

The *sacrospinous ligament* is a thin triangular sheet attached by its broad base to the lateral margins of the sacrum and coccyx. Its apex is attached to the ischial spine. The sacrotuberous and sacrospinous ligaments close the greater and lesser sciatic notches of the ilium to create the greater and lesser sciatic foramina.

The Pubic Symphysis

The pubic symphysis is the joint between the bodies of the two pubic bones. As in all symphyses, a fibrocartilaginous disc is interposed between the articular surfaces of the two bones. Each of these surfaces is covered with a thin layer of hyaline cartilage. The ligaments of this articulation are the superior pubic ligament and the arcuate pubic ligament, or inferior pubic ligament.

The *superior pubic ligament* connects the two pubic bones superiorly and extends laterally as far as the pubic tubercles. The *arcuate pubic ligament,* or *inferior pubic ligament,* is a thick band of fibers uniting the two pubic bones and forming the boundary of the pubic arch (subpubic angle). Its fibers blend with those of the interpubic fibrocartilaginous disc. It attaches to the inferior pubic rami.

Other Ligaments of the Pelvis

In addition to the ligaments associated with the various articulations of the pelvis, there are also important ligaments associated with the attachment of the anterior abdominal wall to the innominate bone. These include the following:

- The inguinal ligament
- The lacunar ligament
- The pectineal ligament
- The iliopectineal band

The *inguinal ligament* is formed by the aponeurosis of the external oblique muscle. It attaches to the anterior superior iliac spine and the pubic tubercle. The medial part of the inguinal ligament is reflected horizontally back and is attached to the pecten pubis as the *lacunar ligament.* Some of the fibers of the lacunar ligament continue laterally along the pectineal line of the pubis. These fibers are known as the *pectineal ligament.*

Connecting the inferior surface of the middle portion of the inguinal ligament to the superior surface of the iliopectineal eminence is the *iliopectineal band.* This band divides the space beneath the inguinal ligament into a more lateral *lacuna musculorum,* for the passage of the iliopsoas muscle and femoral nerve—the floor of this lacuna is the iliopsoas groove of the innominate—and a more medial *lacuna vasorum,* for the passage of the femoral vessels and lymphatics. The lacunar ligament is so called because it demarcates the medial extent of the lacuna vasorum.

The Hip Joint

The *hip (acetabulofemoral) joint* (Figure 7–16) is a spheroidal, or ball-and-socket, joint. As such, it has a great range of motion. In fact, only the glenohumeral joint has a greater range of motion. However, the hip joint has a much deeper bony socket for the reception of the femoral head than does the shoulder joint for the head of the humerus. The hip joint is also surrounded by massive amounts of muscle and a very strong fibrous joint capsule with well-developed intrinsic ligaments relative to the glenohumeral joint. As a result, although the hip joint is more stable and much less subject to displacement or dislocation than is the shoulder joint, its range of motion is somewhat more limited.

The simplest definition of the hip joint is that it is the articulation of the spheroidal head of the femur with the cup-shaped acetabulum. Although that is certainly a straightforward definition, the joint is not quite that simple. The convex femoral head and the concave acetabulum are not quite congruent, in that they do not have exactly the same curvature. Further, the femoral head is not quite spheroid, but slightly ovoid. The joint surfaces approach a nearly spherical form in older age.

Additionally, the femoral head does not present a smooth, uninterrupted articular surface. In fact, near the center of the head of the femur is the roughened *fovea capitis* for the reception of the *ligament of the head of the femur (ligamentum teres capitis*

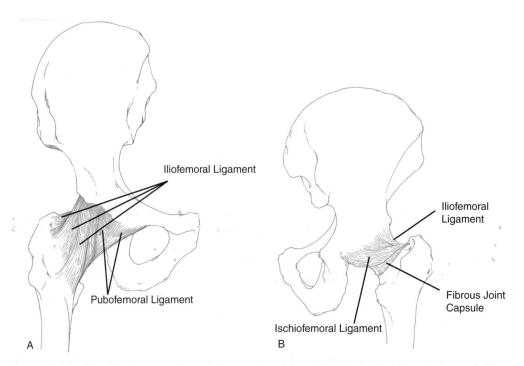

Figure 7–16   The fibrous capsule and ligaments of the right hip joint: (*A*) anterior and (*B*) posterior views.

femoris), a small ligament that runs from the transverse acetabular ligament to the fovea capitis. The articular surface of the femoral head covers more than half a sphere.

The acetabulum does not present a complete complementary articular surface. The articular cartilage of the acetabulum covers only the crescent moon-shaped *lunate surface.* Surrounding the margin of the acetabulum and deepening it is a fibrocartilaginous *acetabular labrum,* which is similar in structure and function to the shoulder's glenoid labrum. The labrum reaches over the head of the femur to a point beyond the greatest circumference of the femoral head. Thus the greatest diameter of the femoral head exceeds the diameter of the opening through the acetabular labrum. This has the effect of making it especially difficult for the head of the femur to be dislocated from the acetabulum.

The entire hip joint is surrounded by a very thick and strong fibrous joint capsule and is reinforced by a number of ligaments, including the following:

- The transverse acetabular ligament
- The ligament of the head of the femur
- The iliofemoral ligament
- The pubofemoral ligament
- The ischiofemoral ligament

The transverse acetabular ligament and the ligament of the head of the femur (ligamentum teres) are intracapsular ligaments, in that they are contained inside the joint's fibrous capsule. The fibrous joint capsule itself contains three very prominent and strong intrinsic ligaments: the iliofemoral, pubofemoral, and ischiofemoral ligaments (see Fig. 7–16).

As noted, most of the acetabulum is surrounded by a fibrocartilaginous labrum. The labrum continues across the gap of the acetabular notch as the *transverse acetabular ligament,* which completes the circumference of the acetabulum. The *ligament of the head of the femur (ligamentum teres capitis femoris)* arises from the transverse acetabular ligament and follows the acetabular notch to reach the fovea capitis of the femoral head. In living persons it is ordinarily compressed into the pad of fat that fills the acetabular fossa. The ligamentum teres is too weak to play an important role in reinforcing the hip joint, but it does carry a small branch of the obturator artery to the head of the femur. This small artery may spare the head of the femur from avascular necrosis in the event of a fracture of the neck of the femur.

The fibrous joint capsule of the hip joint is thick, dense, and strong. It attaches around the margins of the acetabulum, extending 5 or 6 mm beyond the margins of the acetabular labrum. It also attaches to the transverse acetabular ligament and to the margin of the obturator foramen. Inferiorly and laterally it attaches to the neck of the femur. *Anteriorly* on the femur it attaches to the intertrochanteric line, *superiorly* to the base of the neck of the femur, *posteriorly* a centimeter or so medially and superiorly to the intertrochanteric crest, and *inferiorly* to the inferior part of the neck near the lesser trochanter.

The capsule has two zones: an inner *zona orbicularis,* which consists of circular fibers surrounding the neck of the femur, and an outer longitudinal zone. The outer longitudinal fibers run between the acetabulum and femur and are reinforced by the iliofemoral, pubofemoral, and ischiofemoral ligaments.

The *iliofemoral ligament* is a strong, triangular ligamentous band. It lies anterior to the joint and its fibers blend with those of the joint capsule. Its apex attaches to the anterior inferior iliac spine and to the body of the ilium. It then divides into two bands of fibers. One passes laterally and inferiorly to attach to the lower part of the intertrochanteric line of the femur, whereas the other passes more laterally to insert into the more superior part of the intertrochanteric line.

Because of the two bands of fibers, this ligament is sometimes called the Y-shaped ligament because it resembles an inverted Y. The two bands of the ligament are joined by thinner material and often blend tightly together. The iliofemoral ligament defines the limits of hip extension becasue it tightens in extension. It reinforces the anterior part of the fibrous capsule when body weight in the standing position tends to push the trunk backward on the hip joints.

The *pubofemoral ligament* is likewise a strong band of ligamentous fibers that helps reinforce the fibrous joint capsule of the hip joint. Medially it attaches to the pubis near the acetabulum and to the adjoining superior pubic ramus. Its fibers then pass laterally, anterior to the femoral head, to attach to the femoral neck. Its fibers blend with those of the joint capsule and with the nearby medial portion of the iliofemoral ligament. The pubofemoral ligament defines the limits of hyperextension and hyperabduction of the femur.

The *ischiofemoral ligament* is a triangular band of fibers arising from the body of the ischium inferior and posterior to the acetabulum. It blends with the zona orbicularis of the capsule. Its more superior fibers are oriented horizontally across the hip joint, whereas its lower fibers spiral superiorly and laterally to attach to the neck of the femur medial to the greater trochanter. This ligament becomes tense near the limits of extension of the hip joint.

Unique Features of the Human Hip

The human hip is structured to accommodate human habitual bipedality (walking on only the hindlimbs as the principal means of locomotion). Half of the weight above the hip joint is transmitted through each of the femoral heads in the upright position. As a result, the human hip has unique structural components.

Already noted in the discussion of the hip bone is the iliac pillar, the thickened column of trabecular bone running from the cristal tuberosity of the iliac crest to the superior margin of the acetabulum. The iliac pillar becomes increasingly prominent as it approaches its interface with the cristal tubercle. This is a natural consequence of the structure's being the "bony history" of the growth of the cristal tubercle, a thickening of the iliac crest.

The lateral surface of the ilium resists compressive forces generated by the contraction of the gluteus medius and minimus muscles, or hip abductors, in the *single stance* (one-legged) *phase* of human locomotion. Body weight is transferred through the acetabulum and then onto the neck of the femur. A very well developed group of bony trabeculae leads from the femoral head to the inferior cortical bone of the neck of the femur. This is called the *calcar femorale;* it transmits body weight and joint reaction forces from the head of the femur to its shaft.

Likewise, the cortical bone of the femoral neck is uniquely arranged in humans. In many other animals, the cortex of the femoral neck is of uniform thickness all around its perimeter. In humans, the inferior cortex of the femoral neck is much thickened, whereas its superior cortex is very thin (Lovejoy, 1988). The inferior aspect of the femoral neck carries most of the weight from the head of the femur to its shaft.

Ranges of Motion of the Hip Joint

The hip can circumduct; thus movements at the hip joint include flexion/extension, abduction/adduction, and rotation. The range of motion is extensive but not as extensive as those of the glenohumeral joint, being restricted primarily by other body parts. Motions of the hip joint are referred to in relation to the femoral neck. The femoral neck itself is relatively long and meets the shaft of the femur at an angle of approximately 125 degrees. For the thigh to flex and extend, the head and neck of the femur must rotate about their long axes. Likewise, during medial and lateral rotation of the thigh, the junction of the neck and shaft of the femur must swing forward and backward.

Disorders of the Hip Joint

In severe cases of *osteoporosis,* the femoral neck is at great risk of fracture because of its important weight-bearing role. Such fractures in elderly persons are often slow to heal, and complications frequently prove fatal. The head of the femur does not have a rich blood supply. Often in fractures of the neck of the femur, the femoral head loses its blood supply and the bone of the femoral head dies, resulting in *avascular (aseptic) necrosis.*

The hip joint can be subject to severe *osteoarthritis.* Osteoarthritis can cause excessive joint pain because of degeneration of the articular cartilage and the formation of *osteophytes,* pathological bony spicules growing in and around the joint; mobility is often severely limited. Extreme cases may require *joint replacement surgery.*

Snapping hip is a condition in which the iliotibial band or anterior aspect of the gluteus maximus muscle slips over the greater trochanter with an audible popping sound. It may or may not be associated with pain.

Multiple muscles and their tendons are associated with the hip joint, as are multiple bursae. As a result, *tendinitis* and *bursitis* are frequent problems of the hip.

Traumatic dislocation of the hip joint is much less frequent than dislocations of the shoulder because of the hip joint's much stronger and much more restrictive construction. Dislocation of the hip joint occurs most commonly in automobile accidents when a person is sitting with the thighs abducted and laterally rotated.

Congenital dislocation is more common at the hip than elsewhere.

The Knee Joint

The knee is a compound joint (Figure 7–17), consisting of a bicondylar joint between the distal femur and the proximal tibia (tibiofemoral joint) and a sellar joint between the patella and the patellar surface of the femur (patellofemoral joint). The knee also involves several different ligaments and complex motion and is closely associated with the proximal tibiofibular articulation.

Tibiofemoral Articulation

The principal joint of the knee is the *tibiofemoral joint,* or *tibiofemoral articulation.* This joint is sometimes incorrectly referred to as a ginglymus or hinge joint. It is actually, as mentioned, a bicondylar joint between the condyles of the distal femur and the articular surfaces of the proximal tibia. As with all bicondylar joints, the

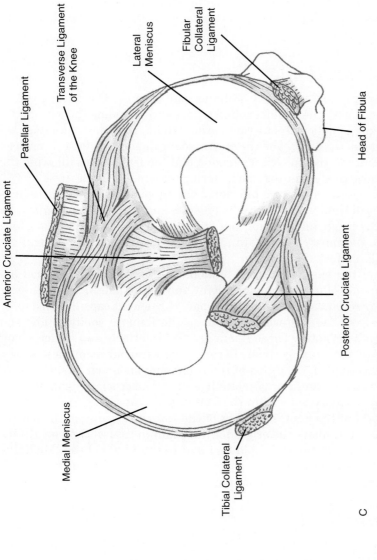

Anterior Cruciate Ligament

Patellar Ligament

Transverse Ligament
of the Knee

Lateral
Meniscus

Fibular
Collateral
Ligament

Head of Fibula

Posterior Cruciate Ligament

Medial Meniscus

Tibial Collateral
Ligament

C

Figure 7–17 Ligaments and menisci of the knee: (A) anterior, (B) posterior, and (C) superior views.

motion occuring between surfaces is not a simple hinge motion, as in a true ginglymus, but a combination of hinge and rotatory motion. As has been described, the distal femur possesses two condyles, the medial and the lateral, with the medial longer than the lateral. That incongruity in length permits lateral rotation of the tibial shaft in knee joint extension and medial rotation in knee joint flexion. A number of ligaments are associated with the tibiofemoral joint and reinforce the fibrous joint capsule. Additionally, because the femoral and tibial joint surfaces are incongruent with one another, menisci (articular discs) separate femoral condyles from the articular facets of the proximal tibia.

THE FIBROUS JOINT CAPSULE

The tibiofemoral joint is surrounded by a fibrous joint capsule. The capsule is partially deficient and blends with the ligaments and tendons surrounding the joint. Anteriorly, the fibrous capsule is deficient superior to the patella, resulting in contact between the synovial lining of the cavity and the tendon of the quadriceps femoris muscle. This reduces friction between the quadriceps tendon and the femur, thus allowing the quadriceps tendon to move freely over the femur during movements of the knee.

At the level of the patella and more inferiorly, the capsule blends with the tendons of the vastus lateralis and vastus medialis muscles and with the *fascia lata,* the broad, thick fascia of the thigh, and its *iliotibial band,* a thickening of the fascia lata laterally that attaches the tensor fascia lata muscle superiorly with the lateral aspect of the proximal tibia inferiorly.

The attachments of the vastus muscles' tendons to the medial and lateral aspects of the fibrous capsule of the tibiofemoral joint and to the patella form the *medial* and *lateral patellar retinacula.* The posterior part of the joint capsule consists of vertical fibers arising from the posterior portions of the femoral condyles and the margins of the intercondylar notch. These fibers proceed inferiorly and attach along the posterior margins of the tibial plateau. Because the synovial membrane of the joint capsule proceeds around the margins of the intercondylar notch in such a way that it passes anteriorly to the anterior cruciate ligament, the cruciate ligaments remain outside the synovial cavity but within the fibrous joint capsule.

On the lateral aspect of the joint, the fibers of the capsule arise from the border of the lateral femoral condyle above the origin for the popliteus muscle and attach inferiorly to the lateral aspect of the tibial plateau and to the fibular head. Medially, the fibrous capsule attaches to the inferior aspect of the medial femoral condyle superiorly and to the medial aspect of the tibial plateau inferiorly.

THE SYNOVIAL MEMBRANE

The *synovial membrane* of the knee joint lines the internal aspect of the fibrous joint capsule. The synovial membrane of the knee joint is the most complicated in the human body. It attaches to the superior border of the patella and then extends upward for a distance beneath the tendon of the quadriceps femoris tendon. This extension is frequently referred to as the *suprapatellar bursa,* but it is not a true bursa; it is actually a continuation of the synovial cavity of the joint. It has its own muscle, the *articularis genu,* to support it during movements of the knee.

The synovial membrane extends to either side of the patella deep to the aponeuroses of the vastus lateralis and vastus medialis muscles, especially under the vastus medialis. Inferiorly, it is separated from the patellar ligament by a fat pad, the *infra-*

patellar fat pad. Two folds, the left and right *alar folds,* of the synovial membrane project from the medial and lateral aspects of the articular surface of the patella. They converge inside the joint to form the *infrapatellar synovial fold* that attaches to the anterior aspect of the intercondylar notch of the femur.

From the superior and posterior aspect of the joint, the synovial membrane forms two pouches, one of which reaches beneath each head of the gastrocnemius muscle as the heads rise from the femur. The synovial membrane covers the superior and inferior surfaces of the menisci. The internal free borders of the menisci are not covered by the synovial membrane. The synovium then continues from the inferior surfaces of the menisci and attaches to the proximal tibia.

A recess of the synovial capsule continues as a small sac between the tendon of the popliteus muscle and the lateral meniscus. This is the *subpopliteal recess.* The synovial membrane in general follows the course of the fibrous joint capsule but is reflected anterior to the cruciate ligaments, which therefore remain outside the synovial cavity. A large number of bursae surround the knee joint to reduce friction between the skin and underlying tissue as the knee moves.

Ligaments

A number of very strong ligaments reinforce the knee joint. Because the knee joints bear all the body weight above the knees and because the highly convex femoral condyles rest somewhat precariously on the relatively shallow articular facets of the proximal tibia, the joint would be highly unstable without a number of strong, cordlike ligaments to help maintain the femur upon the tibial plateau. Even with the presence of these ligaments, the knee is still highly susceptible to injury. Four well-developed ligaments (see Fig. 7–17)—the tibial (medial) and fibular (lateral) collateral ligaments and the anterior and posterior cruciate ligaments—are particularly important to the maintenance of joint integrity. Other ligaments include the oblique popliteal and arcuate popliteal ligaments, the coronary ligament, and the transverse ligament of the knee.

THE FIBULAR COLLATERAL LIGAMENT

The *fibular (lateral) collateral ligament* is a round, dense band, about the diameter of a pencil, extending from the lateral epicondyle of the femur inferiorly to the head of the fibula. (The *proximal tibiofibular joint* lies just lateral and inferior to the knee joint.) The tendon of insertion of the popliteus muscle separates the lateral collateral ligament from the lateral meniscus. The fibular collateral ligament reinforces the lateral side of the knee joint capsule, assisted by the iliotibial band as it passes the lateral aspect of the knee to attach to the proximal tibia.

THE TIBIAL COLLATERAL LIGAMENT

The *tibial (medial) collateral ligament* is composed of two broad bands of fibers arising from the medial epicondyle of the femur just below the adductor tubercle. The deeper band passes inferiorly and posteriorly to insert onto the more posterior and medial part of the border of the tibial plateau. The more superficial band passes inferiorly to attach to the medial and superior aspect of the tibial shaft. The tibial collateral ligament is firmly attached to the margin of the medial meniscus of the tibiofemoral joint. This limits the freedom of the medial meniscus to move about in the joint cavity. Because the medial meniscus is firmly attached to the tibial collateral ligament—unlike the lateral meniscus and collateral ligament, which are *not* joined together—damage to the tibial collateral ligament regularly leads to damage to the medial meniscus.

THE CRUCIATE LIGAMENTS

The anterior and posterior cruciate ligaments are two very strong intra-articular ligaments, each about the diameter of a pencil or larger. They are located in the middle of the joint, but closer to the posterior margin of the tibial plateau than to the anterior margin. They are called *cruciate* ("cross shaped") because they cross one another in a manner resembling a letter X or a tilted cross. The cruciate ligaments help affix the proximal tibia to the distal femur and reinforce the knee joint. They are named according to their points of connection on the tibia.

The *anterior cruciate ligament* attaches to a depression anterior to the intercondylar eminence on the tibial plateau, where it blends with the anterior horn of the lateral meniscus. It passes superiorly, posteriorly, and laterally to insert into the posterior part of the medial surface of the lateral condyle of the femur. The anterior cruciate ligament helps limit hyperextension of the knee and anterior displacement of the tibia relative to the femur. This limits extension of the lateral condyle of the femur and causes medial rotation of the femur on the tibia as the medial condyle continues to full extension. As full extension occurs, the collateral ligaments and the oblique popliteal ligament become taut and eventually prevent any other rotation. This rotation with full extension is often referred to as the "screw home" mechanism of the knee.

The *posterior cruciate ligament* is stronger but shorter and more oblique than the anterior ligament. It attaches to the tibia in a depression posterior to the intercondylar eminence of the tibial plateau and has fibers that proceed onto the posterior aspect of the tibia. It attaches to the posterior horn of the lateral meniscus. It then proceeds superiorly, anteriorly, and medially to insert onto the lateral surface of the medial condyle of the femur, passing medially to the anterior cruciate ligament as it does so. The posterior cruciate ligament defines the limits of both hyperflexion of the knee and anterior motion of the femur relative to the surface of the tibia. This ligament is especially important in walking down steep inclines or steps, where body weight is transferred to the tibia at the same time the knee is flexed.

THE OBLIQUE POPLITEAL LIGAMENT

The *oblique popliteal ligament* blends with and reinforces the posterior portion of the fibrous joint capsule of the tibiofemoral articulation. It attaches laterally and proximally to the margin of the intercondylar fossa and to the posterior aspect of the lateral condyle of the femur. It then passes distally and at an oblique angle medially to insert onto the posterior and medial aspect of the proximal tibia just above the soleal line. Its more superficial fibers blend with the semimembranosus muscle, which passes nearby.

THE ARCUATE POPLITEAL LIGAMENT

The *arcuate popliteal ligament* attaches superiorly to the posterior aspect of the lateral condyle of the femur and then passes medially and inferiorly to cross the posterior aspect of the knee joint articular capsule, passing over the tendon of the popliteus muscle. It attaches to the tibial plateau just posterior to the attachment of the posterior cruciate ligament. It also sends fibers to the posterior aspect of the apex of the fibular head.

THE MENISCI

The medial and lateral menisci (see Fig. 7–17) are two C-shaped fibrocartilaginous articular discs between the femoral condyles and the articular facets on the tibial plateau. The internal borders of the menisci are free, but the external surfaces are bound to the proximal tibia by the *coronary ligament*. The coronary ligament, as the name implies (*coronary* means "crown"), surrounds the top of the proximal tibia. Its fibers are blended with the fibrous joint capsule.

Additionally, the *medial meniscus* is tightly bound to the medial collateral ligament. The two menisci, as noted, are shaped like the letter C. The opening of each C is directed inward toward the center of the joint, and the free ends of each meniscus are attached to the anterior and posterior ends of the tibial intercondylar eminence. The medial meniscus is broader posteriorly than anteriorly. Its anterior end is pointed and attaches anteriorly to the intercondylar eminence of the tibia, in front of the anterior cruciate ligament. Posteriorly it attaches behind the intercondylar eminence, between the attachment of the lateral meniscus and the posterior cruciate ligament. Its outer surface attaches to the fibrous joint capsule of the tibiofemoral joint. It is also firmly attached to the internal aspect of the medial collateral ligament.

The *lateral meniscus* is almost circular, but it is open medially where its anterior and posterior ends attach anteriorly and posteriorly to the intercondylar eminence of the tibia. The anterior end of the lateral meniscus attaches to the tibia lateral and posterior to the anterior cruciate ligament. Its posterior end attaches anterior to the posterior attachment of the medial meniscus. Its outer surface attaches to the fibrous joint capsule of the tibiofemoral joint. The *transverse ligament of the knee* attaches the convex anterior margin of the lateral meniscus to the anterior end of the medial meniscus. It is variable in size and sometimes absent.

The superior surfaces of the two menisci are concave to receive the convex surfaces of the femoral condyles. The inferior surfaces are flat and rest upon the tibial plateau. As a result, the menisci are almost triangular in cross-section. The fibrocartilaginous menisci are somewhat deformable and increase the congruity between the articular surfaces of the femoral condyles and the articular facets of the proximal tibia. They deepen the receptacles for the femoral condyles on the tibial plateau.

Additionally, the curvatures of the femoral condyles are not uniform. Because the menisci are somewhat compliant, they can change shape throughout the range of motion of the joint to maintain their congruency, which is important to joint lubrication. The presence of the menisci in the joint also helps to more evenly distribute the transfer of weight from the femur to the tibia.

Patellofemoral Articulation

The second component of the knee joint is the *patellofemoral articulation,* or *patellofemoral joint*. The patella itself is a large sesamoid bone embedded in the tendon of the quadriceps femoris muscle. It is customary to refer to the band of collagenous tissue that joins the inferior aspect of the patella to the tibial tuberosity as the *patellar ligament,* following the old adage that *ligaments connect bone to bone* (patella to tibia), whereas *tendons connect muscle to bone* (quadriceps femoris to patella).

The patellar ligament is, in fact, the distal continuation of the tendon of the quadriceps femoris muscle, the patella being simply a large sesamoid bone interrupting that tendon. It is therefore also referred to as the patellar tendon. However, we follow convention and refer to it as the *patellar ligament.*

The superficial fibers of the patellar ligament are continuous over the anterior surface of the patella and blend with the quadriceps tendon. The tendons (or aponeuroses) of insertion of the vastus medialis and vastus lateralis give rise to the *medial* and *lateral patellar retinacula* that attach along the medial and lateral aspects of the patella.

The posterior aspect of the patella is its articular surface, which is divided into *medial* and *lateral articular facets.* These articulate with the patellar groove on the anterior and inferior aspects of the femur. The joint itself takes the form of a sellar articulation. The synovial capsule of the patellofemoral joint is simply a continuation of the synovial capsule of the tibiofemoral joint. During flexion and extension of the knee joint, the patella tracks along the patellar groove of the femur.

A principal function of the patella is to move the quadriceps tendon farther anterior to the center of rotation of the knee joint, increasing the moment arm of the quadriceps femoris and giving it greater mechanical advantage in extension of the knee. If the patella is absent, about 30 percent more force is required to extend the knee (Jenkins, 1998).

Unique Features of the Human Knee

Human habitual bipedal locomotion has led to some unique features of the human knee. During normal walking, the body must be supported on one leg while the other is swung forward to take the next step. The body's weight can be better balanced on a single knee joint if that knee joint is under the center of gravity, in the midline. To bring the knees under the midline of the body, the shafts of the femurs angle inward from the hip to the knee, so that the medial aspects of the two femurs nearly meet at the knee. Thus the shafts of the femurs are not vertical but are angled slightly.

The tibial plateaus are approximately horizontal, as are the inferior aspects of the medial and lateral condyles of the femurs in the anatomical position. The angle thus formed between the shaft of the femur and a vertical parasagittal plane is the *bicondylar angle.* In humans, this angle is an average of approximately 9 or 10 degrees, being higher in females because of the greater relative width of the hips (Heiple and Lovejoy, 1971).

The bicondylar angle develops in growing children as they begin to walk. Before that, the condition in human children is much like that in quadrupedal mammals; that is, the knees are vertically aligned with the hips. Because of the presence of a large bicondylar angle, the line of action, or direction of pull, of the quadriceps femoris muscle on the patella is angled, generating both a Y component of force (vertical) and an X component of force (horizontal). As such, it has a tendency to pull the patella laterally.

The patella is prevented from slipping laterally out of the patellar groove by the presence of the medial and lateral patellar retinacula, the lowermost fibers of the vastus medialis muscle, and by the anteriorly projecting lateral lip of the patellar groove on the distal femur. Because women have a larger bicondylar angle than men, the force vector generated by the quadriceps femoris muscle has a relatively greater X (horizontal) component than in men. As a consequence, women have a higher incidence of lateral dislocation of the patella than do men.

Ranges of Motion of the Knee Joint

Movements of the knee joint (tibiofemoral and patellofemoral) are described as *flexion, extension,* and *medial* and *lateral rotation*. As has been noted, the knee is not a simple hinge joint but rather a *bicondylar joint*. As with all bicondylar joints (such as that between the occipital condyles and the atlas, or the temporomandibular joint), hinge motions are coupled with rotation.

As the knee goes through flexion and extension, the tibial articular surfaces do not simply slide forward and backward on the femur. During extension, the tibial shaft undergoes lateral rotation; during flexion, it undergoes medial rotation. With the foot fixed, the last 30 degrees of extension involves medial femoral rotation, whereas early flexion involves lateral femoral rotation. From a vertical femorotibial axis, the extreme range of extension is about 5 to 10 degrees beyond that axis, whereas extreme flexion is about 120 degrees with the hip extended or 140 degrees with the hip flexed. Conjunct rotation at the knee with flexion and extension is about 20 degrees, but passive rotation can be 60 or 70 degrees.

Disorders of the Knee Joint

Like the hip joint, the knee is a frequent site of *osteoarthritis*. Severe cases can result in complete joint replacement surgery, which involves prosthetic replacement of the femoral, tibial, and patellar articular surfaces. Because of the lack of congruity between the articular surfaces of the tibia and femur, joint stability relies solely on the surrounding soft tissues. In ordinary circumstances, surrounding musculature and ligaments maintain the joint, but these can be damaged in trauma.

The tibial (medial) collateral ligament is frequently damaged when a force is applied to the lateral aspect of the knee when the foot is firmly fixed on the substrate and the knee is slightly flexed ("clipping injury"). If the force is strong enough, the medial collateral ligament can rupture. If the force is even greater, it may rupture both the medial collateral and the anterior cruciate ligaments. Because the medial meniscus is tightly bound to the medial collateral ligament, damage to that ligament also frequently results in damage to the meniscus.

If a force is applied to the anterior aspect of the knee in full extension, driving it into hyperextension, the anterior cruciate ligament may rupture. If the force is great enough, the posterior cruciate ligament may rupture as well. A force applied to the anterior aspect of the tibia in a flexed knee may result in rupture of the posterior cruciate ligament.

Runner's syndrome (iliotibial band syndrome) is an overuse syndrome in which the iliotibial band becomes inflamed after repetitive slipping back and forth over the lateral epicondyle of the femur. (For more details, see Edwardson, 1995.)

Tibiofibular Articulations

The fibula does not participate in the knee joint except as the site of attachment of the lateral collateral ligament, but the proximal tibiofibular articulation lies just below the lateral aspect of the knee joint on the lateral and inferior aspect of the tibial plateau. There are three tibiofibular articulations: the proximal, middle, and distal tibiofibular joints.

THE PROXIMAL TIBIOFIBULAR ARTICULATION

The *proximal (superior) tibiofibular articulation* (see Fig. 7–17A and B) is a plane synovial joint. The synovial capsule may communicate with the tibiofemoral joint posterolaterally through the subpopliteal recess, which lies deep to the popliteus tendon. Little movement occurs at this joint in humans, because the fibula's primary role is for muscle attachment and contribution to the lateral wall of the ankle joint. The articular surface of the tibia is located on the lateral and inferior aspects of the tibial plateau; the articular surface of the fibula is located on the fibular head. Both the fibular and tibial articular surfaces are flat, oval, and covered with hyaline cartilage. The joint is surrounded by a fibrous joint capsule that is reinforced by the anterior and posterior ligaments of the head of the fibula. These run from the lateral borders of the tibial plateau to the anterior and posterior aspects of the head of the fibula.

THE MIDDLE TIBIOFIBULAR ARTICULATION

The *middle tibiofibular joint (tibiofibular syndesmosis)* consists of the *crural* (leg below the knee) *interosseous membrane.* Like the interosseous membrane between the radius and ulna, this membrane runs between the interosseous borders (crests) of the two adjacent bones, but in the leg rather than in the forearm. Its superior margin does not quite reach the proximal tibiofibular joint, but it presents a free concave superior edge over which the anterior tibial artery and vein pass.

Distally, it becomes continuous with the interosseous ligament of the distal tibiofibular joint. The membrane helps keep the fibula firmly in articulation with the tibia, separates the anterior and posterior muscular compartments of the *leg (crus),* and gives attachment to the deep dorsiflexor and plantarflexor muscles.

THE DISTAL TIBIOFIBULAR ARTICULATION

The *distal (inferior) tibiofibular* joint (Figure 7–18) exhibits very little motion and is a combination syndesmosis and diarthrosis. The medial aspect of the distal end of the fibula bears a rough, triangular, convex surface that articulates with the rough, concave fibular notch on the lateral aspect of the distal tibia. Most of the joint surfaces are joined to one another by a fibrous interosseous ligament; however, approximately the distal ½ centimeter of the joint consists of a plane synovial joint. Its synovial capsule is continuous with that of the ankle joint. In humans, this joint binds the lateral malleolus of the fibula tightly to the distal tibia to form the bony mortise of the ankle joint.

The distal tibiofibular joint in humans is less mobile than in other hominoid (humanlike) primates, but it does have a special function in humans. During the heelstrike phase of locomotion, the fibula moves downward relative to the tibia, deepening the mortise of the ankle. This puts tension on the interosseous membrane of the middle tibiofibular joint and the interosseous ligament of the distal tibiofibular joint to draw the fibula and tibia more tightly together, reinforcing the ankle mortise. This, in turn, dissipates some of the compressive force of heel strike by means of ligament distention (Weinert et al., 1973).

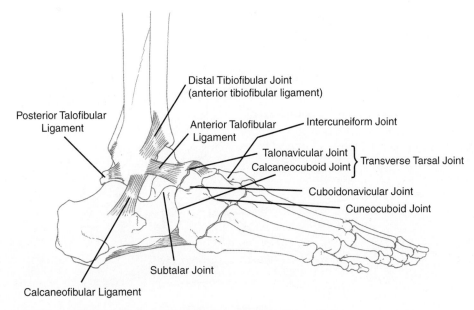

Figure 7-18   Ligaments of the ankle (talocrural joint), lateral view.

The Talocrural Joint

The *talocrural (ankle) joint* (Figure 7–19; refer also to Fig. 7–18 throughout the discussion of the talocrural joint and its ligaments) is the joint between the distal ends of the tibia and fibula superiorly, laterally, and medially, and the superior surface of the talus inferiorly. It is principally a uniaxial joint classified as a ginglymus.

The articular surfaces superiorly are located on the medial aspect of the lateral malleolus of the fibula, the inferior end of the tibia, and the lateral aspect of the medial malleolus of the tibia. The malleoli, the inferior tibia, and the inferior transverse (tibiofibular) ligament complete a deep concavity for reception of the superior surface of the talus. The superior or proximal surface of the talus is highly convex and spool like. This proximal surface articulates with the large facet at the inferior surface of the tibia. Likewise, the talus possesses medial and lateral articular facets that articulate with the facets on the inner aspects of the medial and lateral malleoli.

Capsules and Ligaments

The bones in the talocrural joint are joined by the articular capsule and several ligaments.

THE ARTICULAR CAPSULE

The fibrous *articular capsule* of the talocrural joint attaches superiorly along the margins of the articular surfaces of the tibia and malleoli. Inferiorly, it attaches along the margins of the involved articular facets of the talus. The synovial membrane lines the internal aspects of the capsule and sends a small extension superiorly between the distal ends of the tibia and fibula at the inferior tibiofibular articulation. The articular capsule is thin anteriorly and posteriorly but is reinforced medially and laterally by a number of ligaments.

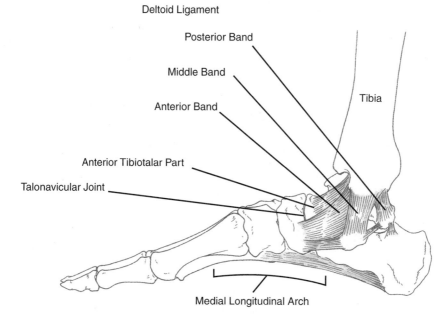

Deltoid Ligament

Posterior Band

Middle Band

Anterior Band

Tibia

Anterior Tibiotalar Part

Talonavicular Joint

Medial Longitudinal Arch

Figure 7-19   Ligaments of the ankle (talocrural joint), medial view.

THE ANTERIOR TALOFIBULAR LIGAMENT

Some describe the anterior talofibular ligament, the posterior talofibular ligament, and the calcaneofibular ligament as three parts of a single *lateral ligament of the talocrural joint.* The *anterior talofibular ligament* is the shortest of these three and runs from the anterior margin of the lateral malleolus to the talus in front of its lateral articular surface.

THE POSTERIOR TALOFIBULAR LIGAMENT

The *posterior talofibular ligament* is both the strongest and the deepest of the three lateral ligaments of the ankle. It runs almost horizontally from the lateral malleolar fossa to the posterior surface of the talus lateral to the groove for the tendon of the flexor hallucis longus.

THE CALCANEOFIBULAR LIGAMENT

The *calcaneofibular ligament* is the longest of the three lateral ligaments of the ankle. It is a narrow rounded cord that extends from the apex of the fibular malleolus. It runs posteriorly and inferiorly to insert into a tubercle on the lateral surface of the calcaneus. The tendons of the fibularis (peroneus) longus and brevis muscles cross over and cover this ligament.

THE DELTOID LIGAMENT

The *deltoid* (or *medial*) *ligament* is a broad, flat, triangular band of ligamentous tissue. It attaches superiorly to the apex as well as to the anterior and posterior borders of the medial malleolus and inferiorly to the tarsal bones by three bands of fibers. It has both superficial and deep fibers.

The *superficial fibers* can be divided into three bands, an *anterior (tibionavicular) band, middle (tibiocalcaneal) band,* and *posterior (posterior tibiotalar) band,* which join with the bones indicated by their names. The *deep fibers* form the *anterior tibiotalar part.* The tendons of the tibialis posterior and flexor digitorum longus muscles cross the deltoid ligament passing from the posterior crural compartment into the sole of the foot.

The Intertarsal Joints

There are a considerable number of *intertarsal* joints. As with the intercarpal joints of the wrist, most of these joints are of the plane synovial type. We do not discuss all the details of each joint but touch upon some of the more important aspects of their anatomy.

The Talocalcaneonavicular Joint

The *talocalcaneonavicular joint* is a compound, multiaxial, spheroidal synovial joint. The head of the talus is rounded and is received by a socket formed by the posterior surface of the navicular, the anterior articular surface of the calcaneus, the *plantar calcaneonavicular (spring) ligament,* and the *calcaneonavicular part of the bifurcate ligament.* Gliding and rotatory movements are permitted at this and at the subtalar joint.

The Subtalar Joint

The talus and calcaneus have two articulations, an anterior and a posterior. The anterior joint takes part in the *talocalcaneonavicular joint,* discussed in the previous section. The posterior, or *subtalar (talocalcaneal) joint,* forms between the posterior concave calcaneal articular facet on the inferior surface of the talus and the convex articular facet on the posterior superior calcaneus. This is a plane synovial joint, surrounded by an articular capsule and reinforced by *anterior, posterior, medial, lateral,* and *interosseous talocalcaneal ligaments.* The interosseous talocalcaneal ligament is the chief union between the talus and calcaneus and forms from the union of the fibrous capsules of the talocalcaneonavicular and subtalar joints. It fills the tarsal sinus, as described with the calcaneus. The synovial capsule of this joint is unique among the intertarsal joints in that it does not communicate with the synovial capsules of the other intertarsal joints.

The Calcaneocuboid Joint

The *calcaneocuboid joint* between the calcaneus and cuboid has the characteristics of a sellar joint but does not produce the wide range of motions usually associated with sellar joints. Ligaments reinforcing the fibrous articular capsule between the more posterior calcaneus and the more anterior cuboid are the dorsal calcaneocuboid ligament; the bifurcate ligament, which consists of the calcaneocuboid part and the calcaneonavicular part; the long plantar ligament (Figure 7–20); and the plantar calcaneocuboid ligament. Movements at this joint accompany those at

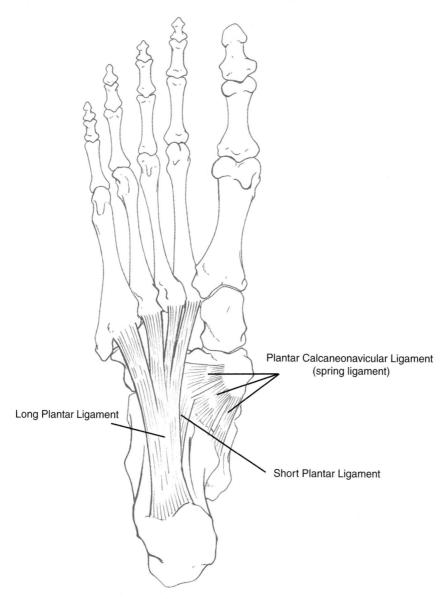

Figure 7–20   Plantar ligaments of the foot.

the subtalar and talocalcaneonavicular joints. They are basically translatory and rotational in nature.

The Transverse Tarsal Joint

The *transverse tarsal joint (Chopart's joint;* see Fig. 7–18) is a term used to describe collectively the *calcaneocuboid* and *talonavicular joints*. Together the joint capsules of these two joints extend transversely, although somewhat irregularly, across the foot. The talus and calcaneus lie posterior to the transverse tarsal joint, whereas the navicular and cuboid lie anterior to it. Some plantarflexion and dorsiflexion of the anterior part of the foot, as well as slight inversion and eversion, is permitted at the transverse tarsal joint. *Pronation* and *supination* of the foot take place principally at this joint.

The Calcaneonavicular Joint

The calcaneus and navicular do not directly articulate but are joined by ligaments. Important ligaments associated with this joint are the *calcaneonavicular part of the bifurcate ligament,* from the anterior calcaneus to the lateral navicular, and the plantar calcaneonavicular (spring) ligament. By supporting the head of the talus, the spring ligament helps maintain the *medial longitudinal arch* of the foot.

The Cuboidonavicular Joint

The *cuboidonavicular joint* is a syndesmosis and consists of *dorsal, plantar,* and *interosseous cuboidonavicular ligaments.* This joint is occasionally synovial; in such a case, its synovial cavity is continuous with the cuneonavicular joint.

The Intercuneiform Joints

The *intercuneiform joints* are plane synovial joints. *Dorsal, plantar*, and *interosseous ligaments* join adjacent bones with one another, reinforcing the joint capsules.

The Cuneocuboid Joint

The cuneocuboid joint is a plane synovial joint. The bones are united by *dorsal, plantar,* and *interosseous cuneocuboid ligaments.*

The Cuneonavicular Joint

The distal surface of the navicular bone articulates with the three cuneiform bones in the *cuneonavicular joint,* a joint that is typically described as a plane synovial joint. However, the navicular's articular surface is transversely convex and divided by faint ridges into three facets, one for each cuneiform bone. Its articular capsule and synovial cavity are continuous with those of the intercuneiform and cuneocuboid joints. *Dorsal* and *plantar cuneonavicular ligaments* join the dorsal and plantar surfaces of the navicular with each of the three cuneiform bones.

Ligaments in the Foot Associated with the Tarsal Bones

THE PLANTAR CALCANEONAVICULAR LIGAMENT

The *plantar calcaneonavicular (spring) ligament* (see Fig. 7–20) is broad and thick and connects the anterior margin of the sustentaculum tali of the calcaneus to the plantar surface of the navicular. The dorsal surface of the ligament has a triangular fibrocartilaginous facet upon which rests the head of the talus. By supporting the head of the talus, the ligament helps maintain the medial longitudinal arch of the foot and thus keeps the "spring" in the step. The plantar surface of the ligament is supported by the tendons of the tibialis posterior, flexor hallucis longus, and flexor digitorum longus muscles. The medial border of the ligament blends with the deltoid ligament.

THE BIFURCATE LIGAMENT

The *bifurcate ligament* is so called because it divides into two major bands or parts. These are the (lateral) *calcaneocuboid ligament* and the (medial) *calcaneonavicular ligament*. The bifurcate ligament is Y-shaped, with the stem of the Y attaching to the anterior superior (or dorsal) calcaneal surface. Distally it divides into its calcaneocuboid and calcaneonavicular parts. The calcaneocuboid ligament is the principal connection between the proximal and distal rows of tarsal bones. The calcaneonavicular ligament attaches to the dorsolateral part of the navicular bone.

THE LONG PLANTAR LIGAMENT

The *long plantar ligament* (see Fig. 7–20) is the longest ligament of the tarsus. It connects the plantar aspect of the calcaneus to the ridge and tuberosity of the plantar surface of the cuboid (deep fibers) and continues on to the bases of the second, third, fourth, and sometimes fifth metatarsals (superficial fibers). With the groove on the plantar aspect of the cuboid, this ligament forms a tunnel for the passage of the tendon of the fibularis (peroneus) longus muscle. The ligament and the tendon of the fibularis (peroneus) longus help maintain the *lateral longitudinal arch* of the foot.

THE PLANTAR CALCANEOCUBOID LIGAMENT

The *plantar calcaneocuboid (short plantar) ligament* (see Fig. 7–20) is deeper than the long plantar ligament and is separated from it by areolar connective tissue. It runs from the anterior calcaneal tubercle to the plantar surface of the cuboid. It also helps maintain the lateral longitudinal arch of the foot.

Arches of the Foot

The foot has three arches: the medial longitudinal arch, the lateral longitudinal arch, and the *transverse arch*. The medial longitudinal arch, as alluded to earlier, is maintained principally by the spring ligament, whereas the lateral arch is maintained by the long and short plantar ligaments.

The medial longitudinal arch is composed of the calcaneus; the talus; the navicular; the three cuneiform bones; and the first, second, and third metatarsal bones. The concavity of the arch is supported by posterior (calcaneal) and anterior (metatarsal) pillars. The anterior pillar is formed by the heads of the three medial metatarsal bones.

The flatter lateral longitudinal arch is composed of the calcaneus, cuboid, and fourth and fifth metatarsals. Its *posterior pillar* is the tuberosity of the calcaneus, and its *anterior pillar* is the heads of the two lateral metatarsals.

The *transverse (metatarsal) arch* is formed by the navicular, the three cuneiforms, the cuboid, and the bases of the five metatarsal bones. It is maintained by the ligaments that bind the cuneiforms and the bases of the metatarsal bones together. All three arches are concave inferiorly.

The resilience and elasticity of the medial arch absorb reaction forces applied to the foot, such as those received in jumping. The lateral arch, which is lower and less resilient, is constructed to transmit forces to the ground, along the lateral aspect of the foot, such as in walking and running.

The Tarsometatarsal Joints

The *tarsometatarsal joints* are plane synovial joints. They include articulations between the medial, intermediate, and lateral cuneiforms and the cuboid proximally and the bases of the five metatarsal bones distally. The *first metatarsal* articulates with the medial cuneiform. The *second metatarsal* articulates with adjacent surfaces of the intermediate cuneiform and on either side with small areas of the medial and lateral cuneiforms. The *third metatarsal* articulates with the lateral cuneiform. The *fourth metatarsal* articulates with the lateral cuneiform and the cuboid, whereas the *fifth metatarsal* articulates with only the cuboid. The five tarsometatarsal joints share only three synovial cavities.

The *medial tarsometatarsal joint cavity* is restricted to the joint between the first metatarsal and the medial cuneiform. The *intermediate tarsometatarsal joint cavity* is between the intermediate and lateral cuneiforms and the second and third metatarsals. The *lateral tarsometatarsal joint cavity* is between the cuboid bone and the bases of the fourth and fifth metatarsals. *Dorsal* and *plantar tarsometatarsal ligaments* join the dorsal and plantar surfaces of the bases of the metatarsals to the adjacent surfaces of the tarsal bones. *Interosseous cuneometatarsal ligaments* pass from the cuneiform bones to the bases of adjacent metatarsals; they are variably present, but the first, between the medial cuneiform and the second metatarsal, is constant.

The Intermetatarsal Joints

The *bases* of the second to the fifth metatarsals articulate at plane synovial joints and are also joined by *dorsal, plantar,* and *interosseous intermetatarsal ligaments.* The *heads* of all the metatarsals are joined syndesmotically to one another on their plantar surfaces by the *deep transverse metatarsal ligaments.*

The Metatarsophalangeal Joints

The *metatarsophalangeal joints* are ellipsoid synovial joints. They have loose fibrous joint capsules. The capsules are reinforced by a *plantar ligament* and by *medial* and *lateral collateral ligaments.* The dorsal surface of the capsules is strengthened by the extensor hoods of the extensor muscles of the toes. The joints are capable of flexion, extension, abduction, and adduction.

The Interphalangeal Joints

The *interphalangeal joints* are ginglymi, or synovial hinge, joints. The distal joint surface of each phalanx is pulley-shaped, and the proximal joint surface of the articulating phalanx has a double concavity to fit these pulley-shaped surfaces. Each joint has an articular capsule and a plantar ligament as well as medial and lateral collateral ligaments.

Ranges of Motion of the Joints of the Ankle and Foot

Motions of the ankle and foot include *plantarflexion* and *dorsiflexion, inversion* and *eversion,* and *pronation* and *supination,* as well as flexion and extension of the phalanges and metatarsophalangeal joints. Movements at the talocrural joint include plantarflexion and dorsiflexion. Dorsiflexion is the action of bringing the top of the foot closer to the shin; plantarflexion is the opposite movement. The human talocrural joint allows about 55 degrees of plantarflexion and 35 degrees of dorsiflexion.

Movements at the subtalar joint and at the talocalcaneonavicular joints permit a wide range of gliding and rotatory movements. Movements at these joints result in inversion and eversion of the plantar surface of the foot. In inversion, the medial border of the foot is raised, whereas in eversion, the lateral border of the foot is raised. Movements at the calcaneocuboid joint accompany those of inversion and eversion at the previously mentioned joints.

Pronation and supination of the foot take place principally at the transverse tarsal joint (composed of the calcaneocuboid and talonavicular joints). Supination of the foot occurs when the anterior aspect of the plantar surface of the fully inverted foot is rotated so that the heads of the metatarsals remain in contact with the substrate. Relative to the inverted foot, this involves lifting the lateral border of the foot. Inversion and supination increase as the feet are spread apart, as in standing with the feet widely separated.

Pronation of the foot is the opposite motion; it also occurs at the transverse tarsal joint. During walking, the suspended foot is held in supination. This maximizes the contact of the plantar surface of the foot following heel strike. As the heel rises, and the foot heads toward toe off (the phase of walking in which the foot pushes off with the big toe), the foot pronates to transmit body weight to the head of the first metatarsal.

Disorders of the Joints of the Ankle and Foot

A *sprained ankle* results from forced inversion (turning inward) or from forced eversion (turning outward) of the foot. Most sprains are of the inversion type. This causes the tearing of ligaments at the lateral aspect of the joint. Eversion sprains are less frequent and cause damage to the deltoid ligament. More frequently, the medial malleolus fractures before the ligament ruptures.

Flat foot results from the loss of the longitudinal arches. In this situation, forces are transmitted through the entire plantar surface of the foot. The flattening is brought on by the excessive elongation of the ligaments of the talonavicular and cuneonavicular joints.

OSSIFICATION OF THE LOWER LIMB BONES
The Os Coxae

The os coxae (Figure 7–21) ossifies from three primary centers, one each in the ilium, the ischium, and the pubis. There are five principal secondary centers of ossification: the iliac crest, the ischial tuberosity, the anterior inferior iliac spine, the dorsal rampart of the pubic symphyseal surface, and centers within the *triradiate cartilage,* the zone of hyaline growth cartilage in the acetabulum that separates the three primary

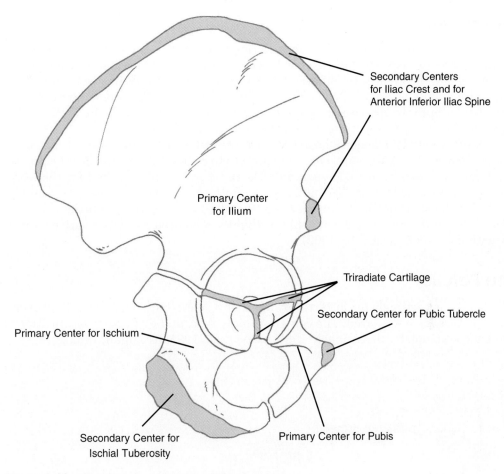

Figure 7-21   Centers of ossification of the os coxae.

centers from one another. There may be additional secondary centers of ossification for the pubic tubercle, pubic crest, and ischial spine.

The primary centers appear in this order: (1) ilium, (2) ischium, (3) pubis. The primary center for the ilium appears at about 8 weeks in utero; for the ischium, at about 3 months in utero; and for the pubis, at about between 4 and 5 months in utero. The centers first appear near the acetabulum, that is, the lower ilium, the body of the ischium, and the superior pubic ramus. By birth, the portions of the three elements of the hip bone nearest the acetabulum have undergone ossification, and only the triradiate cartilage remains cartilaginous. Between ages 8 and 10 years the ischial ramus and the inferior pubic ramus have met (earlier in girls than boys).

Immediately afterward, secondary centers of ossification develop within the triradiate cartilage. The number of these centers may be multiple, and some may fuse with one another as the *os acetabuli* before fusing with the three primary elements of the innominate. The os acetabuli usually appears between the ilium and pubis at about age 12. It fuses with them by age 18 and forms the pubic part of the acetabulum. The other secondary centers of ossification begin to fuse with the remainder of the innominate at or just after puberty, and all are completely synostosed with the remainder of the bone by age 25 (Breathnach, 1965; Krogman, 1962).

The Femur

The femur (Figure 7–22) ossifies from a single primary center for the diaphysis, which begins to ossify at 2 months or less in utero, and four secondary centers: the femoral head, the greater trochanter, the lesser trochanter, and the distal end. There may occasionally be an apophysis for the gluteal tuberosity. The secondary center in the distal epiphysis appears at about 1 year of age and fuses with the distal end of the shaft at about 17 years in girls and 18 to 19 years in boys.

Ossification of the femoral head begins at about 1 year and fuses with the femoral neck between 17 and 18 years, earlier in girls than in boys. The center for the greater trochanter appears at about 3 years in girls and 4 years in boys. That for the lesser trochanter appears between 10 and 11 years. Both the greater and lesser trochanters fuse with the shaft of the femur between 17 and 18 years, usually a little before the head fuses with the neck. Again, this is slightly advanced in girls relative to boys (Breathnach, 1965; Krogman, 1962).

The Patella

The patella is cartilaginous at birth. By age 2 or 3 years (but as late as age 6) several bony centers have appeared. The centers rapidly fuse, and by puberty ossification of the bone is complete (Breathnach, 1965; Gray, 1985, 1995; Krogman, 1962).

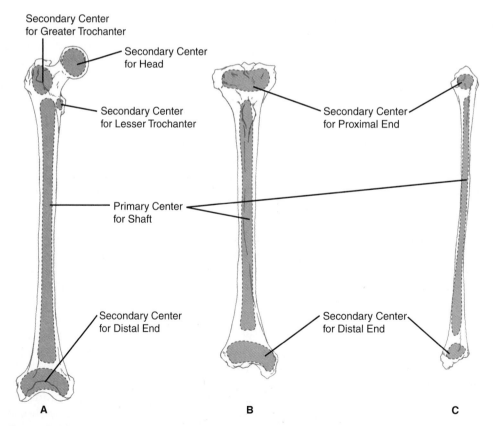

Figure 7-22   Centers of ossification of the (A) femur, (B) tibia, and (C) fibula.

The Tibia

The tibia (see Fig. 7–22) is the classic example of ossification in a long bone. It ossifies from three centers: a primary center for the diaphysis and a secondary center in each of the proximal and distal epiphyses. The center for the diaphysis appears at about 7 weeks in utero; for the proximal epiphysis, shortly before or after birth; and for the distal epiphysis, at about 2 years of age. The distal epiphysis fuses with the shaft of the bone at about 18 years, and the proximal epiphysis fuses at about age 20 (Breathnach, 1965; Gray, 1985; Krogman, 1962).

The Fibula

The fibula (see Fig. 7–22), like the tibia, ossifies from three centers: a primary center for the diaphysis and a secondary center in each of the proximal and distal epiphyses. The center for the diaphysis appears at about 8 weeks in utero; for the proximal epiphysis, at about age 3 or 4; and for the distal epiphysis, at about age 2. The distal epiphysis fuses with the shaft of the bone at about age 20, and the proximal epiphysis fuses at about age 25 (Breathnach, 1965; Gray, 1985; Krogman, 1962).

The Tarsals

All the tarsals ossify from a single center, with the exception of the calcaneus, which has a secondary center for its posterior end. The centers of ossification appear in the following order: (1) calcaneus, 4 to 7 months in utero; (2) talus, 6 months in utero; (3) cuboid, 9 months in utero; (4) lateral cuneiform, 1 year; (5) medial cuneiform, 2 years; (6) intermediate cuneiform and navicular, 3 years. The posterior epiphysis of the calcaneus appears at 8 years and unites with the body of the calcaneus at about puberty (Breathnach, 1965; Gray, 1985; Krogman, 1962).

The Metatarsals

Metatarsals II through V all ossify from two centers: one for the shaft and one for the head (distal end). Metatarsal I (for the hallux) ossifies from two centers as well, but its epiphysis is located at its proximal rather than its distal end. In this regard it follows the pattern of the phalanges (as with the metacarpal for the pollex). The shafts of the metacarpals begin ossification at the 9th or 10th week in utero. At about 3 years of age the center of ossification for the epiphysis of the base of the first metatarsal appears, whereas the centers of ossification for the heads of the other four metatarsals appear between ages 5 and 8. These epiphyses unite with the shafts of the metatarsals between ages 18 and 20 (Breathnach, 1965; Gray, 1985; Krogman, 1962).

The Phalanges

The phalanges, like the first metatarsal, all ossify from two centers: one for a proximal epiphysis and one for the shaft. The ossification centers for the shafts of the proximal and distal phalanges appear between the 8th and 12th weeks in utero and those for the middle phalanges at about 16 weeks in utero. The proximal epiphyses, or phalangeal bases, ossify between 2 and 10 years of age and fuse with the phalangeal shaft by age 18 (Breathnach, 1965; Gray, 1985; Krogman, 1962).

References

Breathnach, AS (Ed) (1965). *Frazer's Anatomy of the Human Skeleton* (6th ed). J and A Churchill, London.

Edwardson, BM (1995). *Musculoskeletal Disorders: Common Problems.* Singular Publishing Group, San Diego.

Gray, H (1985). *Gray's Anatomy* (30th Am ed). CD Clemente (Ed). Lea and Febiger, Philadelphia.

Gray, H (1995). *Gray's Anatomy* (38th Brit ed). PL Williams, LH Bannister, MM Berry, P Collins, M Dyson, JE Dussek, and MWJ Ferguson (Eds). Churchill Livingstone, New York.

Heiple, KG, and Lovejoy, CO (1971). The distal femoral anatomy of *Australopithecus. American Journal of Physical Anthropology, 35,* 75–84.

Jenkins, DB (1998). *Hollinshead's Functional Anatomy of the Limbs and Back* (7th ed). WB Saunders, Philadelphia.

Krogman, WM (1962). *The Human Skeleton in Forensic Medicine.* Charles C Thomas, Springfield, IL.

Krogman, WM, and Iscan, MY (1986). *Human Skeleton in Forensic Medicine* (2nd ed). Charles C Thomas, Springfield, IL.

Lovejoy, CO (1988). Evolution of human walking. *Scientific American, 259,* 82–89.

Soames, RW, and Atha, J (1981). The role of the antigravity musculature during quiet standing in man. *European Journal of Applied Physiology and Occupational Physiology, 47,* 159–167.

Walker, RA, and Lovejoy, CO (1985). Radiographic changes in the clavicle and proximal femur and their use in the determination of skeletal age at death. *American Journal of Physical Anthropology, 68,* 67–78.

Walker, RA, Lovejoy, CO, and Meindl, RS (1994). The histomorphological and geometric properties of human femoral cortex in individuals over 50: Implications for histomorphological determination of age-at-death. *American Journal of Human Biology, 6,* 659–667.

Weinert, CR, McMaster, JH, and Furgeson, RJ (1973). Dynamic function of the human fibula. *American Journal of Anatomy, 138,* 145–150.

Chapter 8

Osteology of the Human Cranium

The skull (Figure 8–1) is divided into two portions: the neurocranium (cranial vault) and the visceral cranium, or splanchnocranium (facial skeleton). The bones of the skull are joined to one another by immovable joints called *sutures*. For all practical mechanical purposes, sutural ligaments and synostosis with advancing age effectively block motion at the sutures and unify the cranium into a rigid structural unit that houses and protects the brain, the sense organs, and the structures associated with speech and mastication. One school of thought in chiropractic and osteopathic medicine is that physiologically important amounts of motion continue at the sutures and that adjustment of the sutures can affect cerebrospinal fluid (Adams et al., 1992; Heisey and Adams, 1993). See Rogers and Witt (1997) for a contrary view.

The *neurocranium* is composed of eight bones that form the cranial vault. Some are paired (one on each side) and some are unpaired (present only in the midline). These eight bones are as follows:

Ethmoid:	Unpaired
Frontal:	Unpaired
Occipital:	Unpaired
Sphenoid:	Unpaired
Temporal:	Paired
Parietal:	Paired

The *visceral cranium* is composed of 14 bones. Like those of the neurocranium, some are paired bilaterally, whereas some are present singly in the midline. These bones are as follows:

Vomer:	Unpaired
Mandible:	Unpaired
Maxilla:	Paired

Figure 8-1   Photograph of the human skull: norma lateralis, or lateral view.

Zygomatic (malar):	Paired
Nasal:	Paired
Lacrimal:	Paired
Palatine:	Paired
Inferior concha:	Paired

In addition to these 22 bones composing the skull proper, several associated bones must be considered. These include the bones associated with the organs of hearing (the auditory ossicles) and speech (the hyoid bone).

THE AUDITORY OSSICLES

The *auditory ossicles* (Figures 8–2 and 8–3) are housed in the petrous portion of the temporal bone. They transmit sound impulses from the *tympanic membrane* (eardrum) to the *cochlea,* the coiled portion of the inner ear containing fluid for transmitting sound impulses to the organ of Corti, which transmits nerve impulses in response to sound vibrations. There are six auditory ossicles, three on each side. They are as follows:

Malleus:	Paired
Incus:	Paired
Stapes:	Paired

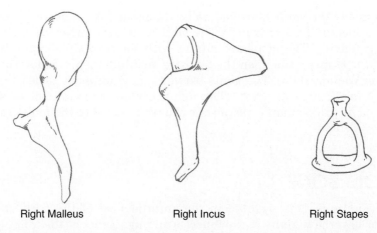

Right Malleus   Right Incus   Right Stapes

Figure 8–2   The auditory ossicles. The largest dimension is approximately 0.5 cm.

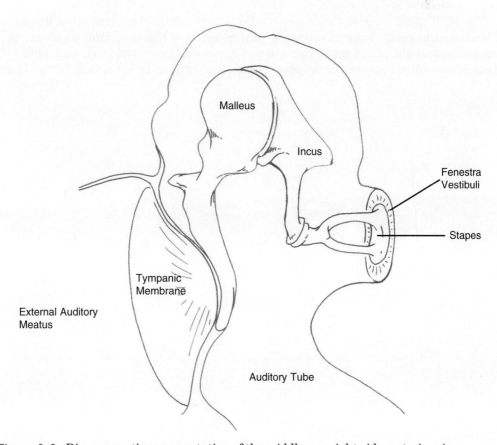

Figure 8–3   Diagrammatic representation of the middle ear, right side, anterior view.

The handle of the *malleus* (colloquially: "hammer") is connected to the tympanic membrane (colloquially: "eardrum"). The malleus in turn articulates with the *incus* (colloquially: "anvil"). The incus articulates with the *stapes* (colloquially: "stirrup"). The base of the stapes rests upon the fenestra vestibuli (oval window) of the cochlea (Greiner and Walker, 1999). The joints between the auditory ossicles are typical, although very small, synovial joints. Through this chain of small bones, sound vibrations received by the tympanic membrane are transferred to the fenestra vestibuli of the cochlea.

THE HYOID BONE

The *hyoid* (Figure 8–4) is situated in the anterior part of the neck inferior to the *mandible,* or lower jaw. Many of the muscles and ligaments of the tongue and larynx attach to the hyoid. It does not articulate with any other bone but it is best considered with the skull.

It is a small bone that consists of a central *body;* a small, superior *lesser cornu* projecting posterosuperiorly from the superolateral aspects of each side of the body; and a larger, inferior *greater cornu,* also projecting posteriorly from the lateral aspect of each side of the body.

The stylohyoid ligament attaches to the lesser cornu. The thyrohyoid ligament attaches to the greater cornu, as do several muscles of the neck and pharynx (the hyoglossus, middle pharyngeal constrictor, digastric, thyrohyoideus, and stylohyoideus muscles). Additional neck, pharyngeal, and oral muscles attach to the body

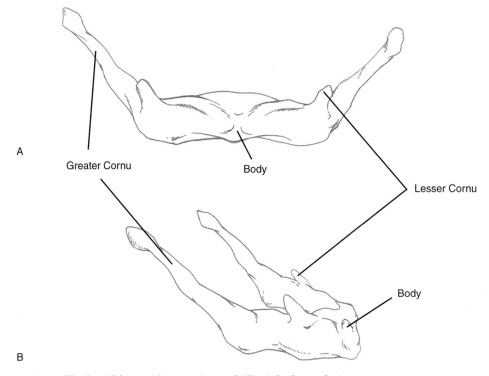

Figure 8–4   The hyoid bone: (*A*) anterior and (*B*) right lateral views.

(the genioglossus, geniohyoideus, mylohyoideus, sternohyoideus, and omohyoideus muscles).

THE SKULL

For ease of studying, the features of the skull are broken down by view: superior, lateral, anterior, posterior, basal (inferior), and interior.

The Superior View of the Skull: Norma Verticalis

The major bones seen in the superior view of the skull, or *norma verticalis* (Figure 8–5), are the *parietals,* the *occipital,* and the *frontal.* Major landmarks are discussed next.

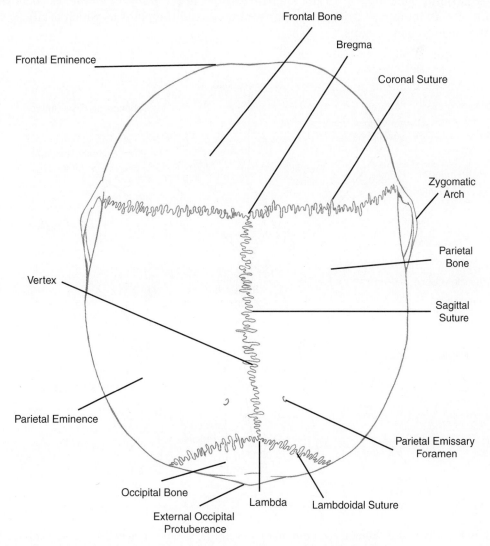

Figure 8-5 The adult human cranium: norma verticalis, or superior view.

Landmarks and Features

The *sagittal suture* lies in the midline between the two parietal bones that form the roof of the cranial vault. The *coronal suture* is located between the two parietal bones posteriorly and the frontal bone anteriorly. The *lambdoidal suture* is found between the two parietals anteriorly and the occipital bone posteriorly.

Bregma is the point at the junction of the coronal and sagittal sutures. In infancy it is the location of the *anterior fontanelle*. The fontanelles are the "soft spots" of the infant cranium, representing areas where the cranial vault bones have not yet grown together at the sutures. *Lambda* is the junction of the sagittal and lambdoidal sutures. In infancy it is the location of the *posterior fontanelle*.

Vertex is the most superior point on the skull when it is oriented in the Frankfort horizontal plane, in which the upper margin of the external acoustic meatus and the lower margin of the left orbit are aligned in a horizontal plane. Vertex usually lies on the sagittal suture about halfway between bregma and lambda. Near the center of each parietal bone, lateral to the sagittal suture, is the *parietal eminence*. It is the point of maximum convexity of the parietal bone and the point at which ossification of the parietal bone begins.

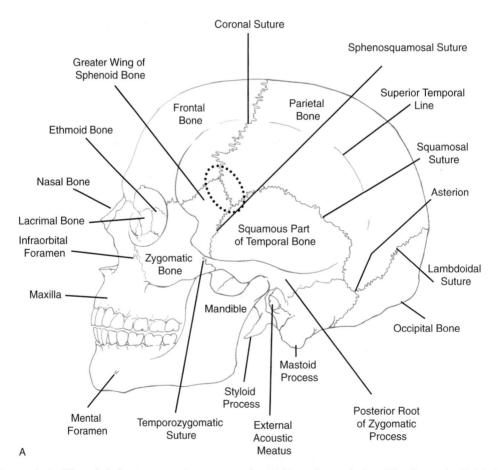

Figure 8–6   The adult human cranium: norma lateralis, or lateral view. The figure is divided into *A* and *B* portions to make the labeling of structures clearer.

The Lateral View of the Skull: Norma Lateralis

Bones visible in the lateral view of the skull, or *norma lateralis* (Figure 8–6), are the frontal, zygomatic, temporal, parietal, occipital, sphenoid, nasal, maxilla, and mandible. The latter three are discussed later. Visible landmarks are discussed next.

Landmarks and Features

The coronal and lambdoidal sutures were discussed in the preceding section. The *squamosal suture* is located between the *squamous part of the temporal bone* and the parietal bone. The *occipitomastoid suture* is located between the occipital bone and the mastoid part of the temporal bone. The *parietomastoid suture* is located between the posteroinferior parietal bone and the mastoid part of the temporal bone.

Pterion is the junction of the greater wing of the sphenoid, the frontal, the parietal, and the temporal bones, found in the region of the temple, superior to the zygomatic arch. It usually represents a region, not a single point. It is the weakest region of the cranial vault. It is the site of the *anterolateral* or *sphenoidal fontanelle* in the skull of the infant.

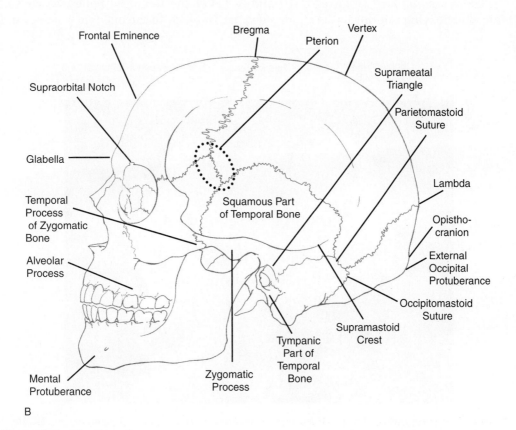

B

Figure 8–6 (*Continued*)

Asterion is the point marking the junction of the occipitomastoid suture, the parietomastoid suture, and the lambdoidal suture. It is the site of the *posterolateral fontanelle* in the skull of the infant. Bregma, lambda, and vertex are all landmarks visible laterally as well as superiorly, as previously described.

The *frontal bone* is the bone of the forehead. It has *zygomatic processes* on either side, projecting to articulate with the zygomatic bones. The *frontal eminences* are the areas of greatest convexity.

The parietal bones each exhibit *superior* and *inferior temporal lines* that arch anteroposteriorly above the squamosal suture. The superior and inferior temporal lines (Figure 8–7) mark the origin of the temporalis muscle; they extend from the zygomatic process of the frontal bone, across the frontal and parietal bones, and then curve anteriorly to become continuous with the *supramastoid crest* and the *posterior root of the zygomatic arch* (Figure 8–8). The parietal eminences are the areas of greatest convexity of the parietal bones.

The *temporal bone* demonstrates several prominent features in the lateral view. The *external acoustic (auditory) meatus* (Figure 8–9) is the bony opening into the ear. In life it is closed by the tympanic membrane, which articulates with the malleus (see Fig. 8–3). The squamous part of the temporal bone is the flat part just inferior to the parietal bone. It exhibits a supramastoid crest, which extends posteriorly from the posterior root of the zygomatic process and superior to the mastoid process. A *suprameatal triangle* and *spine* can also be found between the posterior root of the zygomatic arch and the posterosuperior part of the external acoustic meatus.

The *tympanic part* (Figures 8–10 and 8–11) of the temporal bone is a curved plate of bone lying inferior to the squamous part, anterior to the mastoid process, and

Squamous Part of
Temporal Bone
Inferior Temporal Line
Superior Temporal Line

Figure 8-7   Photograph of the adult human cranium from the right side, demonstrating the superior and inferior temporal lines.

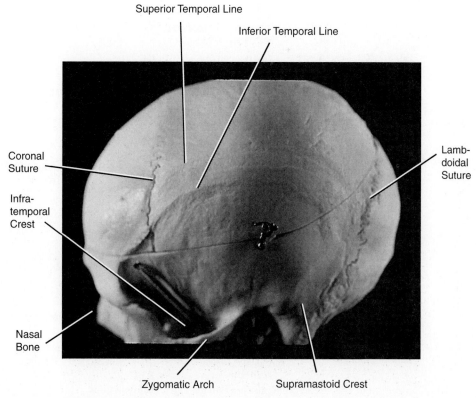

Superior Temporal Line

Inferior Temporal Line

Coronal
Suture

Lamb-
doidal
Suture

Infra-
temporal
Crest

Nasal
Bone

Zygomatic Arch

Supramastoid Crest

Figure 8–8   Photograph of the adult human cranium from the left superior side.

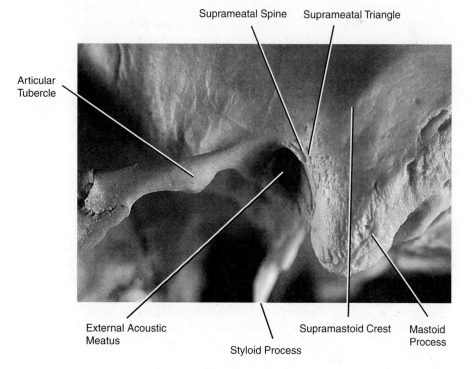

Suprameatal Spine   Suprameatal Triangle

Articular
Tubercle

External Acoustic
Meatus

Styloid Process

Supramastoid Crest

Mastoid
Process

Figure 8–9   The region of the external acoustic meatus, left side.

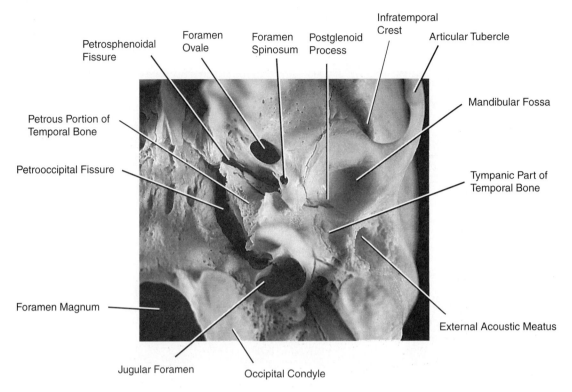

Figure 8-10   The region of the external acoustic meatus, right inferior view.

posterior to the *mandibular fossa (glenoid fossa)*. The mandibular fossa is located between the *articular tubercle* and the tympanic part of the temporal bone. It is divided in two by the *squamotympanic fissure.* The anterior and larger part of the fossa articulates with the condyle of the mandible, which forms the *temporomandibular joint*.

The zygomatic process projects anteriorly from the temporal squama above the mandibular fossa and articular tubercle. Forming the anterior boundary of the mandibular fossa is the bumplike articular tubercle. Posterior to the mandibular fossa is the *postglenoid process,* which is a small, pointed projection of the temporal bone just anterior to the tympanic part of the temporal bone. The *styloid process* is a long, pointed projection that extends inferiorly and anteriorly from the tympanic part and gives attachment to several muscles and ligaments.

The *mastoid portion* of the temporal bone is posterior to the external acoustic meatus. Two structures of interest can be found on this part of the temporal bone. The *mastoid process* (see Figs. 8–6 and 8–9) is a blunt projection for muscle attachments found immediately posterior to the tympanic part and the external auditory meatus. A *mastoid foramen* may be found posterior and/or superior to the mastoid process. It transmits an emissary vein from sigmoid venous sinus inside the skull.

The *zygomatic bone* (see Figs. 8–6 and 8–7) is the bone of the cheek. It presents a *temporal process* that meets the zygomatic process of the temporal bone—a *zygomaticofacial foramen* on its anterolateral aspect and a *zygomaticotemporal foramen* posteriorly. These foramina transmit nerves to the skin of the lateral face and temple, respectively.

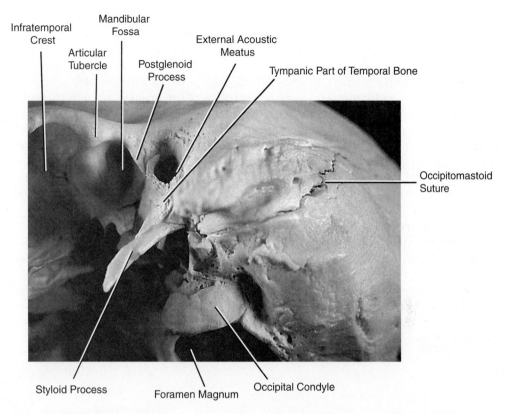

Figure 8–11   The region of the external acoustic meatus, left side, oblique posteroinferior view.

The *zygomatic arch* is formed by the zygomatic process of the temporal bone and the temporal process of the zygomatic bone. The zygomatic process of the temporal arises from two roots. The *anterior root* is directed inward anterior to the mandibular fossa, where it expands and forms the articular tubercle of the temporal bone. A *posterior root* runs posteriorly above the external acoustic meatus and is continuous with the supramastoid crest.

The *sphenoid bone* is found posterior to the frontal and zygomatic bones and anterior to the parietal and temporal bones. The *greater wing of the sphenoid* (see Fig. 8–6) is a superolateral extension of bone that helps form the temple region. At its inferior aspect is a linear roughness or ridge called the *infratemporal crest*. The infratemporal crest lies at about the level of the zygomatic arch. This crest is the point at which the greater wing of the sphenoid bone takes a sharp turn and becomes a part of the base of the skull; it also marks the inferior extent of the temporal fossa and the superior border of the *infratemporal fossa*. The *lateral pterygoid plate* of the sphenoid is a thin plate of bone posterior to the maxilla and inferior to the greater wing of the sphenoid. The lateral pterygoid plate is better observed from the *norma basalis*, or inferior view of the skull.

The *temporal fossa* is formed by parts of the frontal, temporal, sphenoid, and zygomatic bones. This fossa occupies a large part of the lateral aspect of the parietal bone. The temporal fossa is the region bounded by the temporal lines superiorly and posteriorly, the frontal and zygomatic bones anteriorly, and the zygomatic arch and infratemporal crest (on the greater wing of the sphenoid) inferiorly. The bones making up the medial wall of the temporal fossa are the squamous part of the temporal bone, the greater wing of the sphenoid bone, and parts of the frontal and parietal bones.

The *infratemporal fossa* (Figures 8–12 and 8–13) is an irregular space behind the maxilla formed by the infratemporal surface of the greater wing of the sphenoid and part of the temporal squama. This irregularly shaped cavity lies medial or deep to the zygomatic arch. It is bounded anteriorly by the alveolar process and infratemporal surface of the maxilla and the ridge from the maxilla's zygomatic process; posteriorly, by the articular tubercle of the temporal bone and the spine of the sphenoid; superiorly, by the greater wing of the sphenoid and the inferior surface of the temporal squama; medially, by the *lateral pterygoid plate;* and laterally, by the zygomatic arch.

The *foramen ovale, foramen spinosum,* and the *alveolar canals* open into it (discussed later). Two fissures open into the superior and medial part of the infratemporal fossa and meet at right angles: the *inferior orbital fissure* and the *pterygomaxillary fissure.*

The *inferior orbital fissure* opens into the posterolateral part of the orbit. It is bounded by the greater wing of the sphenoid, the lateral border of the orbital surface of the maxilla, the orbital process of the *palatine bone,* and a small portion of the zygomatic bone.

Figure 8–12   The adult human cranium, right side, oblique posteroinferior view.

Pipe Cleaner in Pterygomaxillary Fissure

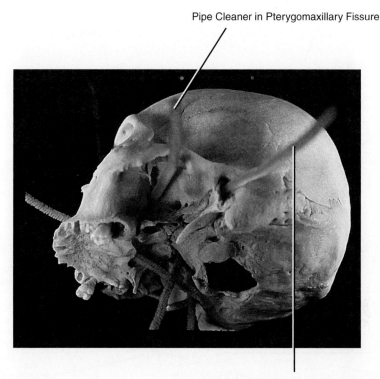

Pipe Cleaner in External Acoustic Meatus

Figure 8–13   Photograph of the adult human cranium, left side, oblique posteroinferior view.

The *pterygomaxillary fissure* is formed by the divergence of the lateral pterygoid plate of the sphenoid from the maxilla. This fissure connects the pterygopalatine fossa with the infratemporal fossa and transmits the terminal part of the maxillary artery and veins.

The Anterior View of the Skull: Norma Frontalis

Major bones visible in the anterior view of the skull, or *norma frontalis* (Figure 8–14), include the frontal, nasals, maxillae, zygomatics, ethmoid, vomer, mandible, and inferior nasal concha. Major visible landmarks are discussed next.

Landmarks and Features

The *frontal bone* (Figures 8–15 and 8–16; see also Fig. 8–14) forms the forehead. The *frontal eminences* are the areas of greatest convexity on the frontal bone. One is located superior to each *superciliary arch,* the bony arch underlying the eyebrow. The *glabella* is the raised area between the two superciliary arches. The *supraorbital margin* is the superior margin of the orbit, formed by the frontal bone. The medial third of the supraorbital margin is rounded; the lateral two-thirds are thin and prominent. At the junction of the medial one-third and the lateral two-thirds is the

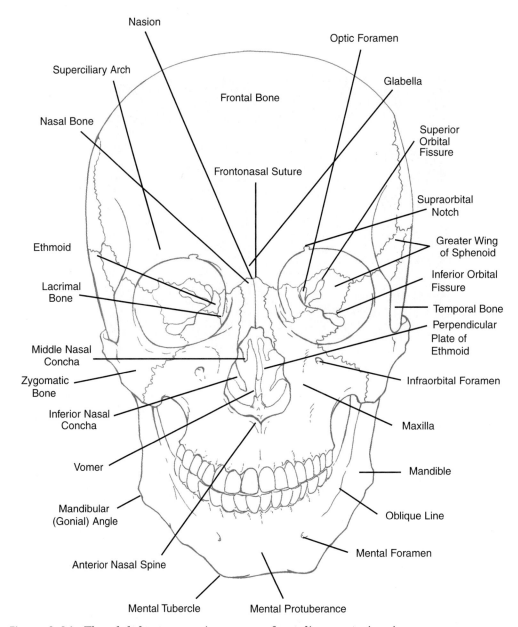

Figure 8–14   The adult human cranium: norma frontalis, or anterior view.

supraorbital notch, or *foramen,* for the transmission of the supraorbital nerve and vessels.

The Facial Skeleton

The *frontonasal suture* (see Fig. 8–14) is located below the glabella. This suture is formed at the junction of the frontal bone with the two small *nasal bones.* The midpoint of this suture is termed *nasion.* The *anterior nasal aperture* is the external opening of the nasal cavity in the skull. The external opening is the external nares.

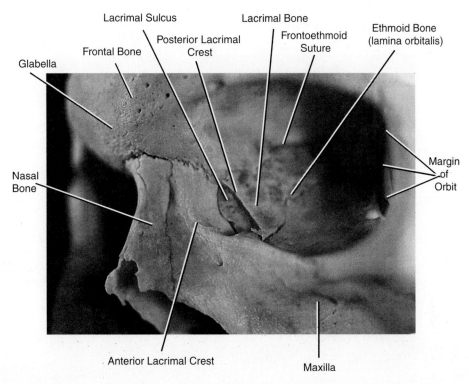

Glabella
Nasal Bone
Frontal Bone
Lacrimal Sulcus
Posterior Lacrimal Crest
Lacrimal Bone
Frontoethmoid Suture
Ethmoid Bone (lamina orbitalis)
Margin of Orbit
Anterior Lacrimal Crest
Maxilla

Figure 8-15   Orbit I: photograph of the left orbit, demonstrating the medial orbital wall and the orbital margin.

At the inferiormost point of the anterior nasal aperture in the midline is the *anterior nasal spine*. Within the nasal cavity, the *bony nasal septum* is visible. The superior and anterior part of the septum is formed by the *perpendicular plate of the ethmoid bone*, whereas the inferior and posterior part is formed by the *vomer*. Projecting medially from the lateral nasal wall on each side is a thin bone called the *inferior nasal concha*.

Below the orbit on the maxilla is the *infraorbital foramen*. The part of the maxilla containing the roots of the upper teeth is the *alveolar process of the maxilla*.

FACIAL SKELETON: THE ORBIT

The *orbits* (see Figs. 8–15 and 8–16) are the conical cavities containing the eyes and associated structures. They are so placed that the medial walls of the two orbits are approximately parallel with each other but their lateral walls are widely divergent. The orbit has a roof, a floor, a medial wall, a lateral wall, a base, and an apex.

The *roof* of the orbit is formed by the orbital plate of the frontal bone and the lesser wing of the sphenoid. The *lacrimal fossa* is located laterally and houses the lacrimal gland. The *floor* is formed by the orbital surface of the maxilla, the orbital process of the zygomatic bone, and the orbital process of the palatine bone.

The *medial wall* of the orbit is nearly vertical and is formed by the frontal process of the maxilla, the *lacrimal bone,* the lamina orbitalis of the ethmoid, and a small part of the body of the sphenoid. Anteriorly lies the *lacrimal sulcus,* which houses the

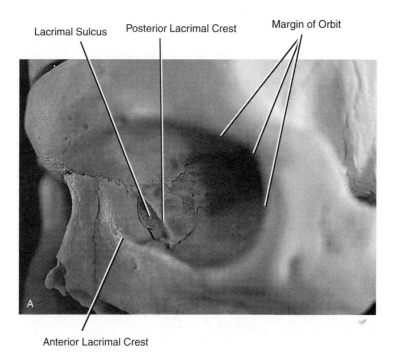

Figure 8–16   Orbit II: photograph showing a broader view of the left orbit, including (A) the lacrimal sulcus and associated structures and (B) the orbital margin and associated structures.

lacrimal sac. The sulcus is bounded by an *anterior lacrimal crest* on the frontal process of the maxilla and a sharper *posterior lacrimal crest* on the lacrimal bone.

In or near the *frontoethmoidal suture* (between the frontal and ethmoid bones) are the anterior and posterior ethmoidal foramina. The *anterior ethmoidal foramen* transmits the anterior ethmoidal nerve, one of the terminal branches of the nasociliary nerve, and anterior ethmoidal vessels. The *posterior ethmoidal foramen* transmits the posterior ethmoidal nerve and vessels.

The *lateral wall* of the orbit is formed by the orbital process of the zygomatic bone and the orbital surface of the greater wing of the sphenoid. Between the roof and the lateral wall near the apex of the orbit—or, more specifically, between the greater and lesser wings of the sphenoid bone—is the *superior orbital fissure*. The oculomotor and trochlear nerves and ophthalmic division of the trigeminal nerve as well as the abducent nerve enter the orbital cavity through this fissure. The *inferior orbital fissure* lies between the lateral wall and the floor of the orbit, inferior to the greater wing of the sphenoid.

The *base* of the orbit is formed by the *orbital margin,* whereas the *apex* of the orbit is formed by the *optic foramen*. The optic foramen is the anterior opening of the *optic canal,* which transmits the optic nerve and the ophthalmic artery. This is an opening that runs through the sphenoid bone.

The zygomatic arch has already been discussed, and the mandible is discussed later.

The Posterior View of the Skull: Norma Occipitalis

The major bones visible in the posterior view of the skull, or *norma occipitalis* (Figures 8–17 through 8–19), are the occipital, the parietals, and the temporals. Landmarks are examined next.

Landmarks and Features

The sagittal and lambdoidal sutures are visible in norma occipitalis as well as in norma verticalis. Occasional small bones, the *sutural* (or *wormian* or *Inca*) bones, may be present in the lambdoidal suture between the parietals and the occipital. They are not a constant feature, and their frequency may vary from population to population. Sutural bones may occur in other sutures of the cranium as well, but they are far more common in the lambdoidal suture than elsewhere. The *parietomastoid suture,* between the parietal bone and the mastoid portion of the temporal bone, is visible in norma occipitalis as well as in norma lateralis. The same is true for the *occipitomastoid suture,* which is between the occipital bone and the mastoid portion of the temporal bone.

Asterion is visible from the posterior view, as well as from the lateral view. Lambda is also visible posteriorly. *Opisthocranion* is the most posterior point on the skull when it is in the Frankfort horizontal plane, described as when the superior border of the external auditory meatus and the inferior margin of the orbit are oriented in the same horizontal plane. It may occasionally lie on the external occipital protuberance but is more often superior to the protuberance. *Inion* is the most posterior point on the external occipital protuberance. Very occasionally opisthocranion may occupy this same location.

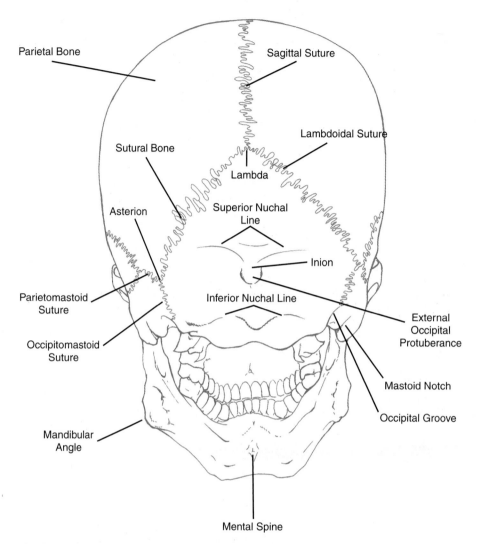

Figure 8–17   The adult human cranium: norma occipitalis, or posterior view.

The *external occipital protuberance* is a prominent raised area at the back of the skull near the midline of the occipital squama. Extending from it laterally on either side are slightly arching ridges that are called the *superior nuchal lines.* Approximately 1 cm above the superior nuchal line may be the faint *highest nuchal line,* for the attachment of the *galea aponeurotica.* The *external occipital crest (median nuchal line)* is a median ridge that extends from *inion* to the *foramen magnum* and gives attachment to the *ligamentum nuchae.* The *inferior nuchal line* begins at the midpoint of the external occipital crest and runs laterally across the occipital bone inferior to the superior nuchal lines.

The *mastoid notch* can be seen on the medial side of the *mastoid process.* This notch is for the posterior belly of the digastric muscle. Medial to the notch is the *occipital groove* for the occipital artery.

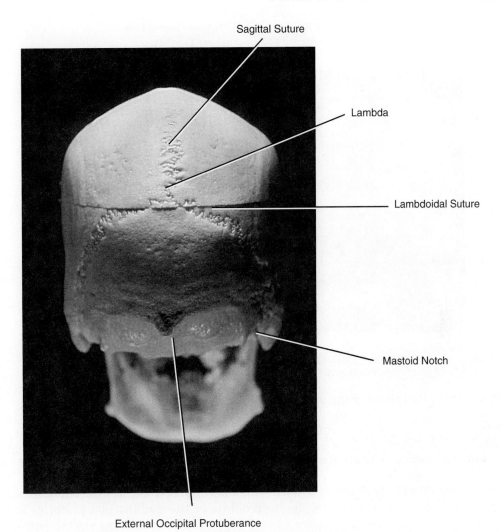

Figure 8-18   Photograph of the adult human cranium in norma occipitalis, or posterior view.

The Basal View of the Skull: Norma Basalis

The major bones visible in the basal (inferior) view of the skull, or *norma basalis* (Figures 8–20 and 8–21), are the occipital, the temporals, the sphenoid, the maxillae, the palatines, the vomer, and the mandible. Visible landmarks are discussed next.

Landmarks and Features

The *hard palate* is formed by the *palatine processes of the maxillae* and the *horizontal plates of the palatine bones*. At the posterior angles of the hard palate, in the palatine bone, are the *greater palatine foramina*. Posterior to these foramina are the *pyramidal processes* of the palatine bones, which are perforated by one or more *lesser*

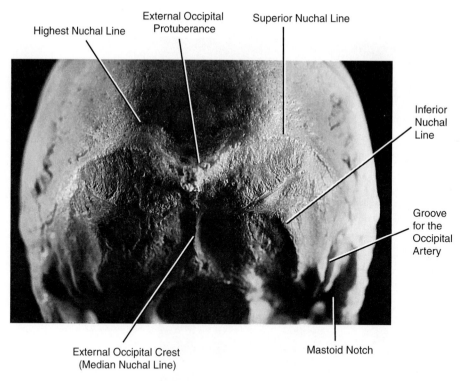

Highest Nuchal Line

External Occipital Protuberance

Superior Nuchal Line

Inferior Nuchal Line

Groove for the Occipital Artery

External Occipital Crest (Median Nuchal Line)

Mastoid Notch

Figure 8-19   Photograph of the nuchal region of the adult human cranium.

palatine foramina. The greater palatine foramen transmits the greater palatine vessels and nerve.

Posterior and superior to the hard palate are the *choanae,* or internal nasal apertures. At the anterior aspect of the hard palate in the midline just posterior to the central incisor teeth is the *incisive fossa.* Deep in the incisive fossa are the paired *incisive foramina* that transmit branches of the nasopalatine nerve. Lateral and anterior to the hard palate are the *alveolar processes* of the maxillae, holding the roots of the upper teeth. On the posterior aspect of the lateral wall of the nasal cavity is the *perpendicular plate of the palatine bone,* at the top of which is an opening called the *sphenopalatine foramen* (Figure 8–22).

Different parts of the sphenoid bone can be seen inferiorly; they include the medial and lateral pterygoid plates, the hamulus, and the pterygoid fossa. The *medial pterygoid plate* is posterior to the palatine bone, and the hook-shaped *pterygoid hamulus* is attached to the posterior part of the free inferior border of the medial pterygoid plate. More laterally is the *lateral pterygoid plate.* The space between the medial and lateral pterygoid plates is the *pterygoid fossa.*

The *pterygoid canal* is a bony tunnel through the sphenoid bone that eventually opens into the *pterygopalatine fossa* (described in detail later). The posterior opening of the canal is located superiorly above the pterygoid fossa at the point where the medial and lateral pterygoid plates meet (Figure 8–23; see also Fig. 8–20B). Another tiny opening to the pterygopalatine fossa is the *palatovaginal (pharyngeal) canal,* which passes anterolaterally through the sphenoid just lateral to the vomer's articulation with the sphenoid. The vomer forms the posterior and inferior part of the bony

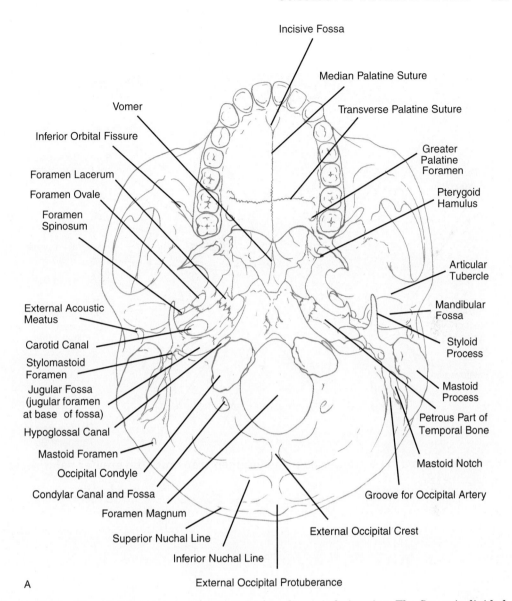

Figure 8-20   The adult human cranium: norma basalis, or inferior view. The figure is divided into *A* and *B* portions to make the labeling of structures clearer.

nasal septum and can be seen through the choanae, separating the nasal cavity into two parts.

More laterally on the sphenoid is the *foramen ovale*. It is an oval opening at the base of the lateral pterygoid plate.

The *sphenoidal spine* is a pointed projection lateral to the foramen ovale. It gives attachment to the sphenomandibular ligament and tensor veli palatini muscle. The sphenoidal spine is pierced by the *foramen spinosum*.

The *pharyngeal tubercle* is located posterior to the vomer on the basilar portion of the occipital bone.

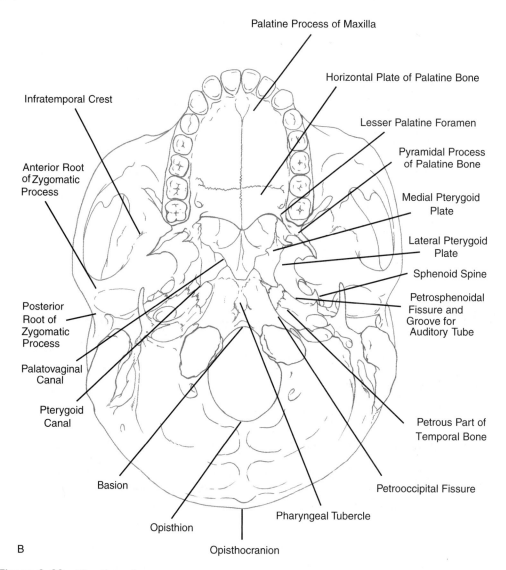

B

Figure 8–20   (*Continued*)

Various parts of the temporal bone are seen in the basal, or inferior, view. These include the squamous and tympanic parts, which have also been seen laterally. The *mastoid process* and *notch* and *occipital groove* (see Figs. 8–20A and 8–21) for the occipital artery are visible in this view as well as in the norma occipitalis. The *styloid process* (Figure 8–24) is visible in this view as well. Lying at its base and separating it from the mastoid process is the *stylomastoid foramen*. Visible in the norma basalis but not in previous views is the *petrous part of the temporal bone* (see Figs. 8–20 and 8–22). This is a wedge-shaped part of the bone that is very dense and "rock hard" (to which *petrous*, meaning "rocklike," refers). It extends between the sphenoid and the occipital bones.

Several foramina and fissures in addition to those mentioned are visible on the base of the skull. The *foramen lacerum* (see Fig. 8–20A) is at the base of the medial

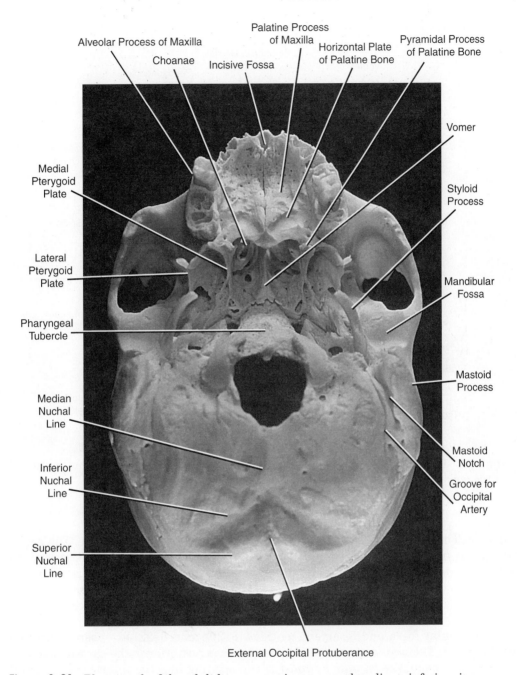

Palatine Process
of Maxilla

Alveolar Process of Maxilla

Pyramidal Process
of Palatine Bone

Choanae

Horizontal Plate
of Palatine Bone

Incisive Fossa

Vomer

Medial
Pterygoid
Plate

Styloid
Process

Lateral
Pterygoid
Plate

Mandibular
Fossa

Pharyngeal
Tubercle

Median
Nuchal
Line

Mastoid
Process

Inferior
Nuchal
Line

Mastoid
Notch

Groove for
Occipital
Artery

Superior
Nuchal
Line

External Occipital Protuberance

Figure 8-21   Photograph of the adult human cranium: norma basalis, or inferior view.

pterygoid plate, between it and the tip of the petrous part of the temporal bone. It usually has very irregular edges. The *carotid canal* (see Figs. 8–20A and 8–22) is a relatively large bony tunnel for the internal carotid artery. Its inferior opening is usually circular, and it passes through the petrous part of the temporal bone.

The *groove for the auditory tube (sulcus tubae auditivae;* see Fig. 8–20B) is located between the petrous portion of the temporal bone and the greater wing of the

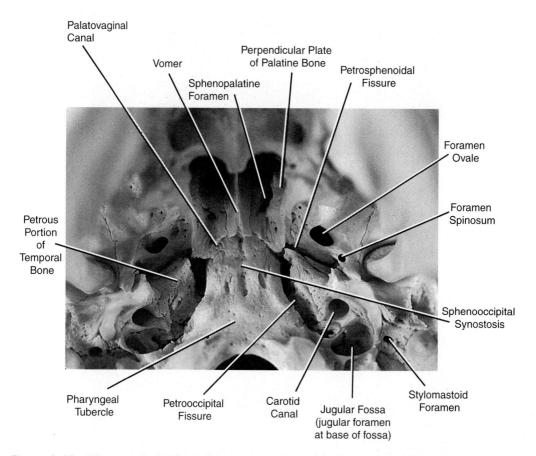

Palatovaginal
Canal

Vomer

Sphenopalatine
Foramen

Perpendicular Plate
of Palatine Bone

Petrosphenoidal
Fissure

Foramen
Ovale

Foramen
Spinosum

Petrous
Portion
of
Temporal
Bone

Sphenooccipital
Synostosis

Pharyngeal
Tubercle

Petrooccipital
Fissure

Carotid
Canal

Jugular Fossa
(jugular foramen
at base of fossa)

Stylomastoid
Foramen

Figure 8–22   Photograph of the adult human cranium: norma basalis, or inferior view. Close-up of the region of the sphenooccipital synostosis.

sphenoid. This groove houses the cartilaginous part of the auditory tube. The *petrosphenoidal fissure* (see Figs. 8–20*B* and 8–22) is at the "bottom" of this groove. In fact, in anatomical position, the fissure is in the superior aspect, or "roof," of the groove. This fissure is the actual space between the petrous part of the temporal bone and the sphenoid, whereas the groove extends a little to either side, making it wider than the fissure.

The jugular fossa and foramen (see Figs. 8–20*A* and 8–22) are posterior to the *carotid canal*. The *jugular fossa* is a depression seen posterior to the carotid canal on the temporal bone; the *jugular foramen* is the opening into the interior of the skull located medially in the fossa between the temporal and occipital bones. The *jugular process* of the occipital bone is an extension of the occipital lateral to the occipital condyles, and its anterior border forms the posterior boundary of the jugular foramen. The *petrooccipital fissure* (see Fig. 8–22) extends anteriorly from the jugular foramen to the foramen lacerum, separating the petrous part of the temporal bone from the occipital.

The *foramen magnum* (Figure 8–25; see also Figs. 8–20*A* and 8–24), which transmits the medulla oblongata (part of the brain stem) and its associated struc-

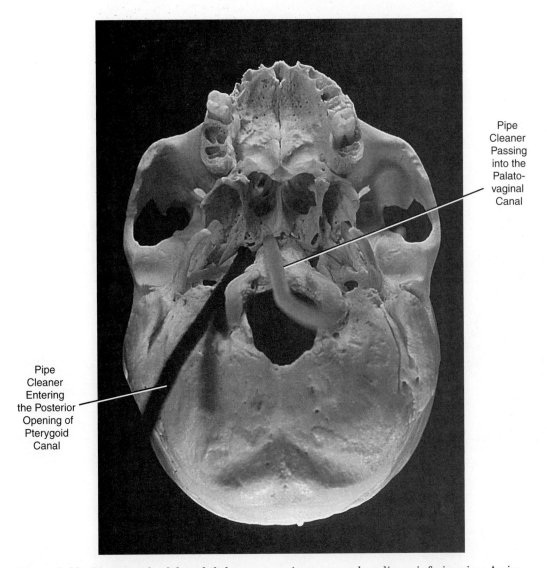

Pipe
Cleaner
Passing
into the
Palato-
vaginal
Canal

Pipe
Cleaner
Entering
the Posterior
Opening of
Pterygoid
Canal

Figure 8–23   Photograph of the adult human cranium: norma basalis, or inferior view. A pipe cleaner is in the posterior opening of the pterygoid canal.

tures, is a very large opening posterior to the basilar portion of the occipital bone. It is bounded laterally by the oval and convex *occipital condyles* (see Figure 8–25; see also Fig. 8–20*A*). These articulate with the superior articular facets of the atlas. Posterior to each condyle is an opening, the *condylar canal,* or a depression, the *condylar fossa* (see Figs. 8–20*A* and 8–24). The canal transmits an emissary vein that connects venous sinuses inside the skull to veins outside the skull. *Basion* is the anteriormost point on the margin of the foramen magnum, whereas *opisthion* is the posteriormost point on its margin. The *hypoglossal canals* (see Fig. 8–20*A*) are openings superior to each occipital condyle. Each transmits a hypoglossal nerve and a meningeal artery.

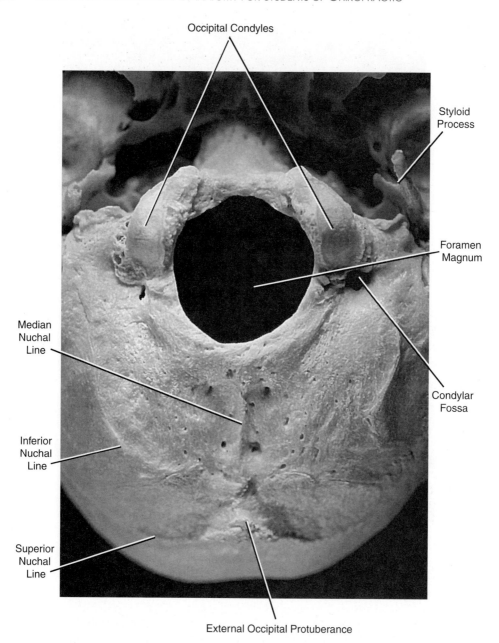

Figure 8-24 Photograph of the adult human cranium: norma basalis, or inferior view. Close-up of the region of the foramen magnum and the nuchal region of the occipital bone.

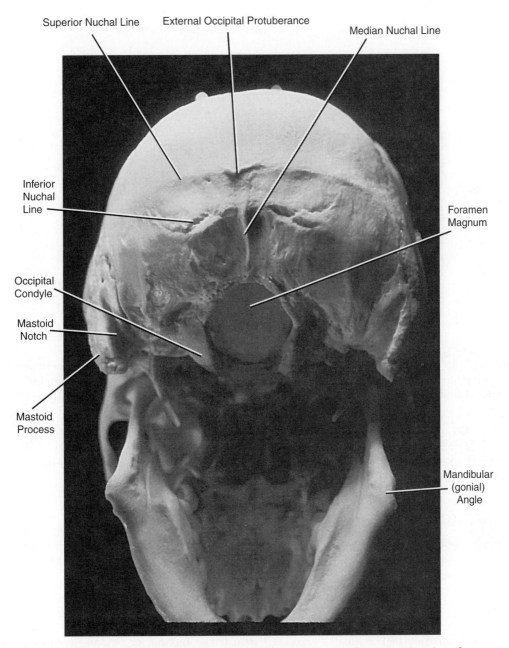

Figure 8-25   Photograph of the adult human cranium, oblique inferoposterior view, demonstrating the region of the foramen magnum and the nuchal region of the occipital bone.

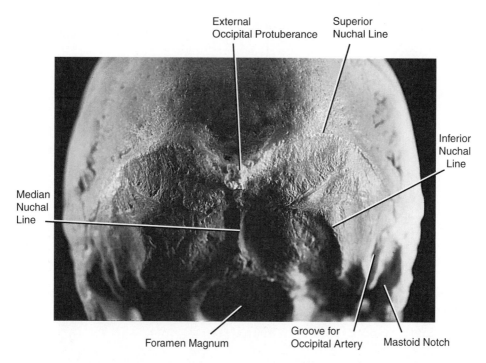

External Occipital Protuberance

Superior Nuchal Line

Inferior Nuchal Line

Median Nuchal Line

Foramen Magnum

Groove for Occipital Artery

Mastoid Notch

Figure 8-26   Photograph of the adult human cranium, oblique inferoposterior view, demonstrating the region of the external occipital protuberance, the median nuchal line, and the superior and inferior nuchal lines.

The external occipital crest (median nuchal line) and the superior and inferior nuchal lines (Figure 8–26; see also Figs. 8–20A, 8–24, and 8–25) are visible in the basilar view as well as from the posterior view of the cranium.

The Interior View of the Skull

Bones visible from the interior of the skull (Figures 8–27 and 8–28) include the frontals, parietals, occipital, temporal, sphenoid, and ethmoid. Landmarks are discussed next.

Landmarks and Features

The interior of the skull is divided into three basins, or fossae—the anterior, middle, and posterior cranial fossae (see Figs. 8–27 and 8–28).

THE ANTERIOR CRANIAL FOSSA

The floor of the *anterior cranial fossa* (see Figs. 8–27 and 8–28) is formed by the *orbital plates* of the frontal bone, the small and much perforated *cribriform plates* of the ethmoid bone, and the lesser wings and body of the sphenoid bone. The floor supports the frontal lobe of the cerebrum. The olfactory nerves run to the nasal cavity through the perforations of the cribriform plates, and the olfactory bulbs of the brain

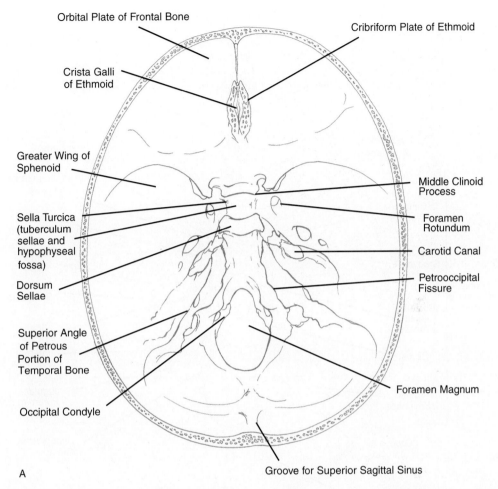

Orbital Plate of Frontal Bone

Cribriform Plate of Ethmoid

Crista Galli of Ethmoid

Greater Wing of Sphenoid

Middle Clinoid Process

Sella Turcica (tuberculum sellae and hypophyseal fossa)

Foramen Rotundum

Carotid Canal

Dorsum Sellae

Petrooccipital Fissure

Superior Angle of Petrous Portion of Temporal Bone

Occipital Condyle

Foramen Magnum

A

Groove for Superior Sagittal Sinus

Figure 8-27 Interior of the adult human cranium, superior views, demonstrating the cranial fossae. The figure is divided into *A* and *B* portions to make the labeling of structures clearer.

sit on these plates. The *crista galli* is a small, perpendicular plate of bone that extends superiorly from the median portion of the superior aspect of the ethmoid bone between the two cribriform plates. It is an anchoring point for the cranial meninges.

THE MIDDLE CRANIAL FOSSA

The *middle cranial fossa* (Figure 8–29; see also Figs. 8–27 and 8–28) is bounded anteriorly by the *posterior margins of the lesser wings of the sphenoid,* the *anterior clinoid processes,* and the ridge forming the *anterior margin of the chiasmatic groove.* This boundary also defines the posterior margin of the anterior cranial fossa. The posterior margin of the middle cranial fossa is formed by the *superior angles of the petrous portions of the temporal bones* and the *dorsum sellae.* This boundary also defines the anterior margin of the posterior fossa.

In the median portion of the middle cranial fossa are the *chiasmatic groove* and the *tuberculum sellae* (Figure 8–30; see also Figs. 8–27 through 8–29). The *chias-*

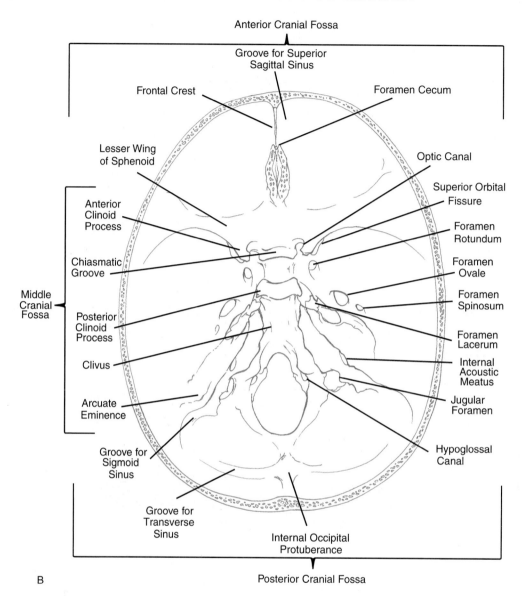

Figure 8–27   (*Continued*)

matic groove extends across the midline and ends on either side at the *optic canal.* The tuberculum sellae is a mild prominence inferior to the groove.

The *anterior clinoid processes* are projections of the lesser wings of the sphenoid located posterior and lateral to the optic canals. Posterior to the tuberculum sellae is the highly concave *fossa hypophyseos* (see Fig. 8–30), which houses the pituitary gland. This fossa is at the center of a structure termed the *sella turcica* (see Figs. 8–29 and 8–30), which is bounded anteriorly by the tuberculum sellae and posteriorly by the dorsum sellae.

To either side on its anterior wall may be the *middle clinoid process.* The middle clinoid processes are highly variable in their presence or absence. They may be entirely absent or they may be present as very small bumps or very well developed pro-

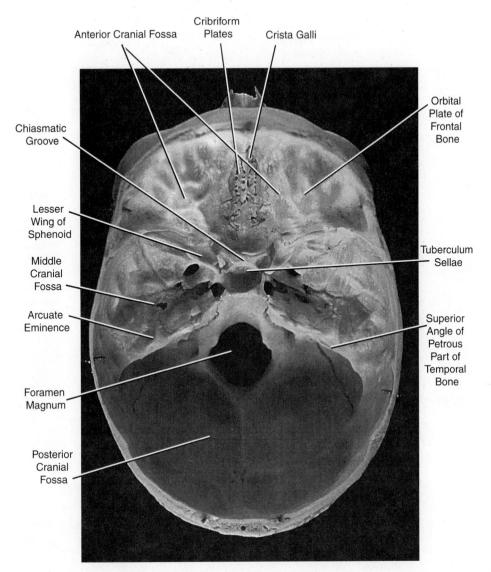

Figure 8–28   Photograph of the interior of the adult human cranium, superior view, demonstrating the cranial fossae.

jections. The posterior margin of the sella turcica is formed by the wall-like dorsum sellae. At the superolateral corners of the dorsum sellae are small projections called the *posterior clinoid processes* (see Figs. 8–27*B* and 8–30). The anterior and posterior clinoid processes provide attachment to a meningeal membrane called the *tentorium cerebelli.*

The lateral deeper portions of the middle fossa house the temporal lobes of the brain. Opening into the middle cranial fossa are the *superior orbital fissure,* the *foramen rotundum,* the *foramen ovale,* the *foramen spinosum,* the *foramen lacerum,* and the *carotid canal* (see Figs. 8–27 and 8–28), most of which are seen in the inferior view.

The internal opening of the carotid canal usually lies more medially, next to the occipital, than does the external opening. The foramen rotundum is not visible

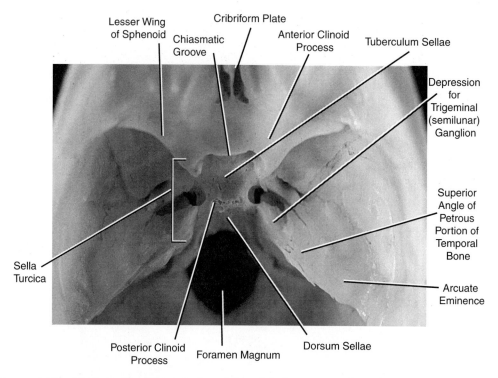

Figure 8-29   Photograph of the interior of the adult human cranium, superior view, demonstrating the middle cranial fossa.

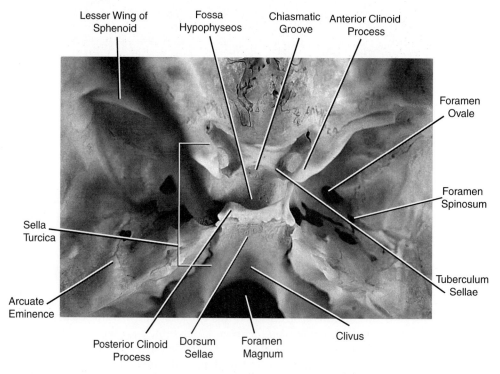

Figure 8-30   Photograph of the interior of the adult human cranium, superior view, demonstrating the sella turcica and associated structures in the middle cranial fossa.

inferiorly. It is a small, usually round opening between the foramen ovale and the superior orbital fissure.

Figure 8–31 demonstrates the isolated sphenoid bone. It is a highly complex bone surrounded by other bones of the cranium. It is, however, a key feature of the middle cranial fossa. Its superior and inferior aspects have been examined. Its principal features visible from its anterior and posterior aspects, including the dorsum sellae, greater and lesser wings, and major foramina, are shown in this figure.

Visible on the anterior surface of the *petrous portion of the temporal bone* (see Fig. 8–27B), within the middle cranial fossa, is a ridge or swelling called the *arcuate eminence*. It is caused by the projection of the superior semicircular canal. Also in the

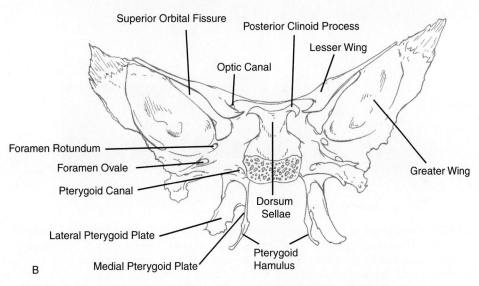

Figure 8–31   The isolated sphenoid bone: (*A*) anterior and (*B*) posterior views.

middle cranial fossa is the *depression for the trigeminal (semilunar) ganglion* of the trigeminal nerve (see Fig. 8–29). This depression is located on the anterior surface of the petrous portion of the temporal bone just lateral to the orifice of the carotid canal.

THE POSTERIOR CRANIAL FOSSA

The *posterior cranial fossa* (Figure 8–32; see also Figs. 8–27 and 8–28) is the largest and deepest of the three fossae. It is formed by the *dorsum sellae,* the antero-superior slope of the *clivus of the sphenoid* and *occipital bones* (see Figs. 8–27 and 8–30), the *petrous* and *mastoid portions of the temporal bone,* the *internal aspect of the squama* (the flat, interparietal portion) *of the occipital bone,* and the *mastoid angles of the parietals.* The latter are the corners of the parietal bones that sit next to the parietomastoid sutures. This fossa houses the cerebellum, pons, and medulla oblongata. The *foramen magnum* pierces the center of this fossa.

Also present in the posterior cranial fossa are the *petrooccipital fissure,* the *jugular foramen,* the *hypoglossal canal,* and the *internal acoustic meatus* (see Fig. 8–27A and *B*). The internal acoustic meatus is an opening on the posterior aspect of the petrous part of the temporal bone. It transmits the vestibulocochlear and facial nerves.

The posterior fossa is bounded posteriorly by the deep *grooves for the transverse sinuses* (see Figs. 8–27B and 8–32). These proceed laterally and then anteriorly to meet the deep, curved *grooves for the sigmoid sinuses,* which run along the internal aspect of the mastoid part of the temporal bone and end at the jugular foramen.

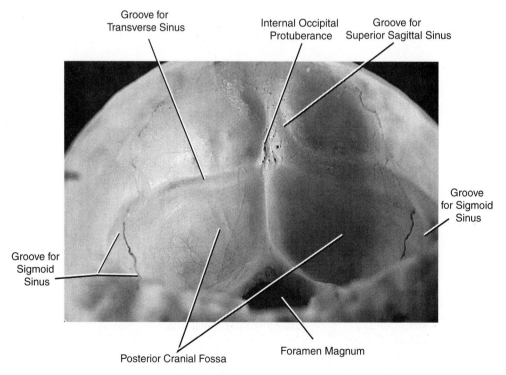

Figure 8-32   Photograph of the internal aspect of the occipital squama, demonstrating the internal occipital protuberance, the confluence of the sinuses (intersection of groove for superior sagittal sinus and grooves for transverse sinuses), and the grooves for the superior sagittal, transverse, and sigmoid sinuses.

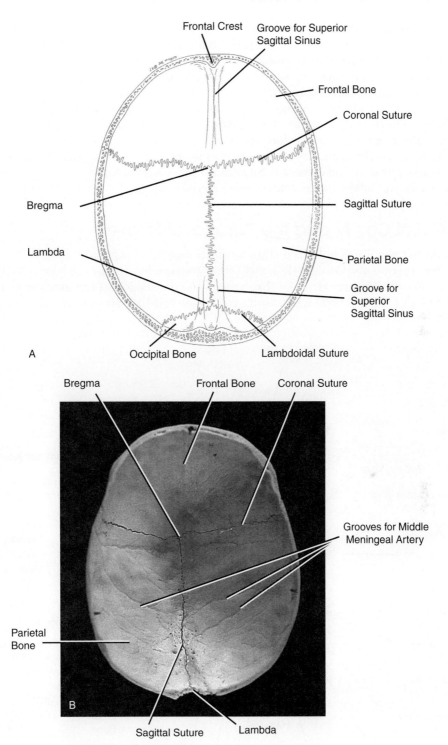

Figure 8–33 (*A*) Line drawing and (*B*) photograph of the internal aspect of the calvarium, or cranial roof.

These are grooves for vascular sinuses, which are part of the venous system of the head, and should not be confused with the bony air sinuses of the frontal, ethmoid, sphenoid, and maxillae. The grooves for the two transverse sinuses meet in the midline posteriorly and groove the surface of the internally projecting *internal occipital protuberance.* At this structure they meet the *groove for the superior sagittal sinus* (Figure 8–33A; see also Fig. 8–32), which lies on the internal aspect of the two parietal bones, where they meet at the sagittal suture. This groove is wider than the sagittal suture and runs posteriorly from the frontal bone to the internal occipital protuberance. The intersection of the grooves for the superior sagittal sinus and the transverse sinuses on the internal occipital protuberance is known as the *impression for the confluence of the sinuses,* or *torcular Herophili.*

The Nasal Cavity and the Paranasal Sinuses

Although not readily visible in a skull that has not been sagittally bisected, a number of important bony, yet very delicate, structures are located in the nasal cavity (refer to Figures 8–34 through 8–36 throughout the discussion of the structures of the nasal cavity). On the lateral nasal wall are three scroll-like projections. These are the

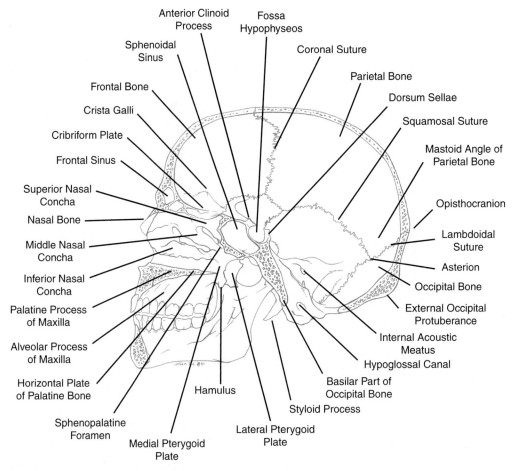

Figure 8-34 Median section of the adult human cranium, right side, demonstrating the nasal conchae as well as the frontal and sphenoid sinuses.

three *nasal conchae.* They include the *superior* and *middle nasal conchae,* which are projections from the labyrinths of the *ethmoid bone.* They form the superiormost portion of the lateral nasal wall.

Inferior to these conchae is the *inferior nasal concha,* a separate, small bone (also known as the *turbinate bone*) that articulates with the maxilla and the perpendicular plate of the palatine bone. The posterior aspect of the lateral nasal wall is also formed by the perpendicular plate of the palatine. The more anterior portion of the lateral nasal wall is formed by the maxilla, along with the inferior nasal concha.

The lacrimal bone and the medial pterygoid plate also contribute to the lateral wall of the nasal cavity. Lateral to and covered by the superior, middle, and inferior nasal conchae are spaces called the *superior meatus, middle meatus,* and *inferior meatus.* Off the superior meatus is the narrow *sphenoethmoidal recess* that separates the superior concha and the anterior aspect of the body of the sphenoid.

In some of the bones surrounding the nasal cavity are mucous membrane-lined spaces called the *paranasal sinuses.* These should not be confused with the vascular sinuses discussed earlier. There are four paranasal sinuses: the *frontal sinus* in the frontal bone, the *sphenoidal sinus* in the body of the sphenoid bone, the *ethmoidal air cells* in the ethmoid bone just medial to the orbit, and the *maxillary sinuses* in the maxillae just lateral to the nasal cavity and superior to the alveolar processes. All of these sinuses drain into the nasal cavity.

The *sphenoidal sinus* opens into the sphenoethmoidal recess. In the middle meatus, hidden lateral to the middle concha, is the bulging *ethmoidal bulla.* This ethmoidal bulla houses the *middle ethmoidal air cells.* Anteroinferior to the bulla is the *uncinate process of the ethmoid,* which descends posteroinferiorly. Between the

Figure 8–35 Parasagittal section of the adult human cranium, demonstrating the bony nasal septum as well as the frontal and sphenoid sinuses.

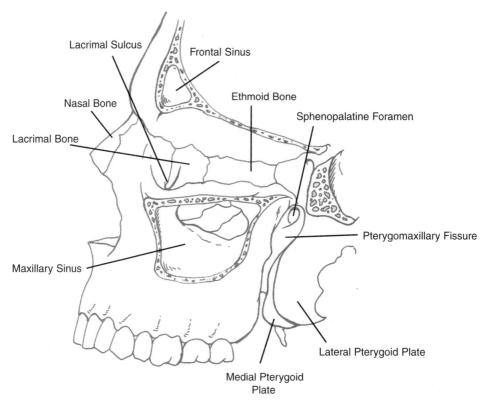

Figure 8–36   The skeleton of the face, left lateral view. The lateral wall of the orbit has been removed to expose the frontal sinus. The lateral wall of the maxillary sinus has also been removed to expose the interior of the maxillary sinus. The pterygomaxillary fissure and the sphenopalatine foramen, both opening into the pterygopalatine fossa, can also be seen.

uncinate process and the ethmoidal bulla is the *hiatus semilunaris,* a crescent-shaped opening that allows communication between the maxillary sinus and the nasal cavity. At its upper end, the hiatus semilunaris is continuous with the *ethmoidal infundibulum,* a funnel-shaped space into which open the *anterior ethmoidal air cells* and sometimes the *frontal sinus.*

The inferior opening of the *nasolacrimal duct,* which is continuous with the *lacrimal sulcus* in the orbit, opens into the inferior meatus lateral to the inferior concha. This passageway drains tears from the eye into the nasal cavity.

In the midline, between the conchae of the left and right side, is the *bony nasal septum,* formed by the vomer and the perpendicular plate of the ethmoid.

The Pterygopalatine Fossa

The *pterygopalatine fossa* (Figures 8–37 and 8–38; refer also to Fig. 8–36 throughout the discussion of the pterygopalatine fossa) is a space in the skull formed at the junction of the *pterygomaxillary fissure,* the *inferior orbital fissure,* and the inferior part of the apex of the orbit. It is bounded by the body, the pterygoid plates and the greater wing of the sphenoid, the infratemporal surface of the maxilla, and the perpendicular plate of the palatine bone. It communicates anteriorly with the orbit

Figure 8–37   Diagrammatic representation of the pterygopalatine fossa.

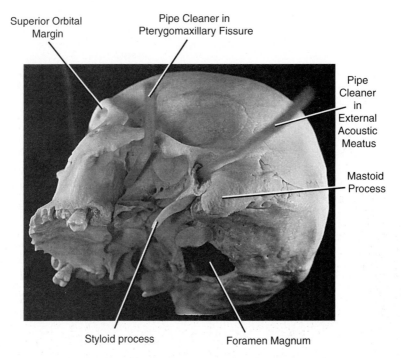

Superior Orbital
Margin

Pipe Cleaner in
Pterygomaxillary Fissure

Pipe
Cleaner
in
External
Acoustic
Meatus

Mastoid
Process

Styloid process

Foramen Magnum

Figure 8–38 Photograph of the adult human cranium, left oblique posteroinferior view. The anterior pipe cleaner is passing into the pterygopalatine fossa through the pterygomaxillary fissure, whereas the posterior pipe cleaner is in the external acoustic meatus. Note the prominent styloid process anteroinferior to the external acoustic meatus.

via the inferior orbital fissure, medially with the nasal cavity via the sphenopalatine foramen, and laterally with the infratemporal fossa by the pterygomaxillary fissure.

Opening into it on the posterior wall are the *foramen rotundum,* the *pterygoid canal,* and the *palatovaginal (pharyngeal) canal.* Opening inferiorly into the pterygopalatine fossa is the *greater palatine (pterygopalatine) canal* (see Figs. 8–35 and 8–37). The fossa contains the maxillary nerve, the pterygopalatine ganglion, the terminal part of the maxillary artery, and various formations connecting with these structures through the openings into this fossa.

The pterygopalatine fossa may be visualized as a small room (see Fig. 8–37) into which open a door (the pterygomaxillary fissure), a window (the inferior orbital fissure), and a number of ducts and pipes.

The Mandible

The *mandible* (Figures 8–39 and 8–40) consists of a U-shaped horizontal *body (corpus)* that bears the teeth and two vertical rami that project superiorly from the posterior portion of the body.

The *body* of the mandible possesses a base or splenium that bears the *alveolar process.* The alveolar process contains the sockets for the teeth. The *external surface (buccolabial surface)* of the mandibular body exhibits several structures. A *mental protuberance* (median) and two *mental tubercles* (lateral) form the *chin.* (The mental protuberance and the two mental tubercles form the *mental trigone.*) The *oblique*

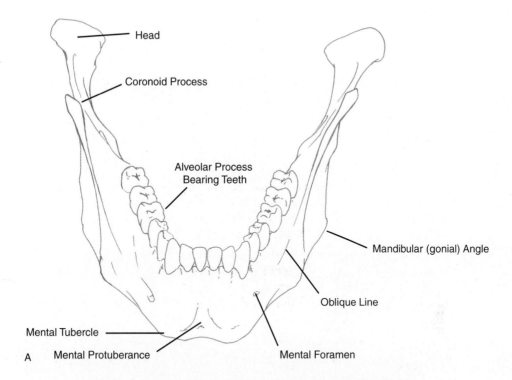

Head

Coronoid Process

Alveolar Process
Bearing Teeth

Mandibular (gonial) Angle

Oblique Line

Mental Tubercle

A   Mental Protuberance

Mental Foramen

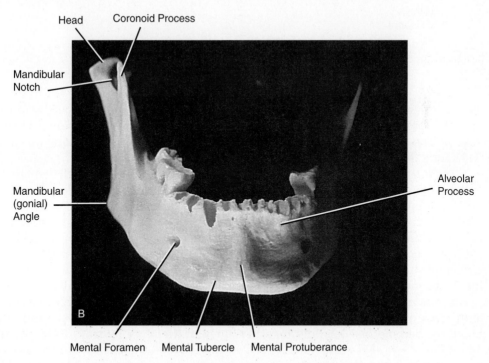

Head   Coronoid Process

Mandibular
Notch

Mandibular
(gonial)
Angle

Alveolar
Process

B

Mental Foramen   Mental Tubercle   Mental Protuberance

Figure 8–39 (*A*) Line drawing and (*B*) photograph of the mandible, anterior view, demonstrating the mental trigone and mental foramina.

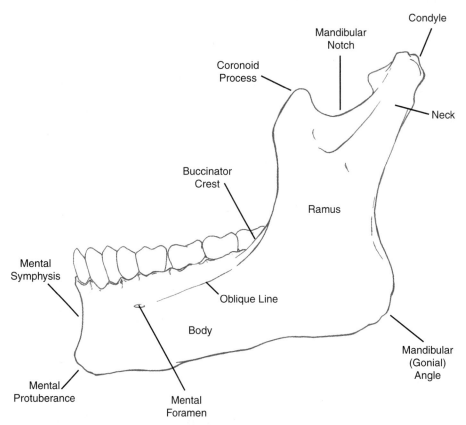

Figure 8–40   The mandible, left external view.

lines of the mandible run from the mental tubercles to the anterior border of the ramus. An opening on either side, the *mental foramen,* transmits the mental nerve and vessels. The *buccinator crest* is a faint ridge running between the oblique line and the teeth. It is for the attachment of the buccinator muscle.

The *internal surface (lingual surface;* refer to Figures 8–41 through 8–43 throughout the remainder of the discussion of the mandible) presents on each side a *mylohyoid line,* a narrow ridge running from the ramus along the body toward the midline. Anteriorly and superiorly from the mylohyoid line is the *sublingual fossa* for the sublingual salivary gland. On the inferior aspect of the chin, anterior and inferior to the mylohyoid line and just lateral to the midline, is the *digastric fossa* (Figure 8–44) for the insertion of the anterior belly of the digastric muscle. Inferoposterior to the mylohyoid line is the much larger *submandibular fossa* for the submandibular salivary gland.

The midline of the mandible is the mandibular symphysis, a fibrocartilaginous joint early in development. The symphysis synostoses and the two halves of the mandible become fused solidly together early in life. Just lateral to the site of the *mandibular symphysis* are small protuberances called the *mental spines (genial tubercles),* which are attachments of the genioglossus and geniohyoid muscles, of the oral cavity.

The *mandibular ramus* exhibits the following features: The *coronoid process* is a beaklike projection directed superiorly and anteriorly. It is for the insertion of the temporalis muscle. The mandibular ramus bears the mandibular *head (articular*

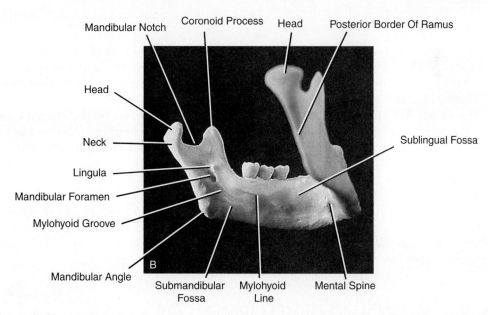

Figure 8–41   (A) Line drawing of the mandible, right internal view, and (B) photograph of left internal view.

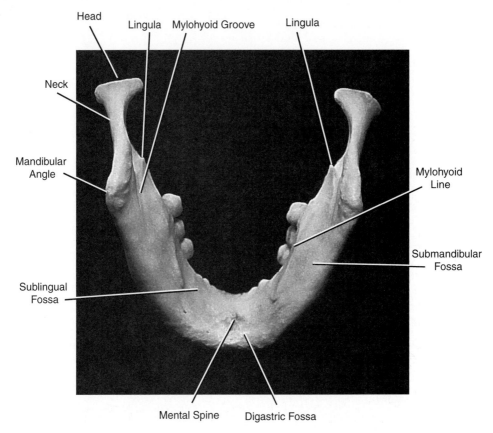

Figure 8–42 The mandible, oblique posteroinferior view, demonstrating the lingulae, mylohyoid lines, mental spines, and fossae for the sublingual and submandibular salivary glands.

condyle) and *neck*. The *head* lies at the superoposterior extremity of the ramus and articulates with the mandibular fossa of the temporal bone to form the *temporomandibular joint*. The neck is the constricted region inferior to the head that joins the head to the ramus.

The *mandibular notch* lies between the coronoid process and the mandibular head. The *medial surface* of the ramus bears the *mandibular foramen*. The medial lip of the foramen is prolonged into the *lingula* for the attachment of the sphenomandibular ligament. The *mandibular foramen* and *canal* (the foramen is the opening of the canal, and the canal runs through the bone) transmit the inferior alveolar nerve and vessels to the mandibular teeth.

The *mylohyoid groove* transmits the mylohyoid nerve and vessels. It originates at the mandibular foramen and extends inferiorly and anteriorly along the medial surface of the mandible. The *mandibular (gonial) angle* is the posteroinferior angle of the jaw, where the ramus and body of the mandible meet.

OSSIFICATION AND DEVELOPMENT OF THE CRANIUM, MANDIBLE, AND HYOID

Vast amounts of literature and research have been devoted to craniofacial growth and development. We touch on the high points here, concentrating especially upon

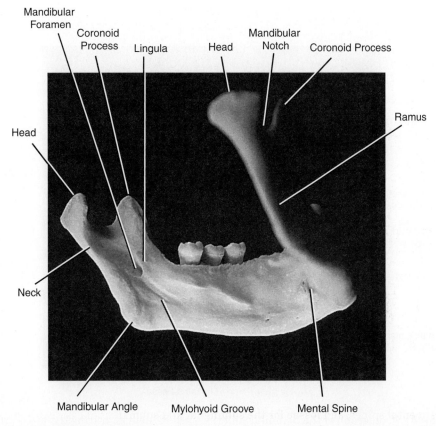

Figure 8–43 Photograph of the mandible, left internal view, demonstrating the lingula, mylo-hyoid line, and mylohyoid groove.

the patterns of ossification within the cranium (Figure 8–45). See a work such as Sperber (1989) or Gray (1985, 1995) for a more detailed discussion of craniofacial embryology and development.

As discussed previously, the cranium is composed of two entities: the neurocranium and the splanchnocranium (the face). Both of these entities have unique developmental characteristics.

The Neurocranium

The *neurocranium* is composed of two elements: the cranial vault and the cranial base). The *cranial vault (calvaria)* is of recent phylogenetic origin and covers the expanded brain. It is also known as the *desmocranium,* because it forms via intramembranous (dermal) ossification. It includes the frontal bone, the parietal bones, the squamous part of the occipital bone, and the squamous part of the temporal bones.

The *cranial base (basicranium)* is phylogenetically much older. It includes the cranial floor and the bony capsules surrounding the nasal and auditory sense organs. It forms via endochondral ossification and is therefore known as the *chondrocranium.* The cranial base includes all the remainder of the cranial bones not included as part of the face or cranial vault, including most of the temporal bones, the basilar part of the occipital bone, the sphenoid, and the ethmoid.

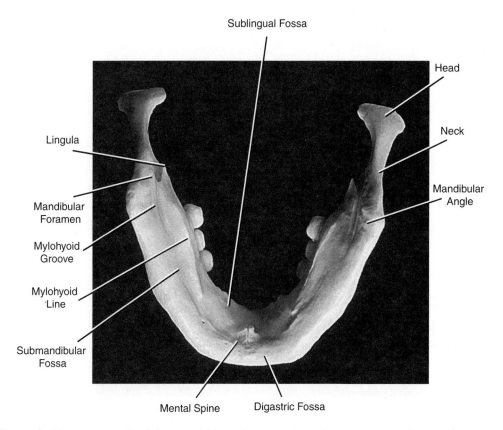

Figure 8-44   Photograph of the mandible, inferior surface, demonstrating the mylohyoid lines and grooves, digastric fossae, mental spines, and submandibular fossae.

The Splanchnocranium

The *splanchnocranium,* also referred to as the *viscerocranium,* is derived from the phylogenetically ancient *branchial arch* structures. Six branchial arches form during development, numbered in cranial to caudal sequence from 1 to 6. However, the fifth branchial arch disappears almost as soon as it develops, leaving only five branchial arches (1 through 4 and 6) to contribute to head and neck structures. Each arch possesses a cartilaginous rod. Although small portions of these cartilages persist and form adult structures, the remainder resorb and are eventually replaced by bone of intramembranous origin. These bones include the *maxillae,* the *mandible,* the *zygomatics,* and the *vomer.*

Also included within the splanchnocranium are the *teeth,* which are not considered in detail here. The teeth are formed from specialized calcified tissue, but they are not bone. They are phylogenetically derived from ectodermal placoid scales. This is reflected in their embryological origin from oral ectoderm. (For further details regarding the development and anatomy of the teeth, see Bhaskar, 1990.)

It is important to note that the alveolar processes of the mandible and maxillae bear a complex developmental relationship with the teeth and that the presence or loss of teeth has important implications for the proper development of the maxillae,

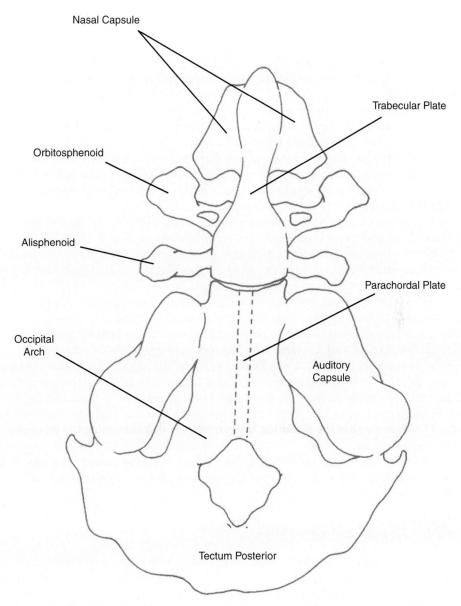

Figure 8–45 Semidiagrammatic representation of the chondrocranium and the capsules forming the anlagen of the cranial base.

mandible, and facial skeleton in general (see Enlow and Hans, 1996). Additionally, dental problems can have serious consequences for general health.

Cranial Anlagen

As we have noted, the cranium develops from both endochondral and intramembranous ossification. We examine here the appearance of the anlagen of the cranial structures.

The Chondrocranium

The portion of the cranium that develops through endochondral ossification includes the base of the skull (the ethmoid and inferior nasal conchae as well as large portions of the sphenoid, occipital, and temporals) and remnants of the first, second, and third branchial arch cartilages.

The *chondrocranium* (see Fig. 8–45) develops from cartilaginous precursors that underlie the developing brain from the interorbitonasal region to the cranial end of the vertebral column. These include the following:

A pair of *parachordal cartilages*, which form the *parachordal plate,* extend from the foramen magnum to the hypophyseal fossa. They are derived from the four occipital sclerotomes, the first cervical sclerotome, and paraxial mesoderm (somitomeric) related to the cranial end of the notochord.

The *hypophyseal cartilages* develop on either side of the hypophyseal stem. They are derived from both paraxial mesoderm (somitomeric) and neural crest.

The *prechordal,* or *trabecular, cartilages* extend anteriorly from the hypophyseal fossa to the developing nasal capsule. At the hypophyseal fossa, these cartilages become continuous with the parachordal cartilages.

As the chondrocranium begions to form, a number of capsules appear, housing the developing olfactory, ocular, and auditory/vestibular sensory systems.

The *cartilaginous nasal capsule* consists of a septum formed by the anterior end of the prechordal plate and a lateral cartilage on either side. Ossification of the upper part of the septum forms the perpendicular plate of the ethmoid and the crista galli. The more inferior and anterior part remains unossified to form the cartilaginous nasal septum. The cribriform plate develops in the upper part of the capsule; the ethmoid labyrinth ossifies in the cartilage of the lateral wall of the cartilaginous nasal capsule. The inferior margin of the lateral cartilage is folded inward to form the inferior nasal concha.

The *auditory (otic) capsule* initially lies lateral to the parachordal plate. It later ossifies to contribute to the formation of the petrous and mastoid portions of the temporal bone.

The Branchial Arch Cartilages

The superior ends of the first and second arch cartilages are closely related to the underside of the auditory capsule. The *cartilage of the first arch* (Meckel's cartilage) forms the incus and the malleus. The *cartilage of the second arch* gives rise to the stapes, the styloid process, and the lesser cornua (horns) of the hyoid bone. The greater cornua and most of the body of the hyoid derive from the cartilage of the *third branchial arch.*

The thyroid cartilage, which sometimes ossifies, most likely derives from the *fourth branchial arch.* Some workers attribute the cricoid cartilage to the *sixth branchial arch.* The *fifth branchial arch* has no skeletal derivatives.

The Membranous Cranium

The portion of the cranium that develops through intramembranous ossification includes the bones forming the roof and walls of the calvarium (frontal, parietals, and squamous portions of the occipital and temporals) and the bones of the face and jaws (maxillae, palatines, nasals, lacrimals, zygomatics, vomer, and portions of the pterygoid plates, greater wings of the sphenoid, and mandible), all of which are derived from the first branchial arch and frontonasal process.

Ossification of Individual Bones of the Cranium

The entirely endochondral ethmoid bone (Figure 8–46) has three centers of ossification: one for the perpendicular plate and crista galli and one for each of the two bony labyrinths. Ossification begins in the ethmoidal (superior and middle) nasal conchae and the orbital plate of the ethmoid at about 4 months in utero. The bony labyrinth of the ethmoid is ossified at birth, but the septum remains cartilaginous throughout the first year. The perpendicular plate and crista galli ossify over the first year and fuse with the labyrinths during the second year. Ethmoidal air cells develop in utero and are rather narrow at birth.

An ossification center for each inferior nasal concha appears at 4 or 5 fetal months; the bone rapidly ossifies. Although derived from the inferior margin of the cartilaginous ethmoid, the inferior concha detaches from the ethmoid to become an independent bone that later synostoses with the maxilla.

The sphenoid bone (Figure 8–47) forms partly from cartilage and partly from membrane. The portions of the sphenoid that undergo endochondral ossification are the body, the lesser wings, and the medial portions of the greater wings. The rest of the bone forms either through intramembranous ossification or through endochondral ossification from secondary cartilages that develop in membrane (e.g., the medial pterygoid hamulus). Up to 19 individual centers of ossification coalesce to form

Figure 8-46   The neonatal cranium: norma lateralis, or lateral view.

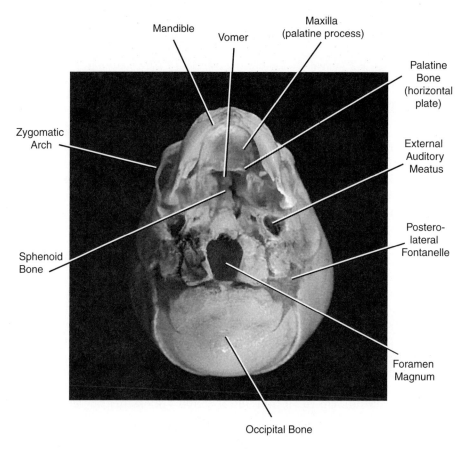

Figure 8-47   The neonatal cranium: norma basalis, or inferior view.

the sphenoid. Initially the sphenoid consists of a presphenoid anterior to the tuberculum sellae and a postsphenoid that includes the sella turcica, the dorsum sellae, and the basisphenoid. The presphenoid and postsphenoid fuse with each other shortly before birth.

Like the sphenoid, the occipital bone (Figure 8–48; see also Figs. 8–46 and 8–47) develops via a combination of intramembranous and endochondral ossification. Most of the occipital bone above the superior nuchal line derives from two intramembranous ossification centers that appear at 8 weeks in utero. The remainder of the occipital bone is derived from five ossification centers that form in the parachordal cartilages. A single, unpaired ossification center forms the basioccipital bone anterior to the foramen magnum as well as the anterior one-third of the occipital condyles. This center appears at about 11 weeks in utero. All remaining ossification centers (two infranuchal centers posteriorly and two exoccipital centers laterally) appear 1 week later. The squamous, exoccipital, and basilar portions fuse to form a single occipital bone by 7 years of age.

Anteriorly the basioccipital is separated from the basisphenoid by the sphenooccipital synchondrosis, a remnant of the chondrocranium, which, like the growth cartilages of long bones, functions as a growth center throughout postnatal ontogeny. Synostosis of the spheno-occipital synchondrosis begins at age 12 to 13 in girls and age 14 to 15 in boys. Complete fusion of the synchondrosis does not occur until age 20.

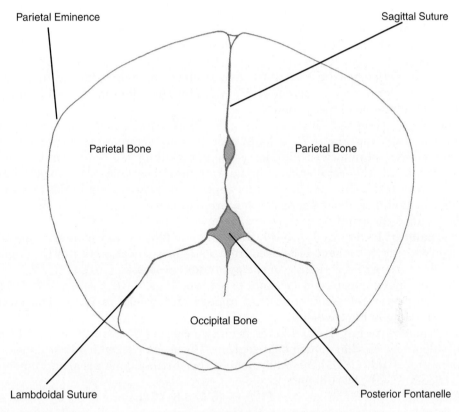

Parietal Eminence

Sagittal Suture

Parietal Bone

Parietal Bone

Occipital Bone

Lambdoidal Suture

Posterior Fontanelle

Figure 8-48 The neonatal cranium: norma occipitalis, or posterior view.

The temporal bone (see Fig. 8–46) follows a complex sequence of ossification. Like the sphenoid and occipital, it is formed from both cartilage and membrane. The squamous part of the bone develops intramembranously from a single ossification center that appears above the root of the zygomatic process at 7 to 8 weeks in utero. The tympanic part of the temporal bone also has an intramembranous origin. It derives from four ossification centers that appear at 12 weeks in utero and form a ring around the external acoustic meatus. The tympanic ring does not fuse with the squamous temporal until after birth.

The remaining petrous and styloid portions of the temporal bone ossify in cartilage from as many as 22 ossification centers that first appear at 5 months in utero. The petrous and squamous portions of the temporal fuse with one another during the first year. The styloid process is derived from two ossification centers that form in the second arch cartilage. The styloid process is initially attached to the temporal bone by cartilage and does not fuse to the bone until middle age. Occasionally the styloid process fails to fuse with the temporal bone.

The hyoid bone has six centers of ossification: two for the body, two for the left and right lesser horns, and two for the left and right greater horns.

The frontal bone (Figure 8–49) derives from two primary ossification centers that appear at 8 weeks in utero in the region of the superciliary arches. At birth the frontal bones are separated by the *metopic suture*. The middle of this suture undergoes synostosis at about 2 years, and by 7 or 8 years the two halves of the frontal are completely fused. On very rare occasions, the two halves of the frontal never fuse and the metopic suture persists into adulthood.

The parietal bones (see Figs. 8–46, 8–48, and 8–49) each form from two centers of ossification that appear at the parietal eminence at 8 weeks in utero. The four corners of the parietal bones remain unossified at birth and help form the anterior, posterior, anterolateral, and posterolateral fontanelles. The fontanelles are completely ossified by the middle of the second year.

The maxilla (Figure 8–50; see also Fig. 8–49) ossifies in membrane from one primary center that appears at 7 weeks in utero at the termination of the inferior orbital nerve. Five secondary ossification centers, including two centers in the incisive region that forms the bone enclosing the four maxillary incisors, appear approximately 1 week later. The maxillary sinus appears as a depression in the lateral wall of the nasal cavity at about 4 months in utero and is well formed by birth. The maxilla grows until the eruption of the third molars.

The palatine bones (see Fig. 8–47) develop in membrane at the inferior margin of the nasal capsule. Each bone is derived from a single ossification center that appears at 8 weeks in utero in the vicinity of the pyramidal process.

The zygomatic, nasal, and lacrimal bones (see Figs. 8–46, 8–49, and 8–50) form from single centers of ossification that appear at 8 weeks in utero. The lacrimal bones are visible in Figure 8–46.

The vomer (see Fig. 8–47) derives from two centers of ossification that form on either side of the cartilaginous nasal septum. These centers, which first appear at 8 weeks in utero, unite with each other behind the cartilaginous nasal septum, where they articulate with the sphenoid.

Each half of the mandible (see Figs. 8–46 and 8–47) begins to ossify in the sixth week in utero from a membranous center appearing at the future location of the mental foramina. This center, lateral to Meckel's cartilage, spreads and gives rise to the body, alveolar process, and most of the ramus. During this process most of Meckel's cartilage is invaded by bone and disappears. Those portions of the cartilage that persist give rise to the incus and malleus, the sphenomandibular ligament, and the accessory endochondral ossicles in the mental symphysis.

The head of the condyle, part of the coronoid process, and the mental protuberance are formed from secondary (membrane) cartilages that appear between the 10th and 12th weeks in utero. At birth, the two halves of the mandible are separated at the mental symphysis. The two halves fuse early in the second year.

The Infant Cranium

As noted, the cranial vault is formed by intramembranous ossification. At birth, the bones of the cranial vault have not completely grown to meet one another, leaving regions of the cranium membranous. This allows the cranium to deform somewhat and makes easier its passage through the birth canal. These regions of membrane remaining at birth are termed *fontanelles,* or "soft spots." Figures 8–46 through 8–50 demonstrate the infant or neonatal cranium. Note the locations of the fontanelles at bregma, lambda, asterion, and pterion. The anterior fontanelle (see Figs. 8–49 and 8–50) is at bregma. The posterior fontanelle (see Fig. 8–48) is at lambda. The anterolateral (or sphenoidal) fontanelle (see Fig. 8–46) is at pterion. The posterolateral fontanelle (see Figs. 8–46 and 8–47) is at asterion. Also note the relatively large neurocranium, the small face, the edentulous mandible and maxilla, and the cartilaginous mandibular symphysis.

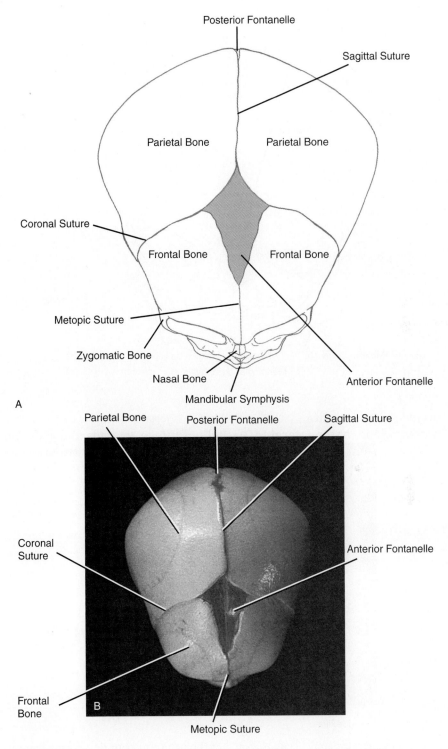

Figure 8–49 (*A*) Line drawing and (*B*) photograph of the neonatal cranium: norma verticalis, or superior view.

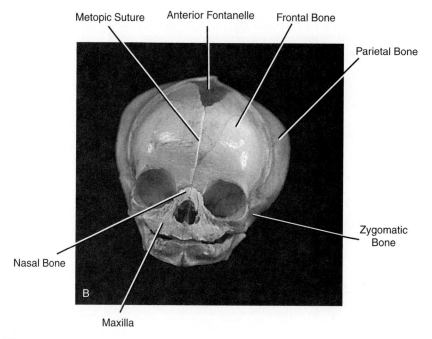

Figure 8-50   (A) Line drawing and (B) photograph of the neonatal cranium: norma frontalis, or anterior view.

The process of deformation of the fetal skull during delivery is called molding. During delivery, one parietal bone slides under the other. This is referred to as the obstetrical hinge joint.

The skull of the neonate does not possess a mastoid process, because it is an apophysis that develops under the origin of the sternocleidomastoid muscle. As a result, the stylomastoid foramen and facial nerve of the infant are very superficial. During delivery, the neonate's facial nerve is very vulnerable to injury. The middle ear cavity at birth is nearly its adult size.

References

Adams, T, Heisy, RS, Smith, MC, and Briner, BJ (1992). Parietal bone mobility in the anesthetized cat. *Journal of the American Osteopathic Association, 92,* 599–600, 603–610, 615–622.

Bhaskar, SN (1990). *Orban's Oral Histology and Embryology* (11th ed). Mosby-Yearbook Publishers, Chicago.

Enlow, DH, and Hans, MG (1996). *Essentials of Facial Growth.* WB Saunders, Philadelphia.

Gray, H (1985). *Gray's Anatomy* (30th Am ed). CD Clemente (Ed). Lea and Febiger, Philadelphia.

Gray, H (1995). *Gray's Anatomy* (38th Brit ed). PL Williams, LH Bannister, MM Berry, P Collins, M Dyson, JE Dussek, and MWJ Ferguson (Eds). Churchill Livingstone, New York.

Greiner, TM, and Walker, RA (1999, April). *Morphometric Variation of the Human Auditory Ossicles.* Paper presented at the 68th annual meeting of the American Association of Physical Anthropologists, Columbus, Ohio (Abstract published in *American Journal of Physical Anthropology,* Suppl 28, p 140, 1999).

Heisey, SR, and Adams, T (1993). Role of cranial bone mobilitiy in cranial compliance. *Neurosurgery, 33,* 869–877.

Rogers, JS, and Witt, PL (1997). The controversy of cranial bone motion. *Journal of Orthopaedic and Sports Physical Therapy, 26,* 95–103.

Sperber, GH (1989). *Craniofacial Embryology.* Williams and Wilkins, Baltimore.

Further Readings and Resources

Textbooks and Anatomic Atlases

Agur, AMR (1991). *Grant's Atlas of Anatomy* (9th ed). Williams & Wilkins, Baltimore.

Aiello, L, and Dean, C (1990). *An Introduction to Human Evolutionary Anatomy.* Academic Press. (Stresses the musculoskeletal anatomy of *Homo sapiens* in relationship to other primates.)

Bass, WM (1995). *Human Osteology: A Laboratory and Field Manual* (4th ed). Special Publications, Missouri Archeological Society, Columbia, MO. (An introductory text geared more toward field archeologists.)

Bennett, KA (1993). *A Field Guide for Human Skeletal Identification.* Charles C Thomas, Springfield, IL.

Breathnach, AS (1965). *Frazer's Anatomy of the Human Skeleton* (6th ed). J and A Churchill, London. (Originally written by J. Ernest Frazer. Long out of print, this work is close in spirit to *Frazer's Anatomy.*)

Clement, JG, and Ranson, DL (Eds) (1998). *Craniofacial Identification in Forensic Medicine.* Edward Arnold, London.

Clemente, CD (1997). *A Regional Atlas of the Human Body* (4th ed). Williams & Wilkins, Baltimore. (A superb anatomical atlas, edited by the editor of the most recent U.S. edition of *Gray's Anatomy.*)

Cormack, DH (Ed) (1987). *Ham's Histology* (9th ed). JB Lippincott, Philadelphia. (Originally by AW Ham, *Ham's Histology* has long been regarded as a classic histology text. Although the text is now out of print, the chapters on tendons and ligaments, bone, and joints are still an excellent introduction to the microanatomy of these structures.)

Cormack, DH (1992). *Essential Histology.* Lippincott-Raven, Philadelphia. (A more recent introductory histology text by the editor of the most recent edition of *Ham's Histology.*)

Currey, J (1984). *The Mechanical Adaptations of Bone.* Princeton University Press, Princeton, NJ.

Edwardson, BM (1995). *Musculoskeletal Disorders: Common Problems.* Singular Publishing Group, San Diego.

Frankel, VH, and Nordin, M (1980). *Basic Biomechanics of the Skeletal System.* Lea & Febiger, Philadelphia.

Gosling, JA, Harris, PF, Humpherson, JR, Whitmore, I, and Willan, PLT (1996). *Human Anatomy: Color Atlas with Integrated Text* (3rd ed). Gower Medical Publishing, London; JB Lippincott, Philadelphia. (This atlas features photographs of actual dissections, accompanied by line drawings to help elucidate those figures.)

Gray, H (1985). *Gray's Anatomy* (30th Am ed). CD Clemente (Ed). Lea & Febiger, Philadelphia. (The American and British versions of *Gray's Anatomy* soon diverged from one another. The American version has remained more conservative, and slightly less expensive, than its British counterpart. The most recent American edition still retains many of the original illustrations prepared for the 1858 edition by H Van Dyke Carter.)

Gray, H (1995). *Gray's Anatomy* (38th Brit ed). PL Williams, LH Bannister, MM Berry, P Collins, M Dyson, JE Dussek, and MWJ Ferguson (Eds). Churchill Livingstone, New York. (The British edition of *Gray's Anatomy* is widely regarded as *the* anatomical reference. Its first edition was published in 1858. Although paperback reprints of century-old editions are widely and cheaply available, they are not recommended for serious study. Although the anatomy of the human body has not changed in the last 100 years, the knowledge about it has grown tremendously and much of the terminology used to describe it has changed drastically.)

Haas, J, Buikstra, JE, and Ubelaker, DH (1994). *Standards for Data Collection from Human Skeletal Remains: Proceedings of a Seminar at the Field Museum of Natural History (Arkansas Archeological Survey).* Arkansas Archeological Survey, Fayetteville, AR.

Hutchings, RT, Marks, SC, and Abrahams, PH (1998). *McMinn's Color Atlas of Human Anatomy* (4th ed). Yearbook Medical Publishers, Chicago.

Iscan, MY (Ed) (1989). *Age Markers in the Human Skeleton.* Charles C Thomas, Springfield, IL.

Jenkins, DB (1998). *Hollinshead's Functional Anatomy of the Limbs and Back* (7th ed). WB Saunders, Philadelphia.

Krogman, WM (1962). *The Human Skeleton in Forensic Medicine.* Charles C Thomas, Springfield, IL. (A classic text in forensic applications of human osteology. A new edition, coauthored with MY Iscan, was published in 1986. Not only is this text a valuable resource in itself, but it includes references to all the important literature on age, gender, and "race" determination from skeletal remains published to that time. Krogman includes detailed descriptions of the time of appearance and fusion of epiphyses in subadults.)

Krogman, WM, and Iscan, MY (1986). *Human Skeleton in Forensic Medicine* (2nd ed). Charles C Thomas, Springfield, IL.

McMinn, RMH, Hutchings, RT, and Logan, BM (1987). *The Human Skeleton/Photographic Manual/Full Size.* Year Book Medical Publishers, St Louis.

Reichs, KJ, and Bass, WM (Eds) (1998). *Forensic Osteology: Advances in the Identification of Human Remains* (2nd ed). Charles C Thomas, Springfield, IL.

Rohen, JW, Yokochi, C, and Lutjen-Drecoll, E (1998). *Color Atlas of Anatomy* (4th ed). Williams & Wilkins, Baltimore.

Ross, HM, Romrell, LJ, and Kaye, GI (1995). *Histology: A Text and Atlas* (3rd ed). Williams & Wilkins, Baltimore. (A profusely illustrated, thorough histology text. Includes an excellent discussion of bone growth and development.)

Saunders, SR, and Katzenberg, MA (Eds) (1992). *Skeletal Biology of Past Peoples: Research Methods.* John Wiley and Sons, New York.

Schwartz, JH (1995). *Skeleton Keys: An Introduction to Human Skeletal Morphology, Development, and Analysis.* Oxford University Press, New York and Oxford.

Shipman, P, Walker, A, and Bichell, D (1985). *The Human Skeleton.* Harvard University Press, Cambridge, MA, and London.

Simon, H (1996). *Dental Anthropology.* Cambridge University Press, London.

Steele, DG (1988). *The Anatomy and Biology of the Human Skeleton.* Texas A&M University Press, Collegeville, TX.

White, TD, and Folkens, PA (1991). *Human Osteology.* Academic Press, San Diego.

Yochum, TR, and Rowe, LJ (1995). *Essentials of Skeletal Radiology* (2nd ed). Williams & Wilkins, Baltimore.

Yokochi, C, Rohen, JW, and Weinreb, EL (1989). *Photographic Anatomy of the Human Body* (3rd ed). Igaku-Shon, Tokyo and New York.

Journal Articles

American Journal of Physical Anthropology

The *American Journal of Physical Anthropology* frequently publishes articles relevant to human osteology; human anatomy; and the determination of skeletal age at death, gender, and "race" of unidentified skeletal remains. Most of the September 1985 edition of the *American Journal of Physical Anthropology* (Vol 68, No 1) was devoted to a series of articles by C. O. Lovejoy and colleagues on the determination of age and gender in unidentified human skeletal material. In subsequent years, the *American Journal of Physical Anthropology* has published a number of articles either confirming or inspired by the research presented by Lovejoy and colleagues. These articles include the following:

Lovejoy, CO (1985). Dental wear in the Libben population: Its functional pattern and role in the determination of adult skeletal age at death. *American Journal of Physical Anthropology, 68*(1), 47–56.

Lovejoy, CO, Meindl, RS, Mensforth, RP, and Barton, TJ (1985). Multifactorial determination of skeletal age at death: A method and blind tests of its accuracy. *American Journal of Physical Anthropology, 68*(1), 1–14.

Lovejoy, CO, Meindl, RS, Pryzbeck, TR, and Mensforth, RP (1985). Chronological metamorphosis of the auricular surface of the ilium: A new method for the determination of adult skeletal age at death. *American Journal of Physical Anthropology, 68*(1), 15–28.

Meindl, RS, and Lovejoy, CO (1985). Ectocranial suture closure: A revised method for the determination of skeletal age at death based on the lateral-anterior sutures. *American Journal of Physical Anthropology, 68*(1), 57–66.

Meindl, RS, Lovejoy, CO, Mensforth, RP, and Carlos, LD (1985). Accuracy and direction of error in the sexing of the skeleton: Implications for paleodemography. *American Journal of Physical Anthropology, 68*(1), 79–85.

Meindl, RS, Lovejoy, CO, Mensforth, RP, and Walker, RA (1985). A revised method of age determination using the os pubis, with a review and tests of accuracy of other current methods of pubic symphyseal aging. *American Journal of Physical Anthropology, 68*(1), 29–45.

Mensforth, RP, and Lovejoy, CO (1985). Anatomical, physiological, and epidemiological correlates of the aging process: A confirmation of multifactorial age determination in the Libben skeletal population. *American Journal of Physical Anthropology, 68*(1), 87–106.

Walker, RA, and Lovejoy, CO (1985). Radiographic changes in the clavicle and proximal femur and their use in the determination of skeletal age at death. *American Journal of Physical Anthropology, 68*(1), 67–78.

Other papers related to the previously mentioned work (by many of the same authors) include the following:

Bedford, ME, Russell, KF, Lovejoy, CO, Meindl, RS, Simpson, SW, and Stuart-Macadam, PL (1993). Test of the multifactorial aging method using skeletons with known ages-at-death from the Grant Collection. *American Journal of Physical Anthropology, 91,* 287–297.

Meindl, RS, Bedford, ME, Russell, KF, Lovejoy, CO, and Simpson, SW (1995). Testing the test of the multifactorial aging method: A reply to Fairgrieve and Oost. *American Journal of Physical Anthropology, 97,* 85–87.

American Journal of Human Biology

Walker, RA, Lovejoy, CO, and Meindl, RS (1994). The histomorphological and geometric properties of human femoral cortex in individuals over 50: Implications for histomorphological determination of age-at-death. *American Journal of Human Biology 6,* 659–667.

Science

Lovejoy, CO, Meindl, RS, Pryzbeck, TR, Barton, TS, Heiple, KG, and Kotting, D (1977). Paleodemography of the Libben site, Ottawa County, Ohio. *Science, 198,* 291–293.

Appendix

Muscle Origins, Insertions, Innervations, Blood Supplies, and Principal Actions

This appendix lists the muscles of the upper and lower limbs, vertebral column, abdomen, and thorax, as well as major muscles of mastication and those attaching to the hyoid bone. These muscle origins and insertions are alluded to in the text and are included here for reference. These muscles all, to a greater or lesser degree, leave marks on the skeleton where their tendons of origin or insertion attach to bone. The muscles are listed regionally, as follows: first, the extrinsic muscles of the back, then the intrinsic muscles of the back, then major muscles of the abdomen and thorax, then those of the upper limb, those of the lower limb, and finally the major muscles of mastication and of the hyoid region. Primary segmental innervation to most muscles is indicated in parentheses at the end of the description of innervation. The following convention is followed in listing segmental innervation: The designations C1 to C8 refer to cervical spinal nerves numbers 1 to 8, T1 to T12 refer to thoracic spinal nerves numbers 1 to 12, L1 to L5 refer to lumbar spinal nerves numbers 1 to 5, and S1 to S5 refer to sacral spinal nerves numbers 1 to 5. Innervations from cranial nerves are referred to by the names of the nerves, followed by their numeric designation, for example, trigeminal nerve (cranial nerve V).

Major Muscles of the Trunk: The Back

The Superficial Back Muscles

The superficial back muscles are extrinsic and hypaxial, innervated by the ventral rami. They act primarily upon the upper limbs.

Trapezius

Origin:	External occipital protuberance; medial one-third of superior nuchal line; ligamentum nuchae; spinous processes of C7 to T12
Insertion:	
Superior fibers:	Lateral one-third of clavicle
Middle fibers:	Spine and acromion of scapula
Inferior fibers:	Base of spine of scapula
Innervation:	Spinal accessory nerve (motor) and ventral rami of third and fourth cervical nerves (sensory and proprioception) (C3, C4)
Blood Supply:	Superficial branch of transverse cervical artery
Action:	Raises, retracts, and rotates scapula; bilateral contraction of superior fibers extends head; unilateral contraction of upper fibers laterally flexes head and cervical vertebral column

Latissimus Dorsi

Origin:	Spinous processes of lower six thoracic, all lumbar and upper sacral vertebrae, from the posterior part of the iliac crest, and from the lower three or four ribs by muscular slips that interdigitate with the external oblique
Insertion:	Crest of the lesser tubercle and floor of the bicipital groove of the humerus
Innervation:	Thoracodorsal nerve (C6–C8)
Blood Supply:	Thoracodorsal artery
Action:	Extension, medial rotation, and adduction of the arm

Levator Scapulae

Origin:	Posterior tubercles of transverse processes of C1 to C3 or C4
Insertion:	Medial border of scapula from superior angle to base of spine
Innervation:	Ventral rami of C3 and C4 from deep branches of the cervical plexus, twig from the dorsal scapular nerve (C5); (C3–C5)
Blood Supply:	Deep branch of transverse cervical artery or dorsal scapular artery
Action:	Elevates and retracts scapula with trapezius, laterally flexes cervical vertebral column if scapula is fixed

Rhomboideus Minor

Origin:	Lower part of ligamentum nuchae and spinous processes of C7 and T1
Insertion:	Medial border of scapula at base (root) of the spine
Innervation:	Dorsal scapular nerve (C4, C5)
Blood Supply:	Deep branch of the transverse cervical artery or dorsal scapular artery
Action:	Elevates the medial border and retracts the scapula (same as rhomboideus major), rotation of scapula

Rhomboideus Major

Origin:	Spinous processes of T2 to T5
Insertion:	Medial border of scapula between base of spine and inferior angle
Innervation:	Dorsal scapular nerve (C4, C5)
Blood Supply:	Deep branch of the transverse cervical artery or dorsal scapular artery
Action:	Elevates the medial border and retracts the scapula (same as rhomboideus minor), rotates scapula

The Intermediate Back Muscles

The intermediate back muscles are extrinsic and hypaxial, innervated by the ventral rami. They are the muscles of respiration.

Serratus Posterior Superior

Origin:	Lower end of ligamentum nuchae, spinous processes of C7 to T2 or T3
Insertion:	Second through fifth ribs lateral to the angles
Innervation:	Ventral rami of second through fifth thoracic nerves (T2–T5)
Blood Supply:	Highest intercostal artery, posterior intercostal arteries
Action:	Elevates upper ribs, muscle of inspiration

Serratus Posterior Inferior

Origin:	Spinous processes of T10 or T11 to L2
Insertion:	Lower three or four ribs lateral to their angles
Innervation:	Ventral rami of lowest four thoracic nerves (T9–T12)
Blood Supply:	Posterior intercostal arteries
Action:	Depresses lower ribs, draws them down and back; muscle of inspiration

The Intrinsic (Deep) Back Muscles: Superficial Layer

The three layers of the intrinsic (deep) back muscles are epaxial, innervated by the dorsal rami.

Splenius Capitis

Origin:	Caudal half of ligamentum nuchae and spinous processes of C7 to T3 or T4
Insertion:	Mastoid process and occipital bone just inferior to lateral one-third of superior nuchal line
Innervation:	Dorsal rami of middle cervical spinal nerves
Blood Supply:	Muscular and descending branches of the occipital artery, superficial branch of the transverse cervical artery

Action:

Unilaterally:	Rotation of head and neck
Bilaterally:	Extension of head and neck

Splenius Cervicis

Origin:	Narrow tendinous band from spinous processes of T3 to T6
Insertion:	Posterior tubercles of transverse processes of upper two or three cervical vertebrae
Innervation:	Dorsal rami of lower cervical spinal nerves
Blood Supply:	Muscular and descending branches of the occipital artery, superficial branch of the transverse cervical artery

Action:

Unilaterally:	Draws head to one side and slightly rotates
Bilaterally:	Extends head

The Intrinsic (Deep) Back Muscles: Intermediate Layer

Erector Spinae: Iliocostalis (Lateral Column of Erector Spinae)

ILIOCOSTALIS LUMBORUM

Origin:	From median sacral crest, spinous processes of T11–5, and iliac and sacral crests via the thoracolumbar fascia
Insertion:	Lower borders of the lower six or seven ribs near the angles
Innervation:	Dorsal rami of lumbar spinal nerves
Blood Supply:	Posterior intercostal arteries, lumbar arteries
Action:	Extension and lateral flexion of vertebral column

ILIOCOSTALIS THORACIS

Origin:	Upper borders of lower six ribs medial to insertions of iliocostalis lumborum
Insertion:	Upper six ribs and sometimes the transverse process of C7
Innervation:	Dorsal rami of thoracic spinal nerves
Blood Supply:	Posterior intercostal arteries
Action:	Extension and lateral flexion of vertebral column

ILIOCOSTALIS CERVICIS

Origin:	Upper six ribs medial to the insertion of iliocostalis thoracis
Insertion:	Transverse processes of the fourth, fifth, and sixth cervical vertebrae
Innervation:	Dorsal rami of spinal nerves C4 to C6 (C4–C6)
Blood Supply:	Posterior intercostal arteries
Action:	Extension and lateral flexion of the vertebral column

Erector Spinae: Longissimus (Middle Column of Erector Spinae)

LONGISSIMUS THORACIS

Origin:	Middle layer of thoracolumbar fascia transverse processes and accessory processes of the lumbar vertebrae
Insertion:	Transverse processes of the lower nine thoracic vertebrae and the lower nine ribs
Innervation:	Dorsal rami of lumbar and thoracic spinal nerves (T1–T12)
Blood Supply:	Posterior intercostal and lumbar arteries
Action:	Extension and lateral flexion of the vertebral column

LONGISSIMUS CERVICIS

Origin:	Transverse processes of the upper four to six thoracic vertebrae medial to the insertion of the longissimus thoracis
Insertion:	Transverse processes of second through sixth cervical vertebrae
Innervation:	Dorsal rami of cervical spinal nerves (C4–C8)
Blood Supply:	Posterior intercostal arteries
Action:	Extension and lateral flexion of the vertebral column

LONGISSIMUS CAPITIS

Origin:	Medial to upper border of longissimus cervicis partly from the tendons of origin of this muscle and from the articular processes of the lower four cervical vertebrae
Insertion:	Posterior edge of the mastoid process

Innervation:	Dorsal rami of cervical spinal nerves (C3–C8)
Blood Supply:	Muscular branches of occipital artery, deep cervical branch of the costocervical trunk

Action:

Unilaterally:	Rotation of face toward same side
Bilaterally:	Extension of vertebral column

LONGISSIMUS LUMBORUM

Although the longissimus lumborum is not traditionally described, a number of workers, including Bogduk (1980) and Bustami (1986), now recognize a lumbar portion of the longissimus, inserting into the transverse processes of lumbar vertebrae.

Erector Spinae: Spinalis (Medial Column of Erector Spinae)

SPINALIS THORACIS

Origin:	Blends with longissimus thoracis and arises from spinous processes of T11 to L2
Insertion:	Spinous processes of upper four to eight thoracic vertebrae
Innervation:	Dorsal rami of thoracic spinal nerves (T1–T12)
Blood Supply:	Posterior intercostal arteries
Action:	Extension of the vertebral column

SPINALIS CERVICIS

Origin:	Often absent from the lower part of ligamentum nuchae and spinous processes of C7 to T2
Insertion:	Spinous processes of C2 to C3 and sometimes C4
Innervation:	Dorsal rami of cervical spinal nerves
Blood Supply:	Posterior intercostal arteries
Action:	Extension of vertebral column

SPINALIS CAPITIS

The spinalis capitis may originate from upper thoracic spinous processes. It usually blends laterally with the semispinalis capitis and is considered with the semispinalis capitis. It is highly variable in its morphology and presence (Greiner et al., 1998).

The Intrinsic (Deep) Back Muscles: Deep Layer

Transversospinalis Group: Semispinalis

SEMISPINALIS CAPITIS

Origin:	Transverse processes of upper six or seven thoracic vertebrae
Insertion:	Occipital bone between superior and inferior nuchal lines
Innervation:	Medial branches of dorsal rami of cervical spinal nerves (C1–C6)
Blood Supply:	Descending branch of occipital artery, deep branch of costocervical trunk

Action:

Unilaterally:	Turns face toward opposite side
Bilaterally:	Extension of neck

NOTE: Spinalis capitis is frequently fused with this muscle and is represented by the more medial fibers of the combined muscle mass. It may have a separate origin from upper thoracic spinous processes (Greiner et al., 1998).

SEMISPINALIS CERVICIS

Origin:	Transverse processes of upper five or six thoracic vertebrae
Insertion:	Second through fifth cervical spinous processes
Innervation:	Medial branches of cervical dorsal rami (C6–C8)
Blood Supply:	Deep branch of costocervical trunk, posterior intercostal arteries

Action:

Unilaterally:	Rotation of vertebral column toward opposite side
Bilaterally:	Extension of vertebral column

SEMISPINALIS THORACIS

Origin:	From the transverse processes of thoracic vertebrae T6–T10
Insertion:	Spinous processes of upper thoracic and lower cervical vertebrae
Innervation:	Dorsal rami of thoracic spinal nerves (T1–T6)
Blood Supply:	Posterior intercostal arteries

Action:

Unilaterally:	Rotation of the vertebral column toward the opposite side
Bilaterally:	Extension of the vertebral column

Transversospinalis Group: Multifidus (Lumborum, Thoracis, and Cervicis Portions)

Origin:	Posterior surface of sacrum, posterior sacroiliac ligament, posterior superior iliac spine, erector spinae aponeurons, mamillary processes of lumbar vertebrae, transverse processes of thoracic vertebrae, and articular processes of cervical vertebrae 4 through 7
Insertion:	Spines of vertebrae two to four segments superior to vertebra of origin
Innervation:	Dorsal rami of all spinal nerves
Blood Supply:	Posterior intercostal and lumbar arteries, deep cervical branch of costocervical trunk
Action:	Extension, lateral flexion, and rotation of vertebral column; extension and lateral motions of pelvis

Transversospinalis Group: Rotatores Longus and Rotatores Brevis

Origin:	From transverse processes of vertebrae
Insertion:	Lamina of vertebra immediately superior (rotatores brevis), or into lamina of the second vertebra above the vertebra of origin (rotatores longus)
Innervation:	Dorsal rami of spinal nerves
Blood Supply:	Posterior intercostal arteries, lumbar arteries
Action:	Rotation of the vertebral column

Segmental Muscles: Levatores Costarum Longus and Levatores Costarum Brevis

Origin:	Twelve pairs, from transverse processes of seventh cervical and first through eleventh thoracic vertebrae
Insertion:	On external surface of rib below vertebra of origin between the tubercle and angle (levator costarum brevis), or into the external surface of the rib two levels below the vertebra of origin between the tubercle and angle (levator costarum longus)
Innervation:	Dorsal rami of lowest cervical and thoracic spinal nerves (C8, T1–T11)
Blood Supply:	Posterior intercostal arteries
Action:	Elevate ribs, assist in inspiration, rotate and laterally flex vertebral column

Segmental Muscles: Interspinales

Origin:	Superiorly on spine of vertebra

Insertion:	Inferiorly on spine of vertebra immediately superior to vertebra of origin; not always present in thoracic region, frequently double in cervical region
Innervation:	Dorsal rami of spinal nerves
Blood Supply:	Muscular branches of the posterior intercostal arteries, lumbar arteries, deep cervical branches of the costocervical trunk
Action:	Extension of vertebral column

Segmental Muscles: Intertransversarii

Origin:	Superiorly on transverse processes of vertebrae
Insertion:	Inferiorly on transverse processes of vertebrae immediately superior to vertebra of origin; most highly developed in cervical and lumbar regions
Innervation:	Dorsal rami of spinal nerves, except lateral intertransversarii in lumbar and lower thoracic, and anterior and posterior intertransversarii in cervical; these exceptions are innervated by ventral rami
Blood Supply:	Muscular branches of posterior intercostal and lumbar arteries
Action:	Lateral flexion of vertebral column

Muscles of the Suboccipital Region

The muscles of the suboccipital region are intrinsic and epaxial. They are innervated by the dorsal rami.

Rectus Capitis Posterior Minor

Origin:	Posterior tubercle of the atlas
Insertion:	Occipital bone below the inferior nuchal line
Innervation:	Suboccipital nerve (dorsal ramus of C1)
Blood Supply:	Muscular branches of the vertebral artery, descending branch of the occipital artery
Action:	Extension of the head

Rectus Capitis Posterior Major

Origin:	Spinous process of axis
Insertion:	Lateral part of inferior nuchal line of the occipital bone
Innervation:	Suboccipital nerve (dorsal ramus of C1)
Blood Supply:	Muscular branches of the vertebral artery, descending branch of the occipital artery
Action:	Extension and rotation of the head

Obliquus Capitis Superior

Origin:	Transverse process of atlas
Insertion:	Occipital bone above inferior nuchal line
Innervation:	Suboccipital nerve (dorsal ramus of C1)
Blood Supply:	Muscular branches of the vertebral artery, descending branch of the occipital artery
Action:	Extension and lateral flexion of the head

Obliquus Capitis Inferior

Origin:	Spinous process of axis
Insertion:	Transverse process of atlas
Innervation:	Suboccipital nerve (dorsal ramus of C1), second cervical dorsal ramus (C1, C2)
Blood Supply:	Muscular branches of the vertebral artery, descending branch of the occipital artery
Action:	Rotation of atlas and skull around dens of axis

Major Muscles of the Trunk: The Neck and Prevertebral Region

Sternocleidomastoid

Origin: Sternal or medial head from the superior and anterior part of the manubrium; clavicular or lateral head from the superior and anterior part of the medial one-third of the clavicle

Insertion: Lateral surface of the mastoid process; lateral half of the superior nuchal line

Innervation: Spinal accessory nerve (cranial nerve XI); branches of the ventral rami of cervical spinal nerves (C2, C3)

Blood Supply: Suprascapular artery; superior thyroid artery, auricular artery

Action:

  Unilaterally: Rotates the head to the contralateral side; laterally flexes head and neck

  Bilaterally: Flexes head and neck

Scalenus Anterior

Origin: Anterior tubercles of transverse processes of cervical vertebrae 3 through 6

Insertion: Scalene tubercle of the superior surface of the first rib

Innervation: Ventral rami of cervical spinal nerves (C4–C6)

Blood Supply: Ascending cervical branch of the inferior thyroid artery

Action: If the neck is fixed, it elevates the first rib; if the first rib is fixed, it flexes and rotates the cervical vertebral column

Scalenus Medius

Origin: Posterior tubercles of transverse processes of cervical vertebrae 2 through 7

Insertion: Superior surface of first rib posterior to the groove for the subclavian artery

Innervation: Ventral rami of cervical spinal nerves (C3–C8)

Blood Supply: Ascending cervical branch of the inferior thyroid artery

Action: If the neck is fixed, it elevates the first rib; if the first rib is fixed, it flexes and rotates the cervical vertebral column

Scalenus Posterior

Origin: Posterior tubercles of transverse processes of cervical vertebrae 4 through 6

Insertion:	External surface of the second rib, deep and posterior to serratus anterior
Innervation:	Ventral rami of cervical spinal nerves (C6–C8)
Blood Supply:	Ascending cervical branch of the inferior thyroid artery
Action:	If the neck is fixed, it elevates the second rib; if the second rib is fixed, it flexes and rotates the cervical vertebral column

Longus Colli

Origin:	Vertical (vertebral) portion from the bodies of last three cervical and first three thoracic vertebrae; inferior oblique portion from the bodies of the first three thoracic vertebrae; superior oblique portion from the anterior tubercles of the transverse processes of cervical vertebrae 3 through 5
Insertion:	Vertical portion into the bodies of cervical vertebrae 2 through 4; inferior oblique portion into anterior tubercles of the transverse processes of cervical vertebrae 5 and 6; superior oblique portion onto the anterior tubercle of the atlas
Innervation:	Ventral rami of cervical spinal nerves (C2–C6)
Blood Supply:	Ascending cervical, ascending pharyngeal, and vertebral arteries
Action:	Weak flexor of the neck; slightly rotates and laterally flexes the cervical vertebral column

Longus Capitis

Origin:	Anterior tubercles of the transverse processes of cervical vertebrae 3 through 6
Insertion:	Inferior surface of the basilar part of the occipital bone lateral to the pharyngeal tubercle
Innervation:	Ventral rami of cervical spinal nerves (C1–C3)
Blood Supply:	Ascending cervical, ascending pharyngeal, and vertebral arteries
Action:	Flexes head and upper cervical vertebral column; assists in rotating cervical vertebral column and head

Rectus Capitis Anterior

Origin:	Anterior surface of the lateral part of the lateral mass of the atlas and root of the transverse process
Insertion:	Inferior surface of the basilar part of occipital immediately anterior to the foramen magnum
Innervation:	Ventral rami of first and second cervical spinal nerves (C1, C2)
Blood Supply:	Vertebral and ascending pharyngeal arteries
Action:	Flexes the head and helps stabilize the atlanto-occipital joint; may assist in rotation of the head

Rectus Capitis Lateralis

Origin: Superior surface of transverse process of atlas

Insertion: Inferior surface of jugular process of occipital

Innervation: Ventral rami of first and second cervical spinal nerves (C1, C2)

Blood Supply: Vertebral, occipital, and ascending pharyngeal arteries

Action: Laterally flexes the head and helps stabilize the atlanto-occipital joint

Major Muscles of the Trunk: The Thoracic Wall

Intercostal Muscles: Intercostales Externi

The intercostales externi consist of 11 pairs of muscles.

Origin:	From inferior and external surface of first 11 ribs from rib tubercles to costochondral junctions
Insertion:	Into superior and external surface of ribs 2 through 12 from rib tubercles to costochondral junctions
Innervation:	Segmentally by ventral rami of first 11 thoracic spinal nerves (intercostal nerves) (T1–T11)
Blood Supply:	Posterior intercostal, anterior intercostal, and musculophrenic arteries; costocervical trunk
Action:	Elevate ribs in inspiration, support intercostal spaces in inspiration and expiration; may be active in early expiration

Intercostal Muscles: Intercostales Interni

The intercostales interni consist of 11 pairs of muscles.

Origin:	From inferior and internal surface of first 11 ribs from the sternal border to the angle of the rib; they arise from the ridge on the medial side of the costal groove
Insertion:	Superior border of ribs 2 through 12
Innervation:	Segmentally by ventral rami of first 11 thoracic spinal nerves (intercostal nerves) (T1–T11)
Blood Supply:	Posterior intercostal, anterior intercostal, and musculophrenic arteries; costocervical trunk
Action:	Prevent the pushing out or drawing in of the intercostal spaces in inspiration and expiration; depress the ribs in forced expiration; the portion attaching the costal cartilages of the upper four or five ribs probably helps in elevation of the ribs with the external intercostals in forced inspiration

Intercostal Muscles: Intercostales Intimi

The intercostales intimi are the innermost intercostal muscles. They consist of 11 pairs.

Origin:	Similar to the internal intercostal muscles but separated from them by the neurovascular plane containing the intercostal nerve and vessels; originate deep to the internal intercostals from ribs 1 through 11, usually extending from the angles of the

ribs posteriorly to about the costochondral junction anteriorly; may be poorly developed or absent

Insertion:	Insert on the superior margin of ribs 2 through 12 deep to the insertion of the internal intercostal muscles
Innervation:	Segmentally by ventral rami of first 11 thoracic spinal nerves (intercostal nerves) (T1–T11)
Blood Supply:	Posterior intercostal, anterior intercostal, and musculophrenic arteries; costocervical trunk
Action:	Probably act with the internal intercostal muscles; conclusive data are lacking

Subcostalis

Origin:	Internal surface of the ribs, usually the lower ones, near the angles
Insertion:	Internal surface of second or third rib below rib of origin; variable in presence and distribution
Innervation:	Ventral rami of thoracic spinal nerves (intercostal and subcostal nerves) (T1–T12)
Blood Supply:	Musculophrenic and posterior intercostal arteries
Action:	Probably depress the ribs and assist the internal and innermost intercostals in expiration

Transversus Thoracis

Origin:	Lower one-third of the posterior surface of the sternum and costal cartilages of lower three or four vertebrosternal ribs
Insertion:	Inferior and internal surfaces of the costal cartilages of ribs 2 through 6; can vary a great deal
Innervation:	Ventral rami of the first six thoracic spinal nerves (intercostal nerves) (T1–T6)
Blood Supply:	Internal thoracic and anterior intercostal arteries
Action:	Depresses the costal cartilages of the ribs to which it is attached; probably acts in expiration

Major Muscles of the Trunk: The Diaphragm

Sternal Part

Origin: Attaches by two slips to posterior part of xiphoid process

Insertion: Central tendon of diaphragm, an aponeurosis of interwoven collagenous fibers; located nearer front of thorax than rear

Innervation: Principal motor innervation is from phrenic nerve (C3–C5) with some peripheral innervation from intercostal nerves (T6–T12)

Blood Supply: Superior and inferior phrenic arteries, musculophrenic artery, and pericardiacophrenic artery

Action: The essential muscle of respiration; contraction of diaphragm results in a lengthening of thoracic cavity, thereby increasing thoracic cavity volume, which increases negative pressure and thereby draws air into the lungs; contraction of diaphragm is responsible for about two-thirds of volume of inspired air

Costal Part

Origin: Attaches to internal surfaces of lower six ribs and costal cartilages; interdigitates with transversus abdominus muscle

Insertion: Central tendon of diaphragm, an aponeurosis of interwoven collagenous fibers; located nearer front of thorax than rear, so muscle fibers are longer posteriorly

Innervation: Principal motor innervation is from phrenic nerve (C3–C5) with some peripheral innervation from intercostal nerves (T6–T12)

Blood Supply: Superior and inferior phrenic arteries, musculophrenic artery, and pericardiacophrenic artery

Action: The essential muscle of respiration; contraction of diaphragm results in a lengthening of thoracic cavity, thereby increasing thoracic cavity volume, which increases negative pressure and thereby draws air into the lungs; contraction of the diaphragm is responsible for about two-thirds of the volume of inspired air

Lumbar Part

Origin: Consists of several parts: medial and lateral arcuate ligaments and right and left crura (singular: *crus*)

  Right crus: Broader and longer than left; attaches to anterolateral aspect of bodies and intervertebral disks of vertebrae L1 through L3

Left crus:	Attaches to corresponding parts of L1 and L2; shorter than right crus
Left and right crura:	Medial tendinous arches of both crura converge over aorta at level of thoracolumbar disc (IVD T12–L1); this constitutes the *median arcuate ligament*
Lateral arcuate ligament:	Thickening of fascia where diaphragm overlies quadratus lumborum muscle; fibers run from ligament to central tendon of diaphragm
Medial arcuate ligament:	Thickening of fascia where diaphragm overlies psoas major muscle; fibers run from ligament to central tendon of diaphragm
Insertion:	Central tendon of diaphragm, an aponeurosis of interwoven collagenous fibers; located nearer front of thorax than rear, so muscle fibers are longer posteriorly
Innervation:	Principal motor innervation is from phrenic nerve (C3–C5) with some peripheral innervation from intercostal nerves (T6–T12)
Blood Supply:	Superior and inferior phrenic arteries, musculophrenic artery, and pericardiacophrenic artery
Action:	The essential muscle of respiration; contraction of diaphragm results in lengthening of thoracic cavity, thereby increasing thoracic cavity volume, which increases negative pressure and thereby draws air into lungs; contraction of diaphragm is responsible for about two-thirds of volume of inspired air

Major Muscles of the Trunk: The Abdomen

Rectus Abdominus

Origin:	By two tendons, one from the pubic symphysis and one from the pubic crest
Insertion:	By three fascicles into the cartilages of ribs 5 through 7; some fibers may attach as well to the xiphoid process and costoxiphoid ligament
Innervation:	Ventral rami of seventh to twelfth thoracic ventral rami (intercostal and subcostal nerves) (T7–T12)
Blood Supply:	Superior and inferior epigastric arteries
Action:	Flexes the vertebral column, particularly the lumbar portion; tenses the anterior abdominal wall and aids in compressing the abdominal contents; with the thorax fixed, it flexes the pelvis

Pyramidalis

Origin:	Variably present; placed anterior to the rectus abdominus in the rectus sheath; arises from the ventral surface of the pubis
Insertion:	Into linea alba, about midway between the pubis and the umbilicus
Innervation:	Subcostal nerve (ventral ramus of 12th thoracic spinal nerve) (T12)
Blood Supply:	Inferior epigastric artery
Action:	Tenses the linea alba, supports abdominal viscera, and is active in forced expiration

Obliquus Externus Abdominus

Origin:	Eight fleshy strips that arise from the external and inferior borders of the lower eight ribs, interdigitating with serratus anterior and latissimus dorsi
Insertion:	Ventral half of the external aspect of the iliac crest, remainder via a wide aponeurosis that helps constitute the rectus abdominus sheath and via the sheath into the linea alba; the lower border of its aponeurosis forms the inguinal ligament
Innervation:	Ventral rami of lower six thoracic and first two lumbar spinal nerves (T7–T12)
Blood Supply:	Superior and inferior epigastric arteries
Action:	Compresses abdomen, supports abdominal viscera, active in forced expiration; via actions on the ribs rotates the vertebral

column to the contralateral side; bilateral contraction helps flex lumbar vertebral column

Obliquus Internus Abdominus

Origin: Thoracolumbar fascia, anterior two-thirds of the iliac crest deep to obliquus externus abdominus, lateral two-thirds of the inguinal ligament

Insertion: Costal cartilages of the last three ribs, and then via its aponeurosis into the rectus sheath and thus into the linea alba

Innervation: Ventral rami of lower six thoracic and first lumbar spinal nerves (T7–T12, L1)

Blood Supply: Superior and inferior epigastric arteries, deep circumflex iliac artery

Action: Compresses abdomen, supports abdominal viscera, active in forced expiration; via actions on the ribs rotates the vertebral column to the ipsilateral side; bilateral contraction helps flex lumbar vertebral column

Transversus Abdominus

Origin: Deep surfaces of the lower six costal cartilages, middle layer of the thoracolumbar fascia, anterior two-thirds of the iliac crest, lateral third of the inguinal ligament deep to the obliquus internus abdominus

Insertion: Via the rectus sheath into the linea alba with the oblique abdominal muscles

Innervation: Ventral rami of the lower six thoracic ventral rami, iliohypogastric nerve, and ilioinguinal nerve (T7–T12, L1)

Blood Supply: Deep circumflex iliac artery; inferior epigastric artery

Action: Compresses abdomen, supports abdominal viscera, active in forced expiration

Quadratus Lumborum

Origin: Iliolumbar ligament and posterior part of the iliac crest

Insertion: Inferior border of the 12th rib, transverse processes of lumbar vertebrae 1 to 4

Innervation: Subcostal nerve (ventral ramus of 12th thoracic spinal nerve); ventral rami of lumbar spinal nerves 1 to 3 (T12, L1–L3)

Blood Supply: Lumbar branch of the iliolumbar artery

Action: Depresses and fixes the 12th rib; acts as a muscle of inspiration by fixing the 12th rib and thereby stabilizing the inferior attachments of the diaphragm; laterally flexes the vertebral column when contracting unilaterally; with the pelvis fixed and both quadratus lumborum muscles contracting bilaterally, they probably help extend the lumbar vertebral column

Upper Limb Musculature:
The Shoulder

Trapezius, Latissimus Dorsi, Levator Scapulae, Rhomboideus Minor, and Rhomboideus Major

These muscles are discussed with the superficial back muscles, beginning on page 298.

Serratus Anterior

Origin:	Fleshy digitations from the external surfaces of the upper eight or nine ribs
Insertion:	Costal surface of the vertebral border of the scapula
Innervation:	Long thoracic nerve (C5–C7)
Blood Supply:	Lateral thoracic artery
Action:	Upward rotation and protraction of the scapula; raises ribs if scapula is fixed

Deltoideus

Origin:	Lateral third of the clavicle, acromion process of the scapula, and spine of the scapula
Insertion:	Deltoid tuberosity on the lateral aspect of the humerus
Innervation:	Axillary nerve from the brachial plexus (C5, C6)
Blood Supply:	Anterior and posterior humeral circumflex arteries, thoracoacromial trunk, subscapular and profunda brachii arteries
Action:	Abduction of the arm; posterior fibers assist with extension of the arm, anterior fibers with flexion of the arm

Supraspinatus

Origin:	Supraspinous fossa of the scapula
Insertion:	Superior facet of the greater tubercle of the humerus
Innervation:	Suprascapular nerve, from brachial plexus (C5–C6)
Blood Supply:	Suprascapular artery and dorsal scapular artery
Action:	Abduction and lateral rotation of the arm, helps keep the humeral head in contact with the glenoid fossa of the scapula; one of the rotator cuff muscles

Infraspinatus

Origin:	Infraspinous fossa of the scapula
Insertion:	Middle facet of the greater tubercle of the humerus
Innervation:	Suprascapular nerve of the brachial plexus (C5, C6)
Blood Supply:	Suprascapular artery
Action:	Lateral rotation of the arm; one of the rotator cuff muscles

Teres Minor

Origin:	Dorsal surface of the axillary border of the scapula
Insertion:	Inferior facet of the greater tubercle of the humerus
Innervation:	Axillary nerve of the brachial plexus (C5, C6)
Blood Supply:	Circumflex scapular and posterior humeral circumflex arteries
Action:	Adducts and laterally rotates the arm; one of the rotator cuff muscles

Teres Major

Origin:	Dorsal surface of the inferior angle of the scapula
Insertion:	Medial lip of the bicipital groove of the humerus
Innervation:	Lower subscapular nerve of the brachial plexus (C6, C7)
Blood Supply:	Posterior humeral and thoracodorsal arteries
Action:	Extension, adduction, and medial rotation of the humerus

Subscapularis

Origin:	Subscapular fossa of the ventral surface of the scapula
Insertion:	Lesser tubercle of the humerus
Innervation:	Upper and lower subscapular nerves of the brachial plexus (C5–C6)
Blood Supply:	Suprascapular axillary and subscapular arteries
Action:	Medial rotation of the humerus; one of the rotator cuff muscles

Upper Limb Musculature: The Pectoral Region

Pectoralis Major

Origin: Sternal half of clavicle (clavicular head) and lateral border of sternum to seventh rib (sternal head)

Insertion: Lateral lip of the bicipital groove of the humerus

Innervation: Medial and lateral pectoral nerves (C5–T1)

Blood Supply: Pectoral branches of the thoracoacromial trunk of the axillary artery, superior thoracic and lateral thoracic arteries

Action: Medial rotation, adduction, and flexion of the arm at the glenohumeral joint

Pectoralis Minor

Origin: Outer surfaces of the anterior aspects of the third, fourth, and fifth ribs (deep to the pectoralis major)

Insertion: Tip of the coracoid process of the scapula

Innervation: Medial and lateral pectoral nerves (Note: only the medial pectoral nerve pierces the muscle; the lateral sends fibers that join with the medial, but the lateral nerve itself passes superior to the pectoralis minor) (C8, T1)

Blood Supply: Pectoral branches of the thoracoacromial trunk of the axillary artery; lateral thoracic artery

Action: Protracts the scapula; aids the levator scapulae and rhomboids in rotating the scapula downward (depression of the glenoid)

Subclavius

Origin: From the junction of the first rib and first costal cartilage anterior to the costoclavicular ligament

Insertion: Subclavian groove on the inferior surface of the middle third of the clavicle

Innervation: Subclavian branch of the brachial plexus (C5, C6)

Blood Supply: Clavicular branch of the thoracoacromial trunk of the axillary artery

Action: Pulls the clavicle, and thus the shoulder, downward and forward

Upper Limb Musculature: The Arm

Anterior Compartment

Coracobrachialis

Origin:	Tip of the coracoid process of the scapula
Insertion:	Medial aspect of the humerus at midshaft
Innervation:	Musculocutaneous nerve of the brachial plexus (C5–C7)
Blood Supply:	Brachial artery
Action:	Flexes and adducts the arm

Brachialis

Origin:	Inferior one-half to two-thirds of the anterior aspect of the humerus
Insertion:	Ulnar tuberosity and coronoid process
Innervation:	Musculocutaneous nerve of the brachial plexus (C5, C6) plus a small branch from radial nerve (C7)
Blood Supply:	Brachial and radial recurrent arteries, anterior ulnar recurrent arteries, and ulnar and radial collateral arteries
Action:	Flexion of the forearm

Biceps Brachii

Origin:	
Long head:	From supraglenoid tubercle of the scapula
Short head:	Coracoid process of the scapula
Insertion:	By a common tendon into the radial tuberosity and by the bicipital aponeurosis to the deep fascia covering the common origin of the forearm flexor muscles
Innervation:	Musculocutaneous nerve of the brachial plexus (C5, C6)
Blood Supply:	Brachial artery
Action:	Supination of the forearm; flexes the forearm, flexes and adducts the arm

Posterior Compartment

Triceps Brachii

Origin:	
Long head:	From the infraglenoid tubercle of the scapula
Lateral head:	Lateral aspect of the humeral shaft
Medial head:	Posterior aspect of the humeral shaft, deep to the other two heads

Insertion:	Olecranon process of the ulna
Innervation:	Radial nerve from the brachial plexus (C6–C8)
Blood Supply:	Profunda brachii artery, posterior humeral circumflex artery, ulnar recurrent arteries, and interosseus recurrenta
Action:	Extension of the forearm; long head aids in adducting the abducted arm; long head extends the humerus at the glenohumeral joint

Anconeus (Sometimes considered a superficial muscle of the posterior compartment of the forearm)

Origin:	Dorsal aspect of the lateral epicondyle of the humerus, appears as an inferior extension of the triceps brachii
Insertion:	Lateral aspect of the olecranon process and superior one-quarter of the dorsal aspect of the shaft of the ulna
Innervation:	Radial nerve from the brachial plexus (C6, C7, C8)
Blood Supply:	Profunda brachii
Action:	Assists in extension of the forearm

Upper Limb Musculature: The Forearm

Anterior Compartment: Superficial Muscles

Pronator Teres

Origin:

   Humeral head: Medial epicondyle of the humerus and common flexor tendon

   Ulnar head: Coronoid process of ulna

Insertion: Middle of the lateral border of the radius

Innervation: Median nerve from brachial plexus (C6, C7)

Blood Supply: Anterior ulnar recurrent artery, ulnar and radial arteries

Action: Pronates the forearm, assists in flexing the forearm

Flexor Carpi Radialis

Origin: Medial epicondyle of humerus via common flexor tendon and the antebrachial fascia

Insertion: Bases of the second and third metacarpal bones

Innervation: Median nerve from the brachial plexus (C6, C7)

Blood Supply: Radial artery, ulnar artery and branches

Action: Flexes and abducts the hand at the wrist; assists in flexing the forearm

Palmaris Longus

The palmaris longus is absent in 3 to 10 percent of the population.

Origin: Medial epicondyle of humerus via common flexor tendon

Insertion: Palmar aponeurosis

Innervation: Median nerve from the brachial plexus (C7, C8)

Blood Supply: Posterior ulnar recurrent artery, ulnar artery and branches

Action: Flexes the wrist, cups the palm via the palmar aponeurosis

Flexor Carpi Ulnaris

Origin:

   Humeral head: Medial epicondyle of humerus via common flexor tendon

   Ulnar head: Olecranon process and posterior border of the ulna

Insertion:	Pisiform (which acts as a sesamoid bone in its tendon), then continues to the base of the fifth metacarpal and to the hook of the hamate
Innervation:	Ulnar nerve from the brachial plexus (C7, C8, T1)
Blood Supply:	Posterior ulnar recurrent artery, ulnar artery and branches
Action:	Flexes wrist, adducts hand, and assists in flexing the forearm

Flexor Digitorum Superficialis

Origin:	
Humeral head:	Medial epicondyle of humerus via common flexor tendon
Ulnar head:	From coronoid process of ulna
Radial head:	From the oblique line of the radius
Insertion:	Bases of the middle phalanges of digits 2 to 5 of the hand
Innervation:	Median nerve from the brachial plexus (C7, C8, T1)
Blood Supply:	Ulnar and radial arteries
Action:	Flexes the middle phalanges on the proximal phalanges; then flexes proximal phalanges on the metacarpal heads; then aids in flexing wrist and forearm

Anterior Compartment: Deep Muscles

Flexor Digitorum Profundus

Origin:	Proximal three-quarters of the anterior surface of the ulna and the interosseous membrane
Insertion:	Bases of the distal phalanges of digits 2 to 5 of the hand
Innervation:	Ulnar nerve (medial half of muscle) and anterior interosseous branch of the median nerve (lateral half of muscle), both from the brachial plexus (C8, T1)
Blood Supply:	Ulnar and anterior interosseous arteries
Action:	Flexes the distal phalanges on the middle phalanges after the flexor digitorum superficialis has flexed the middle phalanges; further contraction aids in flexion of the wrist

Flexor Pollicis Longus

Origin:	Anterior surface of the distal one-quarter of the radius and the interosseous membrane
Insertion:	Base of the distal phalanx of the thumb
Innervation:	Anterior interosseous branch of the median nerve (from brachial plexus) (C7–C8)
Blood Supply:	Anterior interosseous artery and radial artery
Action:	Flexes the thumb

Pronator Quadratus

Origin:	Anterior surface of the distal one-quarter of the ulna deep to the origin of the flexor pollicis longus
Insertion:	Distal one-quarter of the anterior surface of the radius
Innervation:	Anterior interosseous branch of the median nerve (from brachial plexus) (C7–C8)
Blood Supply:	Anterior interosseous artery, radial artery
Action:	Pronates the forearm, helps bind the radius to the ulna

Posterior Compartment: Superficial Muscles

Brachioradialis

Origin:	Proximal two-thirds of the lateral supracondylar ridge of the humerus
Insertion:	Lateral surface of the distal end of the radius
Innervation:	Radial nerve from the brachial plexus (C5–C6)
Blood Supply:	Radial recurrent artery, radial collateral artery
Action:	Flexes forearm after flexion is begun by brachialis and biceps brachii; may also act as a semisupinator and semipronator

Extensor Carpi Radialis Longus

Origin:	Deep to brachioradialis from the lateral supracondylar ridge of the humerus
Insertion:	Base of second metacarpal
Innervation:	Radial nerve (C6, C7)
Blood Supply:	Radial and radial recurrent arteries, radial collateral artery
Action:	Extends the wrist and abducts the hand

Extensor Carpi Radialis Brevis

Origin:	Lateral epicondyle of the humerus via the common extensor tendon
Insertion:	Base of the third metacarpal
Innervation:	Posterior interosseous branch (sometimes called the "deep branch") of the radial nerve (C7, C8)
Blood Supply:	Radial and radial recurrent arteries, radial collateral artery
Action:	Extends the wrist and abducts the hand

Extensor Digitorum

Origin:	Common extensor tendon and the intermuscular septum
Insertion:	Four tendons insert into the extensor expansions

Innervation:	Posterior interosseous branch of the radial nerve (C7, C8)
Blood Supply:	Posterior interosseous artery from ulnar artery
Action:	Extends the proximal interphalangeal, distal interphalangeal, and metacarpophalangeal joints of the medial four digits; assists in extension of the wrist

Extensor Digiti Minimi

Origin:	From the common extensor tendon from the lateral epicondyle of the humerus
Insertion:	Extensor expansion of the fifth digit, often fused with the extensor digitorum
Innervation:	Posterior interosseous branch of the radial nerve (C7, C8)
Blood Supply:	Posterior interosseous artery from ulnar artery
Action:	Extends the proximal interphalangeal, distal interphalangeal, and metacarpophalangeal joints of the fifth digit

Extensor Carpi Ulnaris

Origin:	From the common extensor tendon from the lateral epicondyle of the humerus
Insertion:	Base of the fifth metacarpal
Innervation:	Posterior interosseous branch of the radial nerve (C7, C8)
Blood Supply:	Posterior interosseous artery from ulnar artery
Action:	Extends and adducts the hand at the wrist

Posterior Compartment: Deep Muscles

Supinator

Origin:	From the common extensor tendon from the lateral epicondyle of the humerus; radial collateral and annular ligaments of the elbow, supinator crest and fossa of the ulna
Insertion:	Lateral, posterior, and anterior surfaces of the proximal one third of the radius
Innervation:	Posterior interosseous, or deep branch of the radial nerve (C6–C7)
Blood Supply:	Radial recurrent and posterior interosseous arteries, radial artery
Action:	Supinates the forearm

Abductor Pollicis Longus

Origin:	Deep to supinator, proximal posterior surface of radius and ulna, and interosseous membrane
Insertion:	Base of the first metacarpal

Innervation: Posterior interosseous branch of the radial nerve (C7, C8)

Blood Supply: Posterior interosseous artery from ulnar artery

Action: Abducts and extends the thumb at the carpometacarpal joint

Extensor Pollicis Brevis

Origin: Posterior surface of the radius and the interosseous membrane

Insertion: Base of the proximal phalanx of the thumb

Innervation: Posterior interosseous branch of the radial nerve (C7, C8)

Blood Supply: Posterior interosseous artery from ulnar artery

Action: Extends the proximal phalanx and metacarpal of the thumb at the metacarpophalangeal carpometacarpal joints

Extensor Pollicis Longus

Origin: Posterior surface of the middle one-third of the ulna; interosseous membrane

Insertion: Base of the distal phalanx of the thumb

Innervation: Posterior interosseous branch of the radial nerve (C7, C8)

Blood Supply: Posterior interosseous artery from ulnar artery

Action: Extends the thumb at the interphalangeal joint

Extensor Indicis

Origin: Posterior surface of the distal one-third of the ulna; interosseous membrane

Insertion: Extensor expansion of digit 2 (index finger)

Innervation: Posterior interosseous branch of the radial nerve (C7, C8)

Blood Supply: Posterior interosseous artery from ulnar artery

Action: Extends the second digit; assists in extending the hand at the wrist

Upper Limb Musculature: The Intrinsic Muscles of the Hand

Lumbricals: Four

Origin:	From the tendons of the flexor digitorum profundus
Insertion:	Lateral sides of the extensor expansions of digits 2 through 5
Innervation:	
Lateral two:	Median nerve (C8, T1)
Medial two:	Ulnar nerve (C8, T1)
Blood Supply:	Superficial and deep palmar arches (from radial and ulnar arteries)
Action:	Flex the digits at the metacarpophalangeal joints and extend them at the proximal and distal interphalangeal joints

Thenar Muscles

Abductor Pollicis Brevis

Origin:	Flexor retinaculum, scaphoid and trapezium bones
Insertion:	Lateral side of the base of the proximal phalanx of the thumb
Innervation:	Recurrent branch of the median nerve (C8, T1)
Blood Supply:	Superficial palmar branch of the radial artery
Action:	Abducts thumb and aids in opposition of thumb to digit 5

Flexor Pollicis Brevis

Origin:	Flexor retinaculum, tubercle of trapezium (superficial head—deep to abductor pollicis brevis), also trapezoid and capitate bones—deep head
Insertion:	Lateral side of base of proximal phalanx of thumb; fuses with abductor tendon and contains a sesamoid bone in its tendon
Innervation:	Recurrent branch of the median nerve (C8, T1)—superficial head, deep branch of ulnar nerve (C8, T1)—deep head
Blood Supply:	Superficial palmar branch of the radial artery
Action:	Flexes metacarpophalangeal joint of thumb

Opponens Pollicis

Origin:	Flexor retinaculum, tubercle of trapezium (deep to abductor pollicis brevis and lateral to flexor pollicis brevis)
Insertion:	Anterior and lateral side of first metacarpal

Innervation:	Recurrent branch of the median nerve (C8, T1)
Blood Supply:	Superficial palmar branch of the radial artery
Action:	Opposes the thumb (draws first metacarpal anteriorly and medially) to each of the other digits

Adductor Pollicis

Origin:

Oblique head:	Bases of second and third metacarpals; trapezium, trapezoid, and capitate bones
Transverse head:	Anterior surface of the shaft of the third metacarpal
Insertion:	Medial side of the base of the proximal phalanx of the thumb
Innervation:	Deep branch of the ulnar nerve (C8, T1)
Blood Supply:	Deep palmar arch, princeps pollicis artery
Action:	Adducts thumb and aids in opposition

Hypothenar Muscles

Abductor Digiti Minimi

Origin:	Pisiform bone and tendon of the flexor carpi ulnaris
Insertion:	Medial side of the base of the proximal phalanx of digit 5 (little finger)
Innervation:	Deep branch of ulnar nerve (C8, T1)
Blood Supply:	Deep palmar branch of ulnar artery, dorsal carpal branch of ulnar artery
Action:	Abducts digit 5

Flexor Digiti Minimi Brevis

Origin:	Hook of hamate and flexor retinaculum
Insertion:	Fuses with tendon of abductor digiti minimi and then to base of the proximal phalanx of digit 5
Innervation:	Deep branch of ulnar nerve (C8, T1)
Blood Supply:	Deep palmar branch of ulnar artery, dorsal carpal branch of ulnar artery
Action:	Flexes proximal phalanx of digit 5

Opponens Digiti Minimi

Origin:	From the hook of the hamate and flexor retinaculum deep to short abductor and flexor muscles of digit 5
Insertion:	Medial border of fifth metacarpal
Innervation:	Deep branch of ulnar nerve (C8, T1)

Blood Supply:	Deep palmar branch of ulnar artery, dorsal carpal branch of ulnar artery
Action:	Opposes digit 5; draws metacarpal 5 anteriorly and rotates it to bring palmar surface of digit 5 into opposition with the palmar surface of the thumb

Palmaris Brevis

Origin:	Ulnar side of flexor retinaculum and palmar aponeurosis
Insertion:	Skin on the medial side of the palm
Innervation:	Superficial branch of the ulnar nerve (C8, T1)
Blood Supply:	Superficial palmar arch
Action:	Wrinkles skin on the medial side of the palm, increasing the curvature of the hollow of the palm to aid in gripping

Interosseous Muscles

Palmar Interossei: Three

Origin:	
First:	Ulnar side of second metacarpal
Second:	Radial side of fourth metacarpal
Third:	Radial side of fifth metacarpal
Insertion:	
First:	Ulnar side of proximal phalanx of digit 2
Second:	Radial side of proximal phalanx of digit 4
Third:	Radial side of proximal phalanx of digit 5
Innervation:	Deep branch of ulnar nerve (C8, T1)
Blood Supply:	Deep palmar branch of ulnar artery, deep palmar arch
Action:	Adduct digits 2, 4, and 5 toward the midline of digit 3

Dorsal Interossei: Four

Origin:	The four dorsal interossei originate by two heads, one each from the adjacent sides of the metacarpal bones
Insertion:	
First:	Radial side of the proximal phalanx of digit 2
Second:	Radial side of the proximal phalanx of digit 3
Third:	Ulnar side of the proximal phalanx of digit 3
Fourth:	Ulnar side of the proximal phalanx of digit 4
Innervation:	Deep branch of ulnar nerve (C8, T1)
Blood Supply:	Deep palmar arch, metacarpal arteries
Action:	Abduct the digits away from the midline of digit 3

Lower Limb Musculature: The Hip Joint Flexors

Iliopsoas

The iliopsoas is the term applied to the iliacus and psoas major muscles collectively, as they insert into the lesser trochanter of the femur by a common tendon.

Iliacus

Origin: Superior two-thirds of the iliac fossa; iliac crest; anterior sacroiliac, lumbosacral, and iliolumbar ligaments; ala of sacrum

Insertion: With the tendon of the psoas major into the lesser trochanter of the femur, capsule of the hip joint, and the shaft of the femur

Innervation: Femoral nerve (L2, L3)

Blood Supply: Iliac branch of the iliolumbar artery and the superior gluteal artery

Action: Flexes the thigh, flexes the pelvis when the thigh is fixed

Psoas Major

Origin: Anterior and inferior surfaces of the transverse processes, bodies, and intervertebral discs of all five lumbar vertebrae

Insertion: After passing beneath the inguinal ligament and anterior to the capsule of the hip joint, inserts with the iliacus (as the iliopsoas muscle) into the lesser trochanter of the femur

Innervation: Branches of the lumbar plexus including contributions from the ventral rami of lumbar spinal nerves 1 through 3 (L1–L3)

Blood Supply: Lumbar branch of the iliolumbar artery, lumbar arteries

Action: Flexes the thigh at the hip joint; if both thighs are fixed and both psoas major muscles contract together, they are important flexors of the hip as in sitting up from a supine position; although mechanically it appears to be a medial rotator of the thigh, electromyographic studies show it to be active during lateral rotation

Psoas Minor

The psoas minor is often absent; it is absent bilaterally in half of subjects.

Origin: Sides of the bodies of the twelfth thoracic and first lumbar vertebrae and the intervertebral disc between them

Insertion: Pectineal line and iliopectineal eminence of the innominate bone

Innervation:	Ventral ramus of the first (and sometimes second) lumbar spinal nerve (L1, L2)
Blood Supply:	Lumbar branch of the iliolumbar artery, lumbar arteries
Action:	Flexes pelvis on the vertebral column, assists the iliopsoas in flexing the vertebral column on the pelvis

Lower Limb Musculature: The Gluteal Region

Tensor Fasciae Latae

Origin: Anterior superior iliac spine and the anterior part of the external lip of the iliac crest

Insertion: Into the iliotibial tract and thus into the lateral aspect of the proximal tibia

Innervation: Superior gluteal nerve (L4, L5)

Blood Supply: Lateral femoral circumflex artery, superior and inferior gluteal arteries

Action: Abducts, medially rotates, and flexes the thigh; helps keep the knee extended and steadies the trunk on the thigh

Gluteus Maximus

Origin: External surface of the iliac blades posterior to the posterior gluteal lines, iliac crest; dorsal surfaces of sacrum and coccyx; sacrotuberous ligament

Insertion: Iliotibial tract, gluteal tuberosity of femur

Innervation: Inferior gluteal nerve (L5, S1, S2)

Blood Supply: Superior and inferior gluteal arteries; first perforating branch of the profunda femoris artery

Action: Extends thigh; laterally rotates thigh; steadies the thigh on the trunk; extends trunk; assists in raising trunk from a seated position; active in climbing and running (forceful extension); generally inactive in quiet walking

Gluteus Medius

Origin: Deep to gluteus maximus; from external surface of iliac blade between anterior and posterior iliac lines

Insertion: Lateral surface of the greater trochanter of the femur

Innervation: Superior gluteal nerve (L4, L5, S1)

Blood Supply: Deep branch of the superior gluteal artery

Action: Abducts thigh; medially rotates thigh when hip is extended; steadies hip joint; supports trunk in single stance and swing phases of walking by contracting on the side in which the foot is in contact with the ground

Gluteus Minimus

Origin: External surface of ilium between anterior and inferior iliac lines

Insertion: Anterior surface of the greater trochanter of the femur

Innervation: Superior gluteal nerve (L5, S1)

Blood Supply: Deep branch of the superior gluteal artery

Action: Abducts thigh; medially rotates thigh when hip is extended; steadies hip joint; supports trunk in single stance and swing phases of walking by contracting on the side in which the foot is in contact with the ground

Lower Limb Musculature: The Short Rotators of the Hip

Piriformis

Origin:	Anterior surface of sacrum; sacrotuberous ligament
Insertion:	Superior border of the greater trochanter of femur
Innervation:	Ventral rami of spinal nerves S1 and S2 (S1, S2)
Blood Supply:	Superior gluteal, inferior gluteal, and internal pudendal arteries
Action:	Lateral rotation of the extended thigh, abducts the flexed thigh, steadies the femur head in the acetabulum

Obturator Internus

Origin:	Pelvic surface of obturator membrane and the surrounding margins of the obturator foramen
Insertion:	Medial surface of the greater trochanter of the femur
Innervation:	Nerve to obturator internus (L5, S1)
Blood Supply:	Superior and anterior gluteal and internal pudendal arteries
Action:	Lateral rotation of the extended thigh, abducts the flexed thigh, steadies the femur head in the acetabulum

Gemellus Superior

Origin:	Ischial spine
Insertion:	Blends with the tendon of the obturator internus and then on to the medial surface of the greater trochanter
Innervation:	Nerve to obturator internus (L5, S1)
Blood Supply:	Superior and inferior gluteal artery, internal pudendal artery
Action:	Lateral rotation of the extended thigh, abduction of the flexed thigh, steadies the femur head in the acetabulum

Gemellus Inferior

Origin:	Ischial tuberosity
Insertion:	Blends with the tendon of the obturator internus and then on to the medial surface of the greater trochanter
Innervation:	Nerve to quadratus femoris (L5, S1)
Blood Supply:	Superior and inferior gluteal artery, internal pudendal artery
Action:	Lateral rotation of the extended thigh, abduction of the flexed thigh, steadies the femur head in the acetabulum

Quadratus Femoris

Origin: Lateral border of the ischial tuberosity

Insertion: Quadrate tubercle of intertrochanteric crest and inferior part of
                     crest

Innervation: Nerve to quadratus femoris (L5, S1)

Blood Supply: Medial and lateral femoral circumflex artery, internal pudendal
                     artery

Action: Adduction and lateral rotation of the thigh, steadies the femur
                     head in the acetabulum

Lower Limb Musculature: The Thigh

Anterior Compartment

Quadriceps Femoris

The quadriceps femoris is composed of four parts that insert into the patella and then onto the tibial tuberosity via the patellar ligament.

RECTUS FEMORIS

Origin:

Direct head:	Anterior inferior iliac spine
Reflected head:	Groove superior to the acetabulum
Insertion:	Into the superior aspect of the patella and then onto the tibial tuberosity via the patellar ligament
Innervation:	Femoral nerve (L2–L4)
Blood Supply:	Lateral femoral circumflex artery, profunda femoris artery
Action:	Extends the leg at the knee; steadies the hip joint and aids the iliopsoas in flexing the thigh

VASTUS LATERALIS

Origin:	Greater trochanter, intertrochanteric line, lateral lip of linea aspera, gluteal tuberosity
Insertion:	Into the superolateral aspect of the patella and then onto the tibial tuberosity via the patellar ligament
Innervation:	Femoral (L2–L4)
Blood Supply:	Lateral femoral circumflex artery, lateral superior genicular artery
Action:	Extends leg at knee

VASTUS INTERMEDIUS

Origin:	Anterior and lateral aspects of the shaft of the femur
Insertion:	Into the superior aspect of the patella and then onto the tibial tuberosity via the patellar ligament; blends with the tendons of the rectus femoris and vastus lateralis and medialis
Innervation:	Femoral nerve (L2–L4)
Blood Supply:	Lateral femoral circumflex artery, femoral and profunda femoris arteries
Action:	Extends leg at knee

VASTUS MEDIALIS

Origin:	Intertrochanteric line and medial lip of the linea aspera
Insertion:	Into the superomedial aspect of the patella and then onto the tibial tuberosity via the patellar ligament
Innervation:	Femoral nerve (L2–L4)
Blood Supply:	Femoral artery, profunda femoris artery, superior genicular arteries
Action:	Extends leg at knee; maintains patella in the patellar groove by drawing it medially

Articularis Genu

Origin:	Inferior aspect of the anterior surface of the shaft of the femur
Insertion:	Capsule of the knee joint and walls of the suprapatellar bursa
Innervation:	Femoral nerve (L2–L4)
Blood Supply:	Profunda femoris artery, superior genicular arteries
Action:	Pulls the capsule of the knee joint superiorly during extension of the leg at the knee

Sartorius

Origin:	Anterior superior iliac spine and superior part of notch inferior to the spine
Insertion:	Superior part of medial surface of the tibia (pes anserinus)
Innervation:	Femoral nerve (L2, L3)
Blood Supply:	Femoral artery
Action:	Flexes, abducts, and laterally rotates the thigh at the hip joint; flexes the leg at the knee joint

Posterior Compartment

Hamstring Muscles

BICEPS FEMORIS

Origin:	
Long head:	Ischial tuberosity
Short head:	Lateral lip of linea aspera and lateral supracondylar line
Insertion:	Lateral side of the head of the fibula; tendon is split by the fibular collateral ligament
Innervation:	
Long head:	Tibial division of the sciatic nerve (L5, S1, S2)
Short head:	Common fibular (peroneal) division of the sciatic nerve (L5, S1, S2)

| *Blood Supply:* | Perforating branches of the profunda femoris artery; popliteal artery |
| *Action:* | Both heads flex the leg at the knee and laterally rotate the leg when it is flexed; the long head extends the thigh at the hip joint (e.g., when starting to walk) |

SEMITENDINOSUS

Origin:	Ischial tuberosity
Insertion:	Medial surface of superior part of tibia (pes anserinus)
Innervation:	Tibial division of sciatic nerve (L5, S1, S2)
Blood Supply:	Perforating branches of the profunda femoris artery; popliteal artery
Action:	Extends thigh, flexes leg, rotates leg medially; when thigh and leg are flexed, it can aid in extending the trunk

SEMIMEMBRANOSUS

Origin:	Ischial tuberosity
Insertion:	Posterior part of medial portion of proximal tibia
Innervation:	Tibial division of sciatic nerve (L5, S1, S2)
Blood Supply:	Perforating branches of the profunda femoris artery; popliteal artery
Action:	Extends thigh, flexes leg, rotates leg medially; when thigh and leg are flexed, it can aid in extending the trunk

ADDUCTOR MAGNUS (ISCHIAL COMPONENT)

The ischial component of the adductor magnus is considered a hamstring muscle. The entire muscle is described next with the adductor muscles of the thigh.

Medial Compartment

Adductor Muscles

OBTURATOR EXTERNUS

Origin:	External margins of the obturator foramen, obturator membrane
Insertion:	Trochanteric fossa of the femur
Innervation:	Obturator nerve (L3, L4)
Blood Supply:	Obturator artery and medial femoral circumflex artery
Action:	Laterally rotates thigh, adducts thigh, steadies head of femur in acetabulum

PECTINEUS

| *Origin:* | Pectineal surface of pubis and pecten pubis |

Insertion:	Pectineal line of femur, between lesser trochanter and linea aspera
Innervation:	Femoral nerve and occasionally a branch from the obturator nerve (L2, L3)
Blood Supply:	Medial femoral circumflex artery, obturator artery
Action:	Medially rotates, adducts, and flexes the thigh

ADDUCTOR LONGUS

Origin:	Anterior surface of pubis inferior to the pubic crest
Insertion:	Middle third of linea aspera inferior to the pectineus
Innervation:	Anterior branch of obturator nerve (L2–L4)
Blood Supply:	Medial femoral circumflex artery, obturator artery
Action:	Adducts thigh, assists with flexion and medial rotation of thigh

ADDUCTOR BREVIS

Origin:	Inferior ramus of pubis deep to adductor longus
Insertion:	Pectineal line and proximal part of linea aspera, deep to pectineus and adductor longus
Innervation:	Anterior branch of obturator nerve (L2–L4)
Blood Supply:	Medial femoral circumflex artery, obturator artery
Action:	Adducts and, to a small extent, flexes the thigh

ADDUCTOR MAGNUS

Origin:	
Adductor part:	Inferior ramus of pubis, ramus of ischium
Hamstring part:	Ischial tuberosity
Insertion:	
Adductor part:	Gluteal tuberosity of femur, linea aspera, medial supracondylar line
Hamstring part:	Adductor tubercle of femur
Innervation:	
Adductor part:	Posterior branch of obturator nerve (L2–L4)
Hamstring part:	Tibial portion of sciatic nerve (L2–L4)
Blood Supply:	Medial femoral circumflex artery, obturator artery, popliteal artery, perforating branches of profunda femoris artery
Action:	Adducts thigh; adductor part also flexes the thigh, whereas the hamstring part extends the thigh

GRACILIS

Origin:	Inferior ramus of pubis
Insertion:	Superior part of medial surface of tibia (pes anserinus)
Innervation:	Anterior branch of obturator nerve (L2, L3)
Blood Supply:	Medial femoral circumflex artery, obturator artery, profunda femoris artery
Action:	Adducts thigh, medially rotates leg, flexes leg at knee

Lower Limb Musculature: The Leg

Posterior Compartment: Superficial Muscles

Because during development the upper limb rotates one way and the lower limb rotates in the opposite direction, the posterior surface of the leg is homologous with the anterior surface of the arm, and vice versa.

Triceps Surae

The triceps surae is composed of the two heads of the gastrocnemius along with the soleus.

GASTROCNEMIUS

Origin:

Lateral head:	Lateral aspect of lateral condyle of the femur
Medial head:	Depression on the superior and posterior part of the medial condyle of the femur; larger than the lateral head

Insertion:	Posterior surface of calcaneus via the calcaneal (Achilles) tendon
Innervation:	Tibial nerve (S1, S2)
Blood Supply:	Sural arteries from the popliteal artery
Action:	Plantarflexes foot, raises heel during walking, and flexes knee joint

SOLEUS

Origin:	Posterior aspect of the head of the fibula, superior one-quarter of the posterior aspect of the fibula, from the soleal line and middle third of the medial border of the tibia, and from a tendinous arch between the tibia and fibula
Insertion:	Posterior surface of calcaneus via the calcaneal (Achilles) tendon
Innervation:	Tibial nerve (S1, S2)
Blood Supply:	Posterior tibial artery, fibular (peroneal) artery, sural branches of popliteal artery
Action:	Plantarflexes foot and steadies leg on foot

Plantaris

Origin:	Inferior end of lateral supracondylar line of the femur and the oblique popliteal ligament
Insertion:	Posterior surface of calcaneus via the calcaneal (Achilles) tendon
Innervation:	Tibial nerve (S1, S2)

Blood Supply:	Sural branches of the popliteal artery
Action:	Weakly assists gastrocnemius in plantarflexing foot and flexing knee joint; may function as a sensory organ

Posterior Compartment: Deep Muscles

Popliteus

Origin:	Lateral surface of lateral condyle of femur and lateral meniscus of knee joint
Insertion:	Posterior surface of tibia superior to soleal line
Innervation:	Tibial nerve (L4, L5, S1)
Blood Supply:	Genicular arteries from the popliteal artery, sural arteries
Action:	Weakly flexes knee and medially rotates tibia at beginning of flexion of the knee

Flexor Digitorum Longus

Origin:	Medial part of posterior surface of tibia inferior to soleal line; broad aponeurosis attaches it to fibula
Insertion:	Plantar surfaces of the bases of the distal phalanges of the lateral four digits
Innervation:	Tibial nerve (L5, S1, S2)
Blood Supply:	Posterior tibial artery, fibular artery
Action:	Flexes lateral four digits and plantarflexes foot; supports longitudinal arches of foot

Flexor Hallucis Longus

Origin:	Inferior two-thirds of the posterior surface of fibula and inferior part of interosseous membranes
Insertion:	Plantar surface of the base of the distal phalanx of great toe (hallux)
Innervation:	Tibial nerve (L5, S1, S2)
Blood Supply:	Fibular (peroneal) artery, posterior tibial artery
Action:	Flexes great toe at all joints and plantarflexes foot; supports longitudinal arch of foot

Tibialis Posterior

Origin:	Interosseous membrane, posterior surface of tibia inferior to soleal line, superior two-thirds of medial surface of fibula
Insertion:	Tuberosity of navicular, cuboid, and all three cuneiform bones, and plantar surfaces of the bases of the second, third, and fourth metatarsals
Innervation:	Tibial nerve (L4, L5)

Blood Supply: Fibular (peroneal) artery, posterior tibial artery

Action: Plantarflexes and inverts foot

Anterior Compartment

Tibialis Anterior

Origin: Lateral aspect of the tibial plateau, superior half of lateral surface of the tibia

Insertion: Medial and inferior surfaces of the medial cuneiform bone, base of the first metatarsal bone

Innervation: Deep fibular (peroneal) nerve (L4, L5)

Blood Supply: Anterior tibial artery

Action: Dorsiflexes and inverts foot

Extensor Digitorum Longus

Origin: Lateral aspect of tibial plateau, superior three-quarters of anterior surface of fibula, anterior surface of interosseous membrane

Insertion: Dorsal aspect of the middle and distal phalanges of the lateral four toes through the extensor expansions

Innervation: Deep fibular (peroneal) nerve (L5, S1)

Blood Supply: Anterior tibial artery

Action: Extends the lateral four digits and dorsiflexes the foot

Fibularis (Peroneus) Tertius

Origin: Inferior one-third of anterior surface fibula and interosseous membrane

Insertion: Dorsum of the base of the fifth metatarsal

Innervation: Deep fibular (peroneal) nerve (L5, S1)

Blood Supply: Anterior tibial artery

Action: Dorsiflexes foot and aids in eversion of foot

Extensor Hallucis Longus

Origin: Middle part of the anterior surface of the fibula and interosseous membrane

Insertion: Dorsal aspect of the base of the distal phalanx of the great toe

Innervation: Deep fibular (peroneal) nerve (L5, S1)

Blood Supply: Anterior tibial artery

Action: Extends great toe and dorsiflexes foot

Lateral Compartment

Fibularis (Peroneus) Longus

Origin: Head and superior two-thirds of lateral aspect of fibula

Insertion: Base of first metatarsal and medial cuneiform bone

Innervation: Superficial fibular (peroneal) nerve (L5, S1, S2)

Blood Supply: Anterior tibial and fibular (peroneal) arteries

Action: Everts foot and weakly plantarflexes foot; also helps steady leg when standing on one foot

Fibularis (Peroneus) Brevis

Origin: Inferior two-thirds of lateral surface of fibula

Insertion: Dorsal surface of tuberosity on lateral side of base of fifth metatarsal bone

Innervation: Superficial fibular (peroneal) nerve (L5, S1, S2)

Blood Supply: Fibular (peroneal) artery

Action: Everts and weakly plantarflexes foot

Lower Limb Musculature: The Intrinsic Muscles of the Foot

Dorsum of Foot

Extensor Digitorum Brevis

Origin:	Anterior part of dorsal surface of calcaneus anteromedial to lateral malleolus, inferior extensor retinaculum
Insertion:	One of four tendons attaches to the base of the proximal phalanx of the hallux *(extensor hallucis brevis);* the more lateral three attach to the tendons of the extensor digitorum longus to digits 2, 3, and 4 *(extensor digitorum brevis)*
Innervation:	Deep fibular (peroneal) nerve (L5, S1)
Blood Supply:	Dorsalis pedis
Action:	Extends digits 1 to 4 at the metacarpophalangeal joints

Extensor Hallucis Brevis

See the preceding description of the insertion of the extensor digitorum brevis.

Plantar Aspect of Foot: First Layer

Abductor Hallucis

Origin:	Medial process of the calcaneal tubercle, flexor retinaculum, and plantar aponeurosis
Insertion:	Medial side of the base of the proximal phalanx of the hallux
Innervation:	Medial plantar nerve (S1, S2)
Blood Supply:	Medial plantar artery
Action:	Abducts and flexes the hallux; helps maintain the medial arch of the foot

Flexor Digitorum Brevis

Origin:	Medial process of the calcaneal tubercle, intermuscular septum, and plantar aponeurosis
Insertion:	Both sides of the middle phalanx of the lateral four digits
Innervation:	Medial plantar nerve (S1, S2)
Blood Supply:	Medial plantar artery
Action:	Flexes the lateral four digits at the proximal interphalangeal and metatarsophalangeal joints; helps maintain the longitudinal arches of the foot

Abductor Digiti Minimi

Origin:	Medial and lateral processes of the calcaneal tuberosity, plantar aponeurosis, and intermuscular septum
Insertion:	Lateral side of the base of the proximal phalanx of digit 5
Innervation:	Lateral plantar nerve (S1, S2, S3)
Blood Supply:	Lateral plantar artery
Action:	Abducts and flexes the fifth digit; helps maintain the lateral longitudinal arch of the foot

Plantar Aspect of Foot: Second Layer

Tendon of Flexor Digitorum Longus

The flexor digitorum longus muscle is described in the Posterior Compartment section on page 341.

Quadratus Plantae

Origin:	Medial surface and lateral margin of plantar surface of calcaneus
Insertion:	Posterolateral margin of tendon of flexor digitorum longus
Innervation:	Lateral plantar nerve (S1, S2, S3)
Blood Supply:	Lateral plantar artery
Action:	Assists flexor digitorum longus in flexing the lateral four digits

Lumbricals

Origin:	From the tendons of insertion of the flexor digitorum longus
Insertion:	Medial sides of bases of proximal phalanges of the lateral four digits and extensor expansions of the tendons of the extensor digitorum longus
Innervation:	
Medial (first) lumbrical:	Medial plantar nerve (S2, S3)
Lateral three lumbricals:	Lateral plantar nerve (S2, S3)
Blood Supply:	Plantar metatarsal arteries, lateral plantar artery, plantar arch
Action:	Flex the proximal phalanges at the metatarsophalangeal joint, extend middle and distal phalanges at the proximal and distal interphalangeal joints of digits 2 to 5

Tendon of Flexor Hallucis Longus

The flexor hallucis longus muscle is described in the Posterior Compartment section on page 341.

Plantar Aspect of Foot: Third Layer

Flexor Hallucis Brevis

Origin:	Plantar surfaces of cuboid bone and lateral cuneiform bone, tibialis posterior tendon
Insertion:	Both sides of the base of the proximal phalanx of the great toe
Innervation:	Medial plantar nerve (S1, S2)
Blood Supply:	First plantar metatarsal artery, medial plantar artery
Action:	Flexes the proximal phalanx of the great toe

Adductor Hallucis

Origin:	
Oblique head:	Bases of metatarsals 2 to 4
Transverse head:	Plantar ligaments of the metatarsophalangeal joints
Insertion:	Tendons of both heads insert into the lateral side of the base of the proximal phalanx of the great toe
Innervation:	Deep branch of the lateral plantar nerve (S2, S3)
Blood Supply:	First plantar metatarsal artery, medial plantar artery, plantar arch
Action:	Adducts great toe; assists in maintaining the transverse arch of the foot

Flexor Digiti Minimi Brevis

Origin:	Base of the fifth metatarsal bone
Insertion:	Base of the proximal phalanx of the fifth digit
Innervation:	Superficial branch of the lateral plantar nerve (S2, S3)
Blood Supply:	Lateral plantar artery
Action:	Flexes the proximal phalanx of the fifth digit at the metatarsophalangeal joint

Plantar Aspect of Foot: Fourth Layer

Plantar Interossei: Three

Origin:	Bases and medial sides of metatarsals 3 to 5
Insertion:	Medial sides of bases of proximal phalanges of digits 3 to 5
Innervation:	Lateral plantar nerve (S2, S3)
Blood Supply:	Plantar metatarsal arteries, lateral plantar artery, plantar arch
Action:	Adduct digits 3 to 5; flex the metatarsophalangeal joints of digits 3 to 5

Dorsal Interossei: Four

Origin:	Adjacent sides of metatarsals 1 to 5 (two heads each)
Insertion:	
First:	Medial side of proximal phalanx of second digit
Second to fourth:	Lateral sides of proximal phalanges of digits 2 to 4
Innervation:	Lateral plantar nerve (S2, S3)
Blood Supply:	Dorsal and plantar metatarsal arteries, arcuate artery
Action:	Abduct digits 2 to 4 and flex metatarsophalangeal joints of digits 2 to 4

Major Muscles of Mastication and the Hyoid

Masseter

Origin:	Anterior two-thirds of the inferior border of the zygomatic arch and the medial surface of the zygomatic arch
Insertion:	Lateral surface of mandibular ramus, at the angle and the inferior and posterior parts of the ramus
Innervation:	Masseteric branch of the mandibular division of the trigeminal nerve (cranial nerve V)
Blood Supply:	Superficial temporal artery, maxillary artery, facial artery
Action:	Closes the jaws by elevating the mandible

Temporalis

Origin:	Floor of the entire temporal fossa and deep surface of the temporal fascia
Insertion:	Medial surface, apex and anterior border of the coronoid process of the mandible, superior portion of the anterior border of the ramus of the mandible
Innervation:	Anterior and posterior deep temporal nerves of the mandibular division of the trigeminal nerve (cranial nerve V)
Blood Supply:	Superficial temporal artery, maxillary artery
Action:	Elevates, closes, and retracts the mandible

Pterygoideus Lateralis

Origin:	
Superior head:	From the infratemporal crest and inferolateral surface of the greater wing of the sphenoid bone
Inferior head:	Lateral surface of the lateral pterygoid plate of the sphenoid bone
Insertion:	Depression on the anterior part of the neck of the mandible, and anterior margin of the meniscus of the temporomandibular joint
Innervation:	Lateral pterygoid nerve from the mandibular division of the trigeminal nerve (cranial nerve V)
Blood Supply:	Pterygoid branch of the maxillary artery
Action:	Protrudes mandible, pulls articular disc anteriorly, and assists in rotatory motions of the mandible in chewing

Pterygoideus Medialis

Origin: Medial surface of the lateral pterygoid plate, pyramidal process of palatine bone, and tuberosity of the maxilla

Insertion: Inferior and posterior part of the internal aspect of the mandibular ramus and angle of the mandible

Innervation: Medial pterygoid nerve from the mandibular division of the trigeminal nerve (cranial nerve V)

Blood Supply: Pterygoid branches of the maxillary artery, facial artery

Action: Elevates the mandible, closing the jaws; acts with lateral pterygoids in protruding the mandible; acts with the lateral pterygoids in rotatory motions of the mandible during chewing

Styloglossus

Origin: Anterior border of the styloid process

Insertion: Into the sides of the tongue

Innervation: Hypoglossal (cranial nerve XII)

Blood Supply: Sublingual artery

Action: Elevation and retraction of the tongue

Stylopharyngeus

Origin: Medial side of the root of the styloid process

Insertion: Superior and posterior borders of the thyroid cartilage

Innervation: Glossopharyngeal nerve (cranial nerve IX)

Blood Supply: Ascending pharyngeal artery

Action: Elevates and dilates the pharynx

Pharyngeal Constrictors

Superior

Origin: Lower third of the posterior border of the medial pterygoid plate, alveolar process of mandible superior to the posterior end of the mylohyoid line, pterygomandibular ligament

Insertion: Median raphe of posterior wall of pharynx, pharyngeal tubercle of occipital bone

Innervation: Cranial root of accessory nerve (cranial nerve XI); vagus nerve (cranial nerve X) through the pharyngeal plexus

Blood Supply: Facial and ascending pharyngeal arteries

Action: Contracts the pharynx during swallowing

Middle

Origin:	Greater and lesser cornua of the hyoid bone and stylohyoid ligament
Insertion:	Into median raphe of the pharynx
Innervation:	Pharyngeal plexus
Blood Supply:	Facial and ascending pharyngeal arteries
Action:	Contracts the pharynx during swallowing

Inferior

Origin:	Sides of thyroid and cricoid cartilages
Insertion:	Into median raphe of the pharynx
Innervation:	Pharyngeal plexus, external and recurrent laryngeal branches of the vagus nerve (cranial nerve X), cranial root of accessory nerve (cranial nerve XI)
Blood Supply:	Inferior and superior thyroid arteries
Action:	Contracts the pharynx during swallowing

Hyoglossus

Origin:	Greater cornua of the hyoid bone
Insertion:	Sides of tongue
Innervation:	Hypoglossal nerve (cranial nerve XII)
Blood Supply:	Sublingual and submental arteries
Action:	Draws down sides of tongue and depresses tongue

Mylohyoid

Origin:	Mylohyoid line of mandible
Insertion:	Median raphe from chin to hyoid bone and onto hyoid
Innervation:	Mylohyoid branch of inferior alveolar nerve from trigeminal nerve (cranial nerve V)
Blood Supply:	Lingual, facial, and inferior alveolar arteries
Action:	Elevates hyoid bone and tongue, raises floor of mouth, depresses mandible when hyoid is fixed

Omohyoid

Origin:	
Inferior belly:	Superior border of scapula and suprascapular ligament to a tendon deep to sternocleidomastoid
Superior belly:	Extends superiorly from this tendon
Insertion:	Inferior aspect of the body of the hyoid bone

Innervation:	Ansa cervicalis (C1–C3)
Blood Supply:	Lingual and superior thyroid arteries
Action:	Fixes hyoid bone; depresses and retracts hyoid and larynx

Geniohyoid

Origin:	Inferior genial tubercle on posterior aspect of mental symphysis of mandible
Insertion:	Anterior aspect of the body of the hyoid bone
Innervation:	First cervical spinal nerve through fibers that travel with the hypoglossal nerve (cranial nerve XII) (C1)
Blood Supply:	Sublingual branch of lingual artery
Action:	Elevates hyoid bone and tongue

Genioglossus

Origin:	Superior genial tubercle on posterior aspect of mental symphysis of mandible
Insertion:	Lowest fibers to hyoid bone, middle fibers along inferior surface of tongue, superior fibers to tip of tongue
Innervation:	Hypoglossal nerve (cranial nerve XII)
Blood Supply:	Sublingual and submental arteries
Action:	Posterior fibers protrude tongue, anterior fibers retract tongue; aids in depressing tongue

Digastric

Origin:	
Anterior belly:	Digastric fossa on the anterior and inferior aspect of the mandible
Posterior belly:	From mastoid notch (digastric groove) of the temporal bone
Insertion:	Intermediate tendon between the two bellies that is affixed to the body and greater cornu of the hyoid by a ligamentous loop
Innervation:	
Anterior belly:	Mylohyoid branch of inferior alveolar nerve from trigeminal nerve (cranial nerve V)
Posterior belly:	Facial nerve (cranial nerve VII)
Blood Supply:	
Anterior belly:	Submental artery
Posterior belly:	Occipital and posterior auricular arteries
Action:	Elevates and fixes hyoid bone, assists lateral pterygoid in opening the mouth by depressing the mandible

References

Bogduk, N (1980). A reappraisal of the anatomy of the human erector spinae. *Journal of Anatomy, 131,* 525–540.

Bustami, FMF (1986). A new description of the lumbar erector spinae muscle in man. *Journal of Anatomy, 144,* 81–91.

Greiner, TM, Bedford, ME, and Walker, RA (1998, April). *Variability in the Human M. spinalis capitis et cervicis: Frequencies and Definitions.* Paper presented at the 67th annual meeting of the American Association of Physical Anthropologists, Salt Lake City. (Abstract published in *American Journal of Physical Anthropology*, Suppl 26, p 88, 1998).

Index

Numbers followed by an "f" indicate figures.